D0000654

BY PENELOPE LEACH

The First Six Months (1987)
Babyhood (1974, 1982)
Your Baby and Child (1978)
"Who Cares?" (1979)

BABYHOOD

BABYHOOD

SECOND EDITION, REVISED AND EXPANDED

Stage by stage, from birth to age two:
how your baby develops physically,
emotionally, mentally

PENELOPE LEACH

ALFRED · A · KNOPF *New York*
1 9 8 7

THIS IS A BORZOI BOOK
PUBLISHED BY ALFRED A. KNOPF, INC.

Copyright © 1974, 1976, 1983 by Penelope Leach

All rights reserved under International and Pan-American Copyright Conventions. Published in the United States by Alfred A. Knopf, Inc., New York, and simultaneously in Canada by Random House of Canada Limited, Toronto. Distributed by Random House, Inc., New York. Originally published in Great Britain by Penguin Books Ltd.

Library of Congress Cataloging in Publication Data
Leach, Penelope.
Babyhood : stage by stage, from birth to age two.
Bibliography: p.
Includes index.
1. Infants—Growth. I. Title.
RJ131.L37   1983   612'.65   82-48881
ISBN 0-394-53092-6
ISBN 0-394-71436-9 (pbk.)

Manufactured in the United States of America
First American edition published October 18, 1976
Second edition, revised and expanded, published June 17, 1983
Reprinted Four Times
Sixth printing, November 1987

FOR MELISSA AND MATTHEW:

THE TWO BABYHOODS I KNOW BEST

ACKNOWLEDGMENTS

A BOOK OF THIS KIND relies on knowledge accumulated from so many sources that to thank each individual is impossible. The research work actually reported and therefore listed in the bibliography is only a small part of the whole. I gratefully acknowledge my debt to all the others and especially to the many whose work has confirmed or elucidated issues which were still merely conjectural when this book was first published in 1974.

Friends and colleagues gave most generously of their time and expertise in reading and criticizing drafts of that first manuscript. I thank them all. But the people to whom this new edition owes most are the parents who, over the years, have written to me with their comments.

Without my husband, Gerald Leach, and our friend Mrs. Anne Hurry, this book really would not have been written and would certainly not have been rewritten for this edition. With her long experience in helping troubled children, adolescents on their way to parenthood, and parents themselves, Mrs. Hurry has helped me to sharpen and focus my ideas about normal development and about what is normal in parenthood. With his long experience of shaping and presenting research data, Gerald has constantly helped me find a way through the problems of presenting other people's material without either distorting it or getting all my sums wrong.

As our children have grown up, they too have taken a hand. Both can read a proof or sort an index.

Finally, I owe a very special thank you to Peter Wright of Penguin Books for all his help as friend and perceptive editor. Without him I should never have made the effort to rewrite this book.

Despite all this help, the facts selected and the opinions expressed throughout the book remain my responsibility alone.

Penelope Leach, 1983

PREFACE TO
THE SECOND EDITION

THERE ARE HUNDREDS of books of advice for parents. This is not another one. Such books tell you *what* to do but they seldom tell you *why* you should, or should not, do this, that, or the other with your baby. Often they leave you wondering how the "expert" author can possibly know what is best for a parent-baby unit he or she has never even met.

The "why?" and the "how do they know?" questions both have a single answer: research. Your favorite author of a baby book has not studied you or your child but he or she has probably studied hundreds of others and has certainly had access to the findings of colleagues who have studied thousands more.

Babyhood was written to give parent experts easy access to the research material used by professional experts. Over the years, some parents have found that, given the facts on what is and is not known about infants in general, they could make their own decisions about handling their own children in particular. Still more have found that once they have the answers to those "why?" and "how do they know?" questions, they could choose and use a baby book far more effectively.

But *Babyhood* was written in the early seventies and, since it was published, research into the development, behavior, feelings, and capabilities of the very young has continued apace. Good advisers try to keep up to date. This new edition offers parents the chance to do so too.

A few of the studies reported in that first edition have been shown to have been ill-conceived or ill-conducted. They have been dropped. But most of this new work builds entrancingly upon the old, with questions asked then now answered; seventies suppositions transformed into eighties knowledge and some theories which seemed poles apart bridged by fresh approaches and new findings. Inevitably the book has grown in size but I hope that its increase in usefulness outstrips its new bulk. I also hope that readers, old and new, will share in some of the excitement felt by the writer.

CONTENTS

II. FROM SIX WEEKS TO THREE MONTHS: MAKING PATTERNS

III. FROM THREE TO SIX MONTHS: DISCOVERING PEOPLE

TABLES AND FIGURES

TABLES

FIGURES

INTRODUCTION

THIS BOOK IS ABOUT being a baby and becoming a toddler. It traces the rapid, varied, but always orderly sequence of changes which take any infant from a helpless parceled newborn to a roving chattering child.

Babies have parents. They, or their substitutes, have to care for the child, do for him the myriad things he cannot do for himself, anticipate wishes which he can barely recognize let alone formulate, and keep the environment they provide and the demands they make in step with his growing maturity. This book is intended for them. But it is meant to provide them with something different from a handbook of advice on child rearing. It does not tell parents how to toilet train their baby; rather it sets out what is known about children's acquisition of control and hence the choices of timing and method which parents can make. It does not tell parents whether to give their baby a pacifier; it discusses what sucking seems to mean to infants, and why pacifiers "work" if they do. It does not only tell parents when their baby should sit up; it describes the sequence in which infants gain control of their wobbly necks and weak shoulders, until they reach a point where sitting alone is the next development to be expected.

The book is not only intended for parents or the people who stand in for them. Many groups of people deal with babies or with the parents of babies, in their professional lives. Student doctors, nurses, social workers will all have to cope with families; playgroup leaders and primary-school teachers will devote themselves to people who have only just stopped being toddlers; police and other public servants will find that the nature and needs of young children are relevant to their jobs. Such people already undergo lengthy and rigorous training in their own specialties. They cannot be expected to trace the complex literature on child development from technical journal to obscure book. This book tries to give them a comparatively easy overview of what is known about how infants develop; a feel for what it is like to be a parent in charge of a developing child; and enough acquaintance with research studies to show them how we know what we know, why we do not know more, and where to look for further information on topics that particularly interest them.

I hope that the book will also be valuable to the increasing number of people who are striving to introduce child development as a topic which is, should, or could be of interest to everyone. "Preparation for Parenthood" courses are gaining a foothold in schools and colleges. The Open University is running courses for parents which non-parents are opting for too. The Pre-School Playgroups Association could fill its existing courses many times over if it had the money to run more. We need more and more such efforts because people who are neither personally nor professionally involved in the daily lives of young families seldom think about children as *people* at all. They still take it for granted that infants are mainly the parents' business and, whatever lip service they may pay to the women's movement, still more the business of their mothers. If anyone happens to make them think in detail about the business of child care they assume, with a sort of woolly emotionalism, that "motherhood" is instinctive and that the close emotional tie which they assume exists between every mother and her child automatically makes the whole thing easy for her. The occasional admiring remark, "I don't know how she does it," usually means that the speaker does not propose to think about it too much and has no intention of finding out.

Caring for a baby, in the sense of being his or her permanent and continuous parent-figure, is probably the most exhausting job which exists in Western society. The baby has to have a known adult on duty or on call 24 hours per day so that even when babysitters take over there is no relief from the business of making the arrangements and shouldering the ultimate responsibility. There are no overtime payments, time off in lieu, nor money for unsocial hours spent walking the baby at 3 A.M. Nobody offers you weekend or holiday breaks and you get coffee breaks only if you make the coffee yourself. For most families the pay is atrocious, often amounting to a halving of pre-delivery income. No union would stand for it.

The job has to be done and it is more worthwhile than any other job because without new people none of the other activities of a society would have any meaning at all. But it would be very much easier to do the job well and happily if the rest of the population would recognize it as interesting, difficult, and valuable. At present almost everyone undervalues it. Few men-who-are-fathers boast either of the fact or the prowess of their fatherhood to their colleagues. Many women-who-are-mothering still use that self-deprecating phrase "I'm only a mother" when asked what they do. It is not surprising; only in the oft-derided company of other mothers are women allowed to acknowledge to themselves the value and the skill of their mothering role. If they meet a problem with their babies and spend time, effort, and skill in putting it right they are, in the eyes of society, only doing what is expected of them. Nobody wants to hear about it and certainly nobody is going to look upon them with the kind of respect offered to anyone else who solves any other kind of problem.

Of course mothers usually do love their babies. Of course it is love which makes much of the business of mothering possible and enjoyable. But interest in a baby and loving care for that baby go together. If people could get interested in infant development they would be in a better position to understand the particular concerns of young parents and they might be more inclined to give them the status which is their due. If parents themselves become interested in infant development they will find it far easier to be loving.

Interest in the processes of a new baby's development makes one look and listen closely, and it is by watching and listening that one sees the signs of *his* interest, of his dawning attachment and love, which will reinforce one's own. Interest makes one wonder what will happen if one does this, rather than that, with the baby. That means thinking oneself into his non-existent shoes, and that is close to love. Interest makes one wonder why he is crying and what will make him stop. When the wondering is put into action it is the same, from the baby's point of view, as love. The interest-love connection is even clearer when everything goes wrong, the baby's behavior is intolerable and parenthood an insupportable burden. Why does he behave like that? Do other babies? What will have to happen in other areas of his development before he is likely to stop? The answers are almost always reassuring because while every baby is unique, none of his behaviors are. The answers almost always increase adult sympathy because babies rarely intend to annoy and the search for the answers provides a degree of temporary objectivity which is calming in itself.

Because the book is written from the point of view of the developing child, the impression of parenthood which it gives is an unrealistically dedicated one. The book takes for granted the parents' wish to give their child any kind of care, contact, or communication which he seems to need. But while most parents want to do their best for their children, this is not the whole story. They can be unaware of a child's need. Or they can be aware of the need but decide not to meet it, feeling that in this instance their own or their other children's needs must come first. Or they may be unable to meet known needs. Money, patience, time can all be thinly spread in a family. None of us is an ideal parent any more than we are ideal husbands or wives, children or friends. No child will ever have all his needs met all the time.

But unrealistic though this view of dedicated parenthood may seem, I make no apology for it. In these days of good contraception, world overpopulation, and increased opportunities for women to make full lives without children and/or partners, there is a moral obligation to choose carefully whether or not to have a child. There is then a moral obligation to rear the children we do choose to have as well as we can, but this obligation is backed by a strong, practical, self-interested one too.

As this book will hopefully illustrate, handling of a baby which is sensitively tuned to his developing needs carries a double payoff. All babies demand, but the babies whose needs are met or anticipated do not demand more than the others, they demand less. Unlike a spoiled 4-year-old who can think of a million things he wants and may ask for them by the thousand if the limits are not made clear, a baby wants only what he needs. If he gets it he is content. If he is content he demands no more until he needs more. To double the benefit of sensitive handling, the more the mother meets or anticipates those needs, the more the baby will reward her with smiles, coos, all the special signs of his passionate devotion which she earns by tuning in to him. She not only gets fewer demands made, she also gets emotional payment for what she does. The mother who gets up cheerfully in the night to feed her baby may spend half an hour awake, and go to bed warmed by his toothless grin. The mother who fights his demands for food, staying in bed while he howls, getting up crossly to offer boiled water, will end up feeding him. But she will probably have been awake for 2 hours, and go to bed feeling that motherhood is hell.

So even though this book is not designed to tell people how to rear their babies, but rather how their babies develop, and therefore what they need, it is intended to be helpful too. I hope it will help mothers and fathers and other caretakers to find ways of doing the job so that life is as satisfactory as possible for the infant and therefore as easy as possible for themselves. Bringing up a baby is a tough job. As with any other tough job, interest and job satisfaction go together.

ON USING THIS BOOK

APOLOGIES TO ALL PARENTS of girls and to all fathers who are the primary caretakers for their children. In the interests of clarity this book has used "she" and "her" to refer to the parent and "he" and "him" to refer to the baby. Our language is sexist, my intention is not.

The book is arranged to cover 5 age periods, represented by Parts I–V in the contents list.

Within each section, except the first, similar topics are covered chapter by chapter.

Any reader who wishes to follow a single topic right through from birth to 2 years will find that he or she can do so, simply by picking one relevant chapter from each section. Hence learning to walk would be followed through by starting with Chapter Four and reading the section called "Postures." Chapter Seven "Beginning to Manage His Body" will be found to follow logically. Chapter Fifteen "Getting Control of His Body" would come next, followed by Chapter Twenty-one "Becoming a Biped" and finishing up with Chapter Twenty-eight "Mobility."

Pounds and ounces, feet and inches have been used throughout the book as the basic units of measurement. Metric equivalents are, in all cases, given in parentheses.

On graphs and charts it will be found that either form of measurement can be read off.

The numerals in brackets in the text refer to source material and research studies listed in the bibliography at the back of the book. Casual readers can ignore them. Others will find the bibliography full enough to give them a starting point for further reading on specialist topics.

PART I

THE FIRST SIX WEEKS

Settling into Life

1

OPENING
THE PARCEL

MANY PARENTS REMEMBER the first few weeks after a baby's birth—especially a first baby's—as a unique period. They face a total upheaval in the pattern of their lives, their relationship with each other, the kind of partnership they have established, their expectations of each other, and their social group. And all this when both of them are still churned up by the actual birth: the mother physically and hormonally, the father by fatigue and empathy. However carefully, lovingly, dedicatedly a birth is prepared for, it is a startling, overwhelming event.

Once the birth is over both parents tend to feel that they need time to recover their equilibrium, to think and talk about it, and to rest. But the birth resulted in a baby. And the presence of that baby usually means no recovery period for either parent. They must somehow struggle straight from giving birth to caring for the baby. There is no time to think about the amazing business of *becoming* a parent because *being* one starts straight away.

So these first weeks tend to be remembered as a peculiarly atmospheric mixture of worry and exhaustion, tenderness and concern. Everything seems to be felt too much: the stitches and the pleasure, the responsibility and the pride, selfishness and selflessness. The mother may have moments when she wonders why on earth she ever had the baby, how she will ever again feel like a fully autonomous person, how she will stand the constant demands of this small creature. She may wallow in private agonizing guilt because she does not feel love for the baby; then again she may have times when she is so overwhelmed by the miracle of minute fingernails or the helplessness of a heavy downy head that she finds the weight of her love for the infant almost too great to bear. The father too is liable to violent swings of feeling. He has a difficult and delicate path

3

to walk. He has to concede the prime role to his wife: she, after all, is the one who labored, the one whose breasts begin to hurt. Yet he must make her feel that this is the child of them both, that he is deeply involved too. He must allow his wife to wrap herself in a symbiotic relationship with the new infant, yet he must reserve enough of their adult relationship to carry his wife through those moments when she feels the infant is eating her alive. Many husbands remark wryly that you cannot get it right during these weeks. If you come in and inquire after the infant's well-being, your wife moans that you only care about the baby now, not about her; if you come in and tell her something interesting, she wails that you don't care about the baby.

Much of the anguish of looking after a very new baby arises from the fact that the mother inevitably lacks the first essential for watchful care. She lacks any baseline of appearance and behavior for *this* infant. He is brand new. She knows nothing about him. She does not know how he looks and behaves when he is content and well, and therefore she cannot easily know when he is discontented or unwell. She does not know how much he "usually" cries, so she cannot know whether today's crying suggests something amiss. She has to make judgments as to the baby's well-being, and she cannot feel secure in those judgments until he has been around long enough for those baselines to be established.

The baby has few baselines himself. He has no established patterns of behavior. He is adapting himself—easily or with difficulty—to life in the outside world; he is recovering from the birth experience, getting himself moving into life. So in these first weeks the mother cannot "know" him. He has not yet got himself into predictable, knowable shape. Only as he settles down and begins to pattern his sucking and his crying, his sleeping and waking, his kicking and wriggling, his looking and listening, can the mother begin to feel that he is a person whom she knows and understands.

Some babies take longer than others to reach this stage, and indeed the stage itself is a subjective judgment by the mother. But most mothers begin to feel that their infants are predictable, knowable, at somewhere between a fortnight and 6 weeks after birth.

In the meantime, an infant needs what it is hardest for parents to give him. Calm. His physiological needs are few, simple, and repetitive. He needs food, warmth, tactile comfort, and a modicum of cleanliness. But the fulfillment of every single one of these needs constitutes a novel experience for a brand-new nervous system. The mother may tremble because she has never bathed a newborn before; but this newborn has never known water since he started to breathe for himself. Everything needs to be done for him as gently, as calmly, and as slowly as possible. He needs no extra stimulation from adults, he has all he can cope with in the myriad new sensations of being outside the womb. He will feel changes of temperature on his skin, detect light and darkness; feel fullness and emptiness, wetness, dryness; feel himself moved through the air, held, put down, moved around. He will hear noises; he must suck for food and water; he will feel his own limbs move, experience different textures against his skin, different tastes in his mouth. He is very busy, in these first weeks, just being alive and staying that way.

Once upon a time most Western mothers received their new babies almost literally as parcels. Clean and wrapped, the baby was brought to the mother by a nurse and taken away again to the nursery. The mother discovered the contents of that parcel gradually over a 10-day hospital stay.

A few mothers still learn their way around their infants under medical care, but many do not. In parts of Europe some babies are delivered at home and the parents are expected to cope from the beginning, with the assistance of specially trained nurses who visit mother and baby daily. In other cases mothers are admitted to the hospital for the actual delivery, but provided all is well with the child and the mother they are allowed home again within 48 or even 24 hours, once again receiving medical supervision on a daily basis in the home. Even in the United States, where the usual stay following a normal birth is around 3 days, the parents may be given little opportunity really to get to know the infant or feel that he belongs to them. An increasing number of hospitals have adopted some form of rooming in. Sometimes this means that mother and baby are together 24 hours a day, but in many cases he will spend only a few hours of each day in the mother's room. While even this obviously helps her to get some sense of his sounds, his rhythms, his aliveness, it cannot compare with taking full charge of the infant all day and all night with no floor nurse at the end of a bell. So while that parcel of baby may have been much peeped at, its final unwrapping still takes place at home.

Of course parents know that if the contents of the parcel was not a basically sound baby they would not have been allowed to take it home. Worry is therefore irrational, panic is shameful, yet both are so common in the first couple of weeks that we might as well allow for them.

BIRTHWEIGHT

One of the first things a new mother is told about her infant is his birthweight. Figures 1 and 2 show the weights and lengths of average, large, and small babies, by their sex. Girls tend to be lighter at birth than boys, and first children tend to be lighter than subsequent ones. If the new infant is of roughly average birthweight, his mother is unlikely to be concerned. In the United States, mothers who have very large babies do not usually find that any special care or precautions are taken. But in many parts of Europe, particularly in Britain, heavy babies are regarded as being more prone to difficulties in the newborn period than babies of average birthweight. An 11-pounder may be kept in the hospital longer

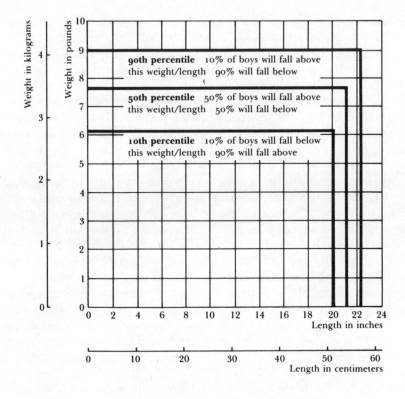

Weight in kilograms

Weight in pounds

90th percentile   10% of boys will fall above
this weight/length   90% will fall below

50th percentile   50% of boys will fall above
this weight/length   50% will fall below

10th percentile   10% of boys will fall below
this weight/length   90% will fall above

Length in inches

Length in centimeters

FIGURE 1. BIRTHWEIGHT AND LENGTH FOR AVERAGE, LARGE,
AND SMALL BOYS

Percentiles are a means of dividing up the population in such a way that 50 percent fall either side of the 50th percentile point, while 10 percent fall above the 90th and 10 percent below the 10th percentile points. Any birthweight or length which falls between the 10th and 90th percentiles is usually regarded as "normal," since that range comprises the weights and lengths of 80 percent of all newborns. Weights and lengths above the 90th percentile would be regarded as high; those below the 10th percentile would be regarded as low.

than the planned 48 hours, so that the medical staff can satisfy themselves that all is well with him. This does not necessarily mean that doctors have noticed anything untoward about the baby. They may well simply be taking precautions on the basis of statistical evidence that such large babies are at slightly greater risk than smaller ones.

Small infants are very seldom allowed home from the hospital until they weigh around 5 1/2 lb. (2.5 kg). Mothers whose babies weigh in at around or below this weight may get confused and worried by the terms "premature" and "small for dates."

Sometimes the term "premature" is used carelessly for any infant who weighs less than 5 1/2 lb. (2.5 kg) at birth. But usually the term is

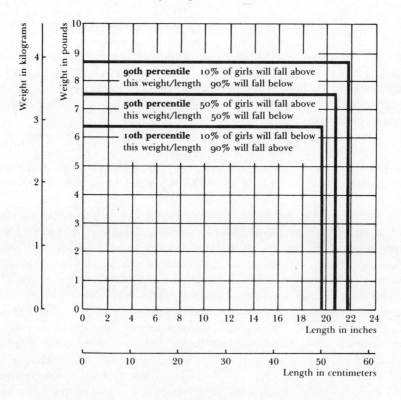

Weight in kilograms / Weight in pounds

90th percentile 10% of girls will fall above
this weight/length 90% will fall below

50th percentile 50% of girls will fall above
this weight/length 50% will fall below

10th percentile 10% of girls will fall below
this weight/length 90% will fall above

Length in inches

Length in centimeters

FIGURE 2. BIRTHWEIGHT AND LENGTH FOR AVERAGE, LARGE,
AND SMALL GIRLS

At birth boys are usually both heavier and longer than girls.

In the absence of prematurity or ill health, the most common reason
for exceptional size is the size of the parents. Small parents tend to have
small babies and large parents large babies.

Size at birth is significantly related to size throughout childhood. Small
babies tend to remain small children, and large babies to be large children,
at least until the growth spurt at puberty.

(Adapted from Tanner, Whitehouse, and Takaishi [213].)

reserved for babies who are born before they have spent their allotted 40
weeks in the womb. Used in this sense, an infant weighing 6 lb. (2.7 kg),
born after 37 weeks' gestation, is premature, but because he is well grown
may need little special care. A 37-week baby weighing 5 lb. (2.3 kg) may
start his life in an incubator, but may be able to suck and to breathe
without assistance from the beginning. With a lighter birthweight and/or
a shorter gestational time, the infant is likely to need very special care,
with a controlled addition of oxygen to the air in the incubator, and
perhaps assisted respiration, and tube-feeding, with accurate monitoring
of his body's biochemistry.

"Small-for-dates" infants are those who have spent the full 40 weeks in the womb, but who nevertheless are born weighing less than 5 1/2 lb., or those whose time in the womb was curtailed, but who weigh even less than would be expected after their gestational period. Sometimes medical staff make careful inquiries of the mother after the birth, in an attempt to establish whether or not her infant is truly "small for dates." If the mother is doubtful about when the pregnancy began the infant may be simply premature.

Both premature and small-for-dates babies start life with a degree of handicap. Both groups are more prone than babies of average birth-weight to neonatal difficulties. Both must be expected to take some time to catch up, developmentally, with babies of similar *birth* date, but greater maturity.

We cannot yet duplicate a uterus in order to give babies born prematurely, or before they have reached an average birthweight, the extra time they need before they face the world. Care in a specialist unit, in an incubator, with assisted breathing and tube-feeding, gives the infant the nearest possible equivalent. For the mother, a tiny frail-looking baby whom she can only see through glass, and who may have a tube down his nose, and various other gadgets attached to his body, is at best a disappointment, at worst a ghastly shock. From the point of view of the infant's development, the period he spends in such special care needs to be regarded as a hiatus, a sort of interim between the delivery and the "real" birth which is the moment when he is strong enough to emerge into independent life. For some months after he leaves the hospital, the baby should be thought of as being the age he would be if he had been born at the expected time or the ordinary sort of weight. Born at 35 weeks gestation, he should not be expected to measure up to other 3-month infants 13 weeks later. He will probably need at least 18 weeks to reach that developmental phase.

But a hiatus in the relationship between baby and parents is not desirable. The mother has "held" the baby in her womb through the long months of pregnancy. As soon as he emerges she needs to hold him in her arms, to explore him, make contact with him, see who it is that she and her partner have made.

After uncomplicated births, most newborn babies are handed straight to their mothers. They are given the opportunity to make this first contact before hospital routine takes over, and they are kept beside the mother's bed 24 hours per day. Premature babies, along with those who have had traumatic births, still tend to be rushed away from the parents to receive the care that they need. If the mother then sees the baby only through glass or plastic, he may not seem like *her* baby at all. Some authorities believe that parents and child may thus miss a critical period in the forging of the bond between them and that in extreme instances there may be real difficulties later on in their learning to love each other. Most agree that although of course the infant's physical well-being must come first, every care should be taken to ensure that the mother "meets" him and that she is allowed to touch him, hold him, and share in his care at the first possible moment [127].

CIRCUMCISION

If the newborn baby is a boy he will almost certainly be circumcised by the hospital staff. Most American parents will take this procedure as much for granted as the cutting of the cord or putting drops in the newborn baby's eyes. Those who do discuss the circumcision with their obstetrician or pediatrician will probably be doing so because they have to arrange a ritual operation as part of their Jewish faith.

Circumcision for religious reasons is beyond the scope of this book; indeed it is beyond the scope of an atheist. Circumcision for deeply felt if less easily describable reasons is beyond this book's scope too. If a father feels that his son should, in this respect, be like himself; a mother feels that she would not like to handle an uncircumcised son; a grandparent would be likely to love the child less because he was left as nature made him, then these are good reasons for having the baby circumcised. But many circumcisions in the United States are carried out without any of these reasons. They are carried out without anybody ever being asked to *think* about their reasons. And that seems a pity. The facts that follow are for people to think about if, having read this far, they find that they are not sure that they feel strongly that boys should be circumcised.

Circumcision has an interesting history. It is practiced by about one sixth of the world's population and dates back at least 6000 years, having been started, according to Herodotus, by the Egyptians. It has been used variously as a secret tribal marking, a way of marking slaves, part of puberty initiation ceremonies, and, of course, a religious rite.

But most people today have none of these reasons for circumcision. The most usual medical reason given is a tight (i.e., a non-retractable) prepuce. But prepuces are not meant to be retractable in infancy. D. Gairdner, in his paper called "The Fate of the Foreskin" [87], found almost no baby boys whose prepuces were retractable in the first 6 months. Only half could be retracted at 1 year, while a fifth were still non-retractable at 2 years.

Normal or not, many people would maintain that an uncircumcised penis is difficult to keep clean; circumcision is more hygienic. If one can manage to separate that argument from thousands of years of powerful tradition, it is a curious one. There are many parts of our bodies which would be easier to keep free of their normal secretions if we opened them up—our nostrils for instance. Yet we do not.

A few years ago the hygiene argument got a powerful boost from research data which suggested that cancer of the penis was less frequent in circumcised males, and cancer of the cervix far less likely in their partners. But these findings are now very much open to doubt. Recent work suggests that the findings of low cancer figures together with high circumcision rates in certain populations are due to chance rather than to cause and effect.

If little boys are not circumcised at the beginning of their lives, a few will, medically, need circumcision later on. On the face of it this is the strongest practical reason for the newborn operation. Upsetting though it can be, physically and psychologically, to a 3-day-old baby, it is far more upsetting to a 5-year-old. But even here the argument is not simple. Doctors who are not basically in favor of circumcising every-body consider that many of these later operations are carried out un-necessarily by doctors who are. Bed-wetting and masturbation are two of the reasons still occasionally given. Neither, of course, could possibly be helped by circumcision. Both would be likely to be made worse by the trauma. Certainly, though, many late circumcisions are caused by parents' attempts to retract the non-retractable prepuce. If such at-tempts are made with any force at all, they tend to make minute splits in the skin between the prepuce and the glans. The splits heal leaving scar tissue which sticks the two together, so that when the prepuce ought to retract in later life it cannot. Attempts at retraction are often the cause of the other main reason for late circumcision: recurrent in-fection under the foreskin. So it does seem that parents who do decide *not* to have a newborn boy circumcised should be very sure they are able to go the whole way with this idea and leave the infant penis strictly alone; simply giving it the ordinary external hygiene the rest of the boy gets. If this is done there is no greater chance of later trouble than of, say, peritonitis. We do not whip out newborns' appendixes in case of that.

Circumcision is not a dangerous operation, but, like all surgical procedures, however small, it carries certain risks. Although the risks are obviously necessary and acceptable where the procedure is *needed* by the patient, few babies *need* circumcision. In many countries, including Brit-ain, doctors long ago decided that while those who felt strongly in favor of circumcision should, of course, be able to arrange it, the operation should no longer be carried out routinely. They saw no benefit to the babies and some bad side effects. They felt that the net sum balanced against routine operation.

Actual figures on side effects are difficult to assess. In a country such as Britain where doctors are largely against the operation, every little problem is recorded. In a country like the United States where it is taken for granted, only serious side effects like real sepsis or hemorrhage will reach the statistics. In fact the actual reported figures for these two countries are 22 percent for Britain and around 6 percent for Amer-ica [155]. An emotionally laden subject produces emotionally biased statistics!

Probably it is only safe to say that while serious side effects are extremely rare, minor ones are quite frequent. The baby is bound to be sore for at least a few days and may be so for much longer if mild infection or diaper irritation set in. Certainly the circumcised baby boy will need much more careful diaper care than his uncircumcised friend. The foreskin protects the delicate end of the penis from the abrasive effects of ammonia in the urine; without it, irritation of the glans is much more likely and will remain so until he abandons diapers for good. Some pain on passing urine, or when bathed, is also likely; it will last until the wound is entirely healed.

But these practical considerations are not the ones which will sway many parents one way or the other. It is hard to see why anyone should have a newborn boy circumcised for *practical* reasons alone, so the basic reasons must be traditional, cultural. I am not concerned to persuade parents one way or the other, but I am concerned to persuade them to *think* about circumcision. At present, in the United States, hospitals circumcise babies because they assume the parents will want it done. Parents accept it perhaps partly because they assume the hospital knows best. There may be a failure in communication here. It may be that the hospitals are taking upon themselves a decision which should really be made, positively, by each set of parents for each son. After all, if you had a baby who was born with a tooth, would you expect the hospital to extract it without asking you whether you would prefer to have it left alone?

If the operation is to be carried out, even as early as the third or fourth day, non-Jewish parents may like to discuss the question of analgesia with their obstetrician. Babies feel pain from birth. Of course they do not *anticipate* pain, nor as far as we know do they *remember* it. But at the time when it is inflicted they feel and respond to it. Many authorities feel that circumcision without pain prevention is thoughtlessly cruel. However, the prevention of the pain is not an easy matter, which is why discussion is necessary. To give a baby of this age a general anesthetic is to introduce well-known if minor dangers. On the other hand, the infiltration of the penis with local anesthetic may well cause as much pain as the removal of the foreskin itself. In some centers techniques have been developed by which the skin which must be removed is frozen with a topical application of local anesthetic spray. It may be that this will become the pain-prevention method of choice in circumcision.

While an unusually low or high birthweight, prematurity whatever the birthweight, together with any neonatal complication, will mean that the new infant is kept in the hospital at least during his first week, many parents may find themselves in full charge of an infant merely hours old.

Many things can worry parents. Newborns are physiologically very different from babies even a few weeks old, and dramatically different from older children or adults. They are prone to all sorts of conditions and appearances which are perfectly normal for *them* but unheard of, or a genuine reason for anxiety, in any other age group. If the mother's own feet suddenly turned bright blue she would be right to feel concerned; how is she to know that the feet of newborn babies often turn blue from time to time while the circulation is adapting to life outside the womb?

The following list of things which parents may notice and worry about during the infant's first week or two is not intended to dissuade them from consulting their doctor about anything that concerns them; rather it is intended to help them get a night's sleep, or pass a reasonably calm day while waiting to consult. The list only covers phenomena which, provided they are noticed in the first 2 weeks after birth, are normal or insignificant, however alarming they may appear. It must be stressed that such signs appearing in an older baby could suggest trouble and would be an indication to seek medical help.

NORMAL PECULIARITIES

Peculiarities of Color

BLUISH HANDS AND/OR FEET   A bluish tinge to the extremities is perfectly normal. It may be continuous or intermittent. If intermittent, it is more likely to be noticed when the infant has been asleep and still for a long period. It does not mean that he is cyanosed (failing to get enough oxygen), it is merely a sign of the immaturity of his circulation. In true cyanosis the tongue is also blue and there are blue-gray shadows to either side of the nose.

HALF RED, HALF PALE   Occasionally the side on which the infant is lying becomes suffused a bright red, while his upper half remains pale. There is a definite line right down his body, marking the junction of red with pale areas. This phenomenon is called the "harlequin color change." It is thought to be due simply to gravity causing the blood to collect in the lower half of the body. It passes as soon as the infant is picked up or turned over, and it has no significance at all.

MONGOLIAN BLUE SPOTS   These are accumulations of pigment, forming spots or patches of a bluish color. They form principally on the buttocks, and are most often seen in infants of African or Mongolian descent. They may also occur in infants of Greek or Italian origin, or in any baby who is going to have a fairly dark skin. They become far less noticeable as the overall skin color darkens.

Mothers are sometimes alarmed by the name, thinking it relates to Mongolism. It does not. They are also sometimes afraid that the blue patches may be bruises, suggesting either ill treatment or a blood disease. They can be reassured.

Other Skin Peculiarities

SPOTS   New babies' skins are liable to a variety of eruptions. The kind that usually cause anxiety are raised red spots with yellow-white centers, which look as if they might be infected. They are called "neonatal urticaria." They usually appear in the first 24 hours and vanish during the first week. They are completely insignificant and require no treatment.

BIRTHMARKS   There are innumerable varieties of these, some of which fade and others of which do not. If there is a mark on the infant's skin which causes anxiety, the doctor will be able to say whether it is a birthmark, and what type it is.

Red marks on the skin, or tiny broken blood vessels in the skin or in the eyes, can arise from pressure during birth—even if the delivery was unassisted. These are quite insignificant, and vanish within a few days.

SKIN PEELING   Most infants' skin peels a little in the first few days. It is usually most noticeable on the hands and the soles of the feet.

SCALY PATCHES ON THE SCALP   Known as "cradle-cap," this is just as normal as peeling of the skin elsewhere. It suggests neither disease nor lack of hygiene. If the scaly patches really cover the scalp, in a cap-shaped thick layer, and the appearance of them is distressing, a doctor can suggest alternatives to simple soap-and-water washing. But from the infant's point of view it is probably best left alone. He is likely to be quite undistressed by his cradle-cap, and thoroughly irritated by having his head cleaned with oil.

Hair

Babies vary in the amount and the type of hair they are born with. Most have very little, very fine hair; a few have a luxuriant growth, and some —especially those born after their expected date of delivery—have coarse, wiry hair. Whatever the hair is like at birth, most of it will fall out during the subsequent few weeks. Some infants will have a period of semi-baldness, while in others the new hair grows in as the newborn hair falls out. Neither the texture nor the color of the newborn hair bears much relation to later hair.

BODY HAIR   In the womb, infants are covered with a fine fuzz of hair. At birth some are still thus covered; others have traces left, usually across the shoulder blades and down the spine; others have no body hair at all. None of it has the least significance. Any excess hair will be rapidly shed in the first week or two.

Swellings

HERNIA   While an umbilical hernia—a small swelling near the navel, which usually becomes more protuberant when the infant cries—cannot be classified as "normal," it is very common. Such hernias are caused by a slight weakness of the muscle wall in the abdomen, or by a failure of the muscle wall to close completely. Most umbilical hernias right themselves by 1 year. Many authorities now believe that they heal more quickly if they are not strapped up. Very few ever require an operation.

SWOLLEN BREASTS   Both male and female babies sometimes develop quite definite breast swelling in the first 3 days. The condition is known as "mastitis neonatorum." It is caused by the pituitary hormone which floods through the mother just before the birth, to stimulate *her* milk secretion. Some passes across the placenta and stimulates the infant's breasts too. There may even be droplets of milk coming from the infant's nipples.

Mastitis neonatorum does not suggest any abnormality, nor require treatment. The breasts should be left strictly alone, as any attempt to squeeze out the milk could lead to infection. The swelling subsides over a few days as the infant's body rids itself of the hormone intended to stimulate his mother and not him.

SWOLLEN GENITALS   Swelling of the genitals in both sexes is equally usual, transient, and insignificant. This too is caused by the mother's hormones reaching the baby across the placenta just before birth.

The Head

MISSHAPEN HEAD   No baby with a significant skull problem will be allowed home from the hospital, or left at home if he was delivered there. So the mother can assume that all is well with her infant's skull, however peculiar it may look.

Even without the use of forceps or vacuum extraction at delivery, the infant's skull may appear lopsided or elongated after birth. The areas of the skull where the bones are not rigid or fully fused allow a considerable degree of this "molding." Without them there would be many more difficult deliveries, as a rigid head tried to get through a narrow birth canal.

Marked degrees of "molding" may take several weeks to right themselves, although they will become less noticeable as the infant grows more hair. Some infants continue to have lopsided skulls for many months, especially if they develop a marked preference for lying on one particular side. The pressure of the skull on the crib mattress can be sufficient to flatten one side of the head slightly. This does not matter in the least, but it can usually be avoided by ensuring that the baby is put down to sleep on alternating sides or on his tummy, at least for as long as he will accept it.

THE FONTANELLES   The most noticeable of these soft areas on a baby's head lies toward the top of the back of his skull, roughly at the crown. This fontanelle does not close up and become hard for months. With normal handling there is absolutely no danger of damaging it, for it is covered by an extremely tough membrane. Often, especially in a baby with little hair, a pulse can be seen beating under the fontanelle. This is perfectly normal. If the infant becomes dehydrated, during illness, fever, starvation, or even extremely hot weather, the fontanelle may appear sunken. This is a useful sign that the infant needs more fluids immediately. If the fontanelle should ever appear tense and bulging, a doctor should see the infant.

Elimination and Secretions

STOOLS   The first substance passed by the new infant is usually the grayish-white "meconium plug." Over the next two or three days, he passes meconium stools, which are greenish-black and very sticky—very *unlike* a normal stool. These must be passed before ordinary digestion can commence. About 70 percent of newborns pass their first meconium stool in the first 12 hours after birth. About 95 percent do so in the first 24 hours. Failure to pass meconium in the first day or two needs investigation, and may be a reason for the infant being kept in the hospital for longer than was planned.

Once the intestine has cleared itself of the meconium with which it was filled in the womb, the infant passes what are known as "changing stools." As their name suggests they are simply the stools produced as the infant adapts to milk feeding from the transfusion feeding of his time in the womb. These stools are greenish-brown. After this the stools settle into the normal "milk stools" which are described on page 45.

BLOOD IN STOOLS   Occasionally this is noticed in the first day or two. It is usually due to maternal blood swallowed during delivery.

URINE   Most infants pass urine in the first hours after birth. About 10 percent do not pass any for the first 36 hours due, it is thought, to passing urine during delivery.

In both boys and girls very early urine may contain a substance called "urates." This appears red on the diaper and may resemble blood.

Once the urine flow is established the infant may urinate as often as 20–30 times in the 24 hours. This is entirely normal; indeed few mothers will actually know how often the baby urinates—all they will know is that his diaper is always wet, however often he is picked up.

A newborn infant who is *dry* for as long as 6 hours should be seen by a doctor. There is a possibility of some obstruction causing retention of the urine.

VAGINAL BLEEDING   A small amount of bleeding from the vagina is common in girls at any time from birth to about 7 days. It is due to the rapid excretion of maternal or placental estrogens transmitted to the infant before birth.

A clear discharge, which may become thicker and whiter in appear-

ance, is also common. It ceases in a couple of days. There is no significance in such vaginal secretions.

NASAL DISCHARGE   Many infants accumulate enough mucus in the nose
to cause snuffles and sneezing. This need not imply a cold or other
infection, and has no significance unless the infant is otherwise unwell.

TEARS   Most newborn babies cry without tears until they are 3–6 weeks
old. About 10 percent produce tears within the first week. This is of no
importance either way.

SWEATING OF THE HEAD   Many infants sweat copiously around the head,
so that the sparse hair appears soaking. This is quite normal and unimportant unless the infant gives other indications of being feverish or
unwell. It is, however, a good reason for frequent rinsing of the hair and
scalp, as the salt in the sweat can cause skin irritation (especially around
the back of the neck) if it is allowed to accumulate.

VOMITING   When infants suck, they take in air as well as milk. Once the
milk reaches the stomach gravity ensures that it settles to the bottom,
leaving the air at a higher level. The infant then brings up his "gas" in
a series of burps and belches. Very often he brings up some of the milk
with the gas. This "spitting up" has no real relation to vomiting in the
sense this word is used in older people. Mothers often believe that the
quantity of milk brought up is much larger than it really is. They worry
that the infant is keeping down too little for adequate nourishment. Even
a dessertspoonful of milk, mixed with a little saliva, looks like a great deal
if it is spilled all over somebody's shoulder.

A very few infants do suffer from projectile vomiting, in which the
milk is literally shot back, as if from a water pistol, sometimes hitting a
wall some feet from the infant's mouth. Such infants should see a doctor,
who will probably want to see a feeding, and therefore the vomiting, for
himself.

Vomiting partially digested milk, an hour or more after a feeding,
does count as true vomiting, and may indicate anything from maldiges-
tion to the beginnings of a cold or other feverish illness.

The Mouth

TEETH   About 1 in 2,000 infants is born with a tooth already through.
Julius Caesar, Hannibal, Louis XIV, and Napoleon are supposed to have
been among them.

The roots of such a tooth are not firmly fixed, so the tooth bends out
of the way when the infant sucks and there is little danger of him hurting
the mother's breast or puncturing the nipple. If left alone such teeth
become firmly fixed and part of the normal dentition. Some authorities
prefer to remove them. There is a very small risk of bleeding attached
to such an extraction, but later dentition will replace the tooth in the normal way.

TONGUE TIE Occasionally a mother notices that her baby's tongue is attached to the lower jaw over a much greater proportion of its length than is her own or that of any other older member of the family. Such a mother may worry in case her baby is tongue tied and will have difficulty later in talking. In fact this is one of the instances where newborn anatomy just looks different from how it will look later. Babies' tongues are meant to have a comparatively long attachment to the jaw. True tongue tie is extremely rare and never requires any action in the first year of life.

WHITE TONGUE A tongue which is uniformly white all over is perfectly normal in a purely milk-fed infant. It clears in a few weeks. Infection does not give a uniform whiteness, but produces patches of white on an otherwise pinky-red tongue.

BLISTERS ON THE UPPER LIP These are produced by sucking and are therefore known as "sucking blisters." They can occur at any time while the infant is purely milk-fed. They may recede between feedings and re-occur. They are of no significance.

The Eyes

SWOLLEN OR PUFFY EYES Often occur soon after birth as a result of pressure during delivery. The puffiness resolves over 2 or 3 days.

BROKEN VEINS IN THE EYES Broken veins may make tiny streaks or patches of red on the white of eye. Again these arise during delivery and rapidly resolve afterward.

"STICKY EYE" A slight yellowish discharge, or collection of yellow matter in the corners of the eyes, suggests this very common neonatal infection. The infant should be seen by the doctor, who may prescribe drops or a solution for bathing the eyes.

"WANDERING EYE" Many newborns appear to squint. Often this is because of the fold at the inner corner of the eyes which can give them a squinting appearance when in fact they are entirely normal.

Sometimes one of a baby's eyes tends to wander away from the focus of the other eye, so that having been focusing on an object with both eyes the baby holds only one steady. This usually rights itself without any treatment by 6 months. Occasionally, though, a baby seems unable to focus both eyes together at all. One is permanently looking off from the direction in which the other is focusing. A fixed squint of this kind should be reported to the doctor as soon as it is noticed. Early treatment is both extremely important and highly successful.

The Ears

DISCHARGE Discharge from the ears is not normal and should always be referred to a doctor whether or not the infant appears ill. It is very unusual in the neonatal period.

STICKING-OUT EARS   Opinions differ as to whether the mother can usefully do anything about ears that stick out. The ears of a new infant are
very soft, and some authorities suggest that they can be persuaded to
grow flatter to the head if they are strapped back with adhesive tape. Most
authorities would agree, however, that there is little point in this procedure which, to do any good, would have to be continuous over months
and might well lead to sore skin from the tape. It is worth making sure
that when the infant is put to lie on his side his ear is not bent forward
under his head.

Ears which appear to stick out to the point of deformity often cease
to be noticeable as the infant grows and acquires more hair.

Even the calmest parents, with the least worrisome infants, need medical
advisers whom they really trust. They need them at this early stage because they can advise the parents on the basis of their experience of
hundreds of infants, while the parents are finding their way around this
one particular infant. However healthy the child turns out, they will
continue to need such medical help, because there are immunizations to
be carried out, childhood infections to be got through, developmental
checks to be made.

In the United States, parents who can afford it will probably register
their new baby with a private pediatrician, and will follow his recommended schedule of routine checkups. If the choice of pediatrician is a
happy one, the parents will find that over the weeks, months, and years,
they strike a relationship with that pediatrician which enables them to
take to him a variety of problems ranging perhaps from feeding difficulties in the early weeks, to adolescent difficulties at puberty. But the right
pediatrician does not only mean a pediatrician who is expert at his stated
job. It is vital that the parents should not be too shy to ask advice, should
not be afraid of "looking silly" to the doctor. It is most unlikely that
anything disastrous will happen to the new infant, but any doctor would
rather a mother ask unnecessarily than take the slightest risk. The kind
of doctor the parents need would also rather the mother asked than
worried herself into a depression, which is quite an easy thing to do
immediately after giving birth. While routine consultations or calls made
because of illness are obviously charged for, many American pediatricians do have stated hours at which parents can telephone to ask for
advice or reassurance. Often the best way to find a sympathetic pediatrician is to ask around among friends and neighbors with very young
children and find the one who is most universally regarded as kind and
helpful.

If parents do not wish to register the baby with a private pediatrician,
or cannot afford the fees, there will be local access to the welfare clinic
or to baby clinics or community health centers. Such centers have

schedules for regular checkups and immunizations. And it is obviously important that parents should take advantage of these. If such regular routine visits are made the parents should be able to strike up the same kind of relationship with the clinic staff which they might be able to have with a private pediatrician. It is only in this way that they can be sure that if something should go wrong, or some anxiety should suddenly strike them, the staff at the center will be in a position to see what, if any, deviation from the normal for *this* baby has taken place. It cannot be too strongly emphasized that a doctor or nurse will be able to be far more helpful to parents if he or she has seen the baby at regular intervals from birth. Unfortunately many parents only use welfare clinics when they are already worried about the baby or, worse, tend to use the emergency room of their nearest hospital instead of a pediatrician or community health center. While the physical care given to a sick baby under these conditions will in most cases be excellent, and while in many cases the staff will try to carry out routine immunization procedures while dealing with the emergency that has persuaded the parents to bring the baby to the hospital, such a way of using the medical services is ideal neither for babies nor for the services themselves. Emergency rooms of hospitals are not designed to cope with babies with feverish colds; they are better occupied in dealing with genuine emergencies. Furthermore, an exhausted young doctor after long hours of emergency duties is not the best person to consult about a possible change in formula or a sleeping problem.

However good and consistent the medical advice which parents have available, there are still going to be times in these early weeks when they wonder if the infant is all right or not. Later on they will go by whether his behavior and appearance are different from usual. But at this stage there is no usual.

Rule-of-thumb methods can give some guidance as to whether or not any infant is in trouble; they all concern his basic behaviors. The baby must eat, sleep, and eliminate. Inability to do any of these things is a signal; it means something. How much it means depends on how it relates to the baby's general appearance and behavior. So to begin with, whatever a baby's symptoms, he is unlikely to be very ill if he is eating well, sleeping peacefully, and eliminating. He can wait to see the doctor at the next office appointment. Equally, if he has no appetite, cries continuously so that he does not sleep and has diarrhea he should probably see a doctor at the first possible opportunity. In between these extremes the infant may refuse his meals, but sleep neither too little nor too much, cry no more than usual, and have no digestive disturbance. In circumstances like these the mother has to decide whether he *seems* ill. This "seeming ill" is a very unscientific, subjective matter—one which becomes second nature to mothers with practice. Largely it is a matter of whether the baby seems floppy, whether he *feels* wrong in her arms, whether his head seems heavier than usual, his crying sounds peculiar, his interest seems less than the day before. If the mother finds herself worried about the infant in some way, even if she cannot exactly specify to herself what she thinks is wrong, she should probably take him to the doctor. After all, she chose the doctor because he did not make her feel she was a bother.

FEEDING

METHOD

THE FIRST EDITION of this book stated that "remarkably few babies in the Western world are breast-fed." Studies published in the United States between 1969 and 1973 had shown that fewer than 25 percent of babies were ever put to the breast at all while two studies in the United Kingdom had reported only 14 percent and 8 percent, respectively, of babies breast-fed to 1 month of age. Figures of this kind were in sharp contrast to those of the immediate post-war period. A National Survey in Britain in 1946, for example, had shown that 60 percent of infants were breast-fed to 1 month, 42 percent to 3 months, and 30 percent to 6 months.

During the seventies, strenuous efforts were made by government advisory bodies and voluntary welfare organizations on both sides of the Atlantic to popularize breast-feeding and to influence mothers to use this method with their infants. Many people believe that these efforts have been successful and that there has been a large increase in the number of babies who are breast-fed. The increase is more apparent than real. Enthusiasm for breast-feeding among health professionals has led to changes in ante-natal teaching and in hospital policy so that a higher percentage of babies are *started* on the breast. A famous lying-in hospital on the East Coast of the United States recently informed the author that "our breast-feeding figures approach 100 percent following normal deliveries. . . ." But few of those babies spend more than three days in the hospital; few of their mothers even have their full milk supply before they go home (for which "reason" many newborns are given bottles by the staff), and a very different percentage carry on with breast-feeding once they leave the hospital. Mothers who do carry on with breast-feeding tend to be of high socioeconomic status. They both supply and are sensitive to the enthusiastic media coverage in favor of breast-feeding, and

they are willing and able to find and use the advice and help of organizations such as the La Leche League. The behavior and expectations of
comparatively vocal and self-aware women may eventually affect the behavior of a majority of mothers; but where breast-feeding is concerned,
they certainly have not done so yet.

Reliable statistics are hard to come by and hard to interpret. Many
surveys use mailed questionnaires because personal interviews are
prohibitively expensive for a sample large enough to yield interesting
results. But mail surveys seldom produce adequate and comprehensible
data. Most respondents know that breast-feeding is socially approved and
therefore tend to over-estimate their own use of the method by, for
example, endorsing "fully breast-fed at x months" despite the fact that
their child is already receiving most of his nourishment from bottles of
formula and/or solid foods. Furthermore, reasons for weaning—either
from breast to bottle or from milk-only to milk-plus-solid foods—are
difficult to elicit by mail. Many mothers will state that they had an "inadequate milk supply" or that they suffered from breast problems. Without
personal follow-up it is impossible to tell whether such perceived problems were objective indications for a change in the baby's feeding or
simply convenient reasons for a change that those mothers wanted to
make anyway.

The best recent available statistics come not from the United States
but from the United Kingdom, where a large national sample of mothers
and babies was studied during 1975 and 1976. Information was collected
in repeated personal interviews between mothers and researchers and the
resulting report [153] gives a remarkably clear and internally consistent
picture of infant-feeding practices. Although no comparable survey has
recently been carried out in the United States, its findings are closely
comparable with those of two smaller-scale American studies published
in 1974 [108].

The British survey showed that while 51 percent of infants were
breast-fed immediately after birth, numbers dropped dramatically after
they were taken home from the hospitals. At 1 week 42 percent were still
being breast-fed, 35 percent at 2 weeks, 24 percent at 6 weeks, 15 percent
at 3 months, and only 9 percent at 6 months.

Those percentages conceal marked regional and educational differences among British families. Where 28 percent of babies living in London or the South-East of Britain were still breast-fed at 6 weeks, only 19
percent of the 6-week-old babies who lived in the industrial North of the
country were still breast-fed. Where 53 percent of 6-week-old babies of
mothers who had continued in full-time education until after their eigh-
teenth birthdays were breast-fed, only 16 percent of this age group were
breast-fed if their mothers had left full-time education by their sixteenth
birthdays. Similar educational trends can be seen in Huenemann's survey
of 448 American babies, together with marked differences in breast-
feeding rates for different racial groups: 17 percent of the Caucasian

group were never breast-fed; 36 percent of the Oriental group were never breast-fed; 58 percent of the Negro group were never breast-fed. Looking at socioeconomic score irrespective of race, 61 percent of Group 1 mothers had either never started breast-feeding or had stopped before the baby was 1 month old, whereas only 22 percent of the more privileged Group 3 mothers were not breast-feeding babies when they reached 1 month of age. Such large differences between groups make it clear that "national" figures, even for a country as small as Britain and certainly for one as large and diverse as the United States, are almost meaningless.

The term "breast-fed" itself conceals wide variations in infant feeding. In the United Kingdom survey a baby was counted as "still breast-fed" if he was offered the breast at all, irrespective of whether or not he was also given formula from a bottle and/or other foods. Only 58 percent of the babies who were being breast-fed at 6 weeks received no bottles at all; 73 percent of the babies who were still being breast-fed at 4 months were given no bottles but by this time most of them were receiving solid foods (see page 78). Both Huenemann's survey [108] and Basedon's survey of largely Negro and Puerto Rican families [15] show that irrespective of breast-feeding, almost half the babies receive cereals in the first month of life. Figures for *complete and exclusive* breast-feeding cannot be extracted from these American surveys, but it is unlikely that a re-analysis of the raw data would show higher numbers than those available from the United Kingdom statistics: 4 percent completely and exclusively breast-fed at 6 weeks and fewer than 1 percent at 4 months.

If most babies are not breast-fed for more than a couple of weeks, few new mothers will take breast-feeding for granted. The majority of children, young people, and parents-to-be today have probably never even *seen* a baby put to the breast. Of course a pregnant woman would be unlikely to decide to breast-feed her coming baby simply because she watched a friend doing so (indeed the survey cited above showed that this experience made no difference to pregnant women's decisions about feeding). But parents who are expecting their own child who neither see nor meet anyone who is breast-feeding, and instead find that bottle-feeding is taken for granted in their area and social group, will have to make a decision to breast-feed very positively and adhere to it in the face of surprise or even, sometimes, derision. Data from this survey, as well as from other sources, clearly suggest that decisions about breast-feeding tap a whole layer of often subconscious feelings in both sexes: feelings which have more to do with breasts and sexuality than breasts and baby-feeding. In the mothers surveyed, the views of their sexual partners were the biggest single influence in their decisions about breast-feeding, a stronger influence even than that of health visitors or other health professionals.

While the sexual relationship between parents is of obvious importance and discussion between them valuable, it is perhaps surprising to find the psychiatrist author of a current book on baby care actually advising women to take careful account of their husbands' feelings about their breasts before embarking on breast-feeding their mutual child [51]. If both sexes are to reach maturity and parenthood able to think rationally about breast-feeding, information and education must clearly start in infancy and continue through childhood and adolescence. If couples are to be influenced toward breast-feeding, positive attitudes need to be formed before their *first* baby is born. Data from the survey showed that while a mother who started to breast-feed her first baby might well change to bottle-feeding and then bottle-feed subsequent children, a mother who started by bottle-feeding the first child almost never attempted to breast-feed subsequent children. The interpretation must surely be that while a woman can try breast-feeding and be disappointed, if she does not try it she will never know what she might be missing.

Some mothers like breast-feeding, finding it obvious and easy. Others do not like it, finding it neither obvious nor easy. Others like the idea of breast-feeding but nevertheless find it difficult. Partisan supporters, while undoubtedly right in their efforts to ensure babies their birthright, have nevertheless done those babies a disservice by maintaining that breast-feeding is a natural function and *therefore* easily possible for all mothers. This is as much wishful thinking as it is wishful thinking to maintain that there is no such thing as constipation. In an ideal (and perhaps more "natural") world, both statements would be true. But in the real (and perhaps especially in the highly industrialized) world neither statement fits the facts.

Such partisan supporters make much of the fact that in past times babies were always fed from the breast and that in many parts of the world they still are. They ignore cultural acceptance of wet-nurses, whether employed or family. They ignore the unknown number of infants who did, and still do, die because breast-feeding fails. They ignore the number who are, and always have been, malnourished because the mother's diet and/or health were poor; they ignore the number of mothers who suffer and have suffered from sore nipples, breast abscesses, and so forth. Any difficulties with breast-feeding in so-called "natural societies" are largely ignored simply because there is no viable alternative. People only begin to debate the pros and cons of different methods of doing anything when they have a choice as to how they should do it.

Western parents do have a choice but, while we should be thankful that happy, healthy babies can be reared either by satisfactory breast-feeding or by careful bottle-feeding, it is a pity that so many mothers still opt for the latter. In recent years more and more differences between the milk intended for babies and the milk intended for calves have been documented; indeed Jelliffe [114] has pointed out that with the exceptions of water and lactose, it is difficult to find any similarities at all. Unmodified cow's milk is totally unsuitable for human infants. Goat's milk, although popularly considered less likely to provoke allergic reactions, is just as unsuitable as are the various evaporated milks, which are still popular among Negro mothers in the United States.

Most Western babies who are not breast-fed are given specially adapted formula "milks," and manufacturers have been quick to respond to demands for new formulae to avoid newly recognized biochemical hazards or to meet special infant needs. It was only in 1977 that Britain's subsidized infant feed "National Dried Milk" was finally withdrawn because of its overload of sodium, potassium chloride, calcium, and phosphorus. An overload of minerals can be dangerous to young babies whose kidneys are too immature to excrete them reliably. The danger is now so well recognized that all infant formulae, fed at the correct dilution, provide a "low-solute feed."

The fats in human and cow's milk are very different. Human milk fat is largely polyunsaturated while butter fat is, of course, saturated. Manufacturers attempt to correct for this difference by substituting some or all vegetable fats or oils for the butter fat, but while this may allow an infant to take sufficient calories without saturated fats, the substitution is not perfect. Babies absorb breast-milk fat better than they absorb any other type and this means a better absorption of fat-soluble vitamins.

All milks are low in iron: breast milk is no exception. But for reasons which are still obscure, the small amount of iron which occurs naturally in human milk is so well-absorbed that breast-fed babies require no iron supplements until much later in their first year than babies fed on iron-fortified formula. The vitamin D in human milk is similarly well-absorbed so that rickets is almost unknown in breast-fed babies, even where there is little sunshine and no supplementation [132]. In these and many other instances, the little that is in breast milk is a little of what is perfect and is therefore enough. Manufacturers can add trace elements and vitamins to their formulae, but they cannot always add what an infant can best utilize.

Cow's milk contains too much of the wrong type of protein for human babies. The total protein content of a feed is reduced in all infant formulae, and various procedures are used during manufacture to render the casein more digestible. But as long as the feed is even based on cow's milk, its protein will include some amino acids which do not occur in human milk. It is these amino acids which are thought to be responsible for sensitizing babies to cow's-milk protein (and therefore, of course, to all dairy products). A large number of allergic disorders are currently attributed to intolerance of cow's milk. This diagnosis is especially common in the United States, where many "disorders" which are regarded as behavioral rather than medical in other parts of the world are attributed to subclinical allergic reactions [13]. Much research remains to be done, but there is certainly some evidence that strict avoidance of *any* foreign antigens in the first half year of life can reduce the incidence of recognized allergic disorders such as eczema [9]. Many American baby milks are now manufactured entirely from vegetable sources, using soy protein instead of cow's-milk protein. These are designed to assist mothers who cannot, or do not want to, breast-feed but who nevertheless want to avoid exposing their babies to cow's-milk protein either because they are anxious to avoid possible allergic reactions or because they want to feed their children a strictly vegetarian diet. While American food technology is arguably the most advanced in the world and parents have a wider choice in the United States than anywhere else, a word of caution is in order. Once milk, human or animal, is excluded from an infant feed, a completely artificial product is being offered and the one chosen should be carefully checked out with a doctor. Some such products require particular dilutions or supplements or may be in some way unsuitable for a particular infant.

Even the most sophisticated manufacturers cannot replicate the protective function of breast milk which contains antibodies and other anti-infective substances. Breast-feeding passes protection from the mother's body to that of her baby during the vulnerable months during which he is building up his own immunities. Many people believe that bottle-fed babies are more liable to illness only because of lack of hygiene in the preparation of feedings. Knowing that their own hygienic precautions will be excellent, they anticipate no problems. A recent survey in Syracuse [80] therefore makes gloomy reading. Over 20 percent of bottle-fed babies—including many whose home care was classified as excellent—suffered from bacterial infections as compared with none among breast-fed babies. Taking pediatric hospital admissions as a whole, children who were breast-fed accounted for only 11 percent where all children in their age group were expected to account for 25 percent.

It seems likely that current research will eventually describe even subtler benefits which infants derive from breast-feeding. Studies comparing breast milk with formulae are usually carried out using pooled samples of breast milk. But the individual mother's milk varies considerably in composition not only from day-to-day or feeding-to-feeding but also during the course of a feeding. The significance of these changes is still not fully understood, but many authorities believe that they are related to the control of the infant's intake by his own appetite, helping him to want to stop eating when his body has received the optimal amount of nourishment. Artificial replication of such a delicate system would obviously be impossible.

Clearly, given what we know and what we do not yet understand about breast milk, it would be ideal if all babies could be fed on it exclusively in their early months. Unfortunately, those who seek to persuade all mothers to breast-feed their infants make far more of the emotional than of the physical gains. Here, the arguments in favor of breast-feeding are much weaker.

The mother who breast-feeds easily and with pleasure probably offers her baby the ultimate in warmth and physical comfort, and the very position in which the baby feeds makes affectionate bodily and eye contact almost inevitable. There is no doubt that breast-fed infants quickly learn to recognize and prefer the very smell of their own mothers [150]; the regularly repeated feeding process automatically encourages bonding between mother and child. But there is no reason why the mother who bottle-feeds should not provide, consciously, what the breast-feeding mother provides without thought. A baby can be held just as warmly for a bottle; he too can be stroked and looked at, talked to and loved. He too can learn his mother's smell from her skin if not from her milk. The same view can be applied to other "advantages" in breast-feeding. Much is made, for example, of the likelihood of a bottle-fed baby being kept waiting for food because he demands it unexpectedly or while the family car is stuck in a traffic jam. Of course it is true that it is *easier* for breast-feeding mothers to meet unpredictable demands but that does not mean that the bottle-feeding mother cannot do so with forethought and care. Any implication that bottle-feeding *per se* indicates, or leads to, lesser love between mother and child is insulting to the many mothers who choose this method and heartbreaking to the many others who can manage nothing else. If a mother finds breast-feeding an easy, enjoyable, and obvious function, then she is fortunate and so is her child. But if she dislikes both the idea and the actuality; tries it only because her advisers insist; suffers from sore nipples; faces a continual struggle to keep up her supplies in the face of a too-busy life; and longs to be able to leave the baby with her husband or a caretaker from time to time, then emotive arguments are likely to be counter-productive. Her relationship with her child and his satisfaction in feeding are both likely to be better if she is able to feed him from a bottle without guilt.

TECHNIQUE

So much has been written about the vital pleasure infants get from sucking food that people sometimes forget that the *newborn* has no experience of sucking his food, and therefore no expectations of pleasure. All he has is an instinctive reaction to being touched on the cheek—turning his head toward the touch—and an instinctive sucking response to the nipple or a similarly shaped object. At the very beginning these instinctive reactions have no backing in experience. The baby does not know that he is crying because he is hungry, that the preliminaries of a feeding mean food, and that food will stop the hunger pain. Some babies, crying for food, will indeed go through the reflex actions, and take a hearty suck, only to continue bawling. Even the first gush of milk does not tell them that the sooner they stop crying and suck the sooner they will feel better. How could it? Other babies seem to have the approved reflexes only to a very limited extent. It is difficult to persuade them to latch on to the breast or bottle, and difficult to persuade them to suck once they have. But there are others who seem to be born suckers; there is even some evidence that these may be the ones who have practiced sucking their fingers in the womb. They learn the lesson, that sucking = food = cessation of hunger pain, so rapidly that it is difficult to realize it ever was a learning process.

The infant has to have food, and he has to have it by sucking. He has to learn the relation between sucking his food and being comfortable. His instincts are there; relating them to satisfactory experience is up to the mother.

The infant's very first feedings may be supervised by a nurse, or the mother may be left to manage mostly on her own. Even where help is offered it may not in fact prove very useful. The nurse would undoubtedly feed the baby expertly *herself;* but she may be far less good at helping the mother to do so. Especially in breast-feeding, it is as difficult to help somebody get an infant comfortably sucking as it is to help somebody tie his tie. You can do it for them, or let them do it, but the two of you doing it together tend to get in a muddle. Feeding a baby is a very one-one procedure. There is really no room for a third party except as demonstrator or admiring audience.

Whether he is easy or difficult to teach about sucking milk, the baby will learn fastest if all concerned keep a clear picture in their minds of the instinctive reactions he already has, and which they must use in the early feedings.

The baby turns his head *toward* a gentle touch on the cheek. It follows that if both cheeks are held, however gently, in an attempt to steer him to breast or bottle, he is confused and angry. In breast-feeding this gentle touch usually happens automatically. The breast brushes against the baby's cheek as the mother gathers him toward her. He then turns inward, toward the breast, and if the nipple then touches his mouth, the mouth purses ready to suck. Timing is therefore important; if he turns inward toward the breast and the mother is not ready to present the nipple, the optimum moment for him to latch on may have been lost.

In bottle-feeding, there is often no preliminary touch to the cheek. The bottle may be presented straight on, so that the first the baby knows of it is the mother's attempt to put the nipple in his mouth. He may accept it, but his natural head-turning and mouth-pursing reflexes have been by-passed, and he may not. In summary, the best chance of a successful feeding, in the early days, lies in giving the baby cues to turn toward the food and purse his lips to receive it before giving it to him.

Unfortunately both mothers and nurses tend to be so concerned over the new infant's need for milk, and so frustrated by his apparent inefficiency in taking it, that they often create difficulties. A very new baby who is distressed and crying will seldom settle easily to a feeding, yet because the adults know he is crying because he is hungry, they try to force him to accept the nipple. The angrier and more desperate he gets, the harder they may try to force him to suck. A situation which should never have arisen in the first place is made worse. If tactful attempts to slip the nipple into the baby's mouth fail, some other way of calming him

—such as wrapping him tightly and rocking him—ought to be tried first, and then the whole cheek-stroking, head-turning, mouth-pursing routine tried again when he is calmer.

Often, too, they have a distorted picture of what the very new infant *ought* to take, and when he ought to take it. Very sleepy babies, who suck 1/4 oz. (7 ml) and fall asleep again, and wake half an hour later to repeat the process, are wearing for the mother, but they will grow out of this pattern in a few days as they become more awake. In the meantime they are probably not getting less food from those minuscule bottle-feedings than they would be getting if they were taking colostrum from the breast. It is arguable that they do not in fact *need* food at all during the first 3–5 days, but only some liquid. Certainly the continual jouncing, flicking, and general shaking around that goes on in an attempt to wake the baby enough to suck some more has nothing to recommend it.

Bottle-fed babies are often wildly frustrated in their early feedings by the hole in the nipple being too small. Recent research involving 122 babies who were 6 days old showed that they took 50 percent of the milk from each breast in 2 minutes and 80–90 percent in 4 minutes. To equal this rate, the milk should drip out of an inverted bottle at several drops per *second* without any shaking. It is no use testing the nipple with water, which, being thinner, comes out faster. Holes that are too small can be enlarged with a sterilized needle.

QUANTITY

People vary in how much they need to eat. They vary at birth and they go on varying. They end up as adults with differing food needs too. One man eats ravenously, does a sedentary job, and still weighs at 50 what he weighed as an athletic 18-year-old. Another diets constantly, exercises more than he wants to and still puts on unwanted pounds. So all people vary both in the amount of food they feel they need—their hunger and appetite—and in the efficiency with which they use what they eat—the number of calories they need to hold their weight steady with a given amount of activity.

Despite all this very real variability most people find it useful to have some idea of the *average* food requirements of the groups of people for whom they have to care and cook, and to know something about the calorie contents of some of the foods they serve. But this is usually information which is given for older children or for adults. With babies, the American trend has been away from any such "weighing and measuring," whether of the baby or his food. A relaxed, "give him what he wants and he'll do fine" attitude has been cultivated instead. While such an attitude is fine as long as parents genuinely *feel* relaxed about infant feeding, it becomes extremely frustrating as soon as any cause for concern shows up. And shameful though it may be in the current state of opinion, a great many parents do worry about what their infants eat and don't eat.

Breast milk has an average caloric value of 20 per fluid ounce, although, as we have seen, the composition of an individual mother's milk will vary during and between feedings.

Proprietary infant milks, whether liquid or dried, are manufactured so that when they are made up exactly according to instructions, they provide a feed of this strength. As long as a baby is being fed either on breast milk or an infant-formula milk, all calculations concerning his intake can be made on the basis of the same figures.

A different basis for calculations would be needed only if an infant were being fed on a dilution of unmodified milk—liquid whole cow's milk or canned evaporated milk, for example—or if he was being fed on a specially prescribed milk-substitute such as soybean "milk" for medical reasons.

In their first few months most infants seem to need about 55 calories for each pound of their bodyweight per day (110 calories per kilogram per day). This works out at around 2 3/4 oz. of made-up milk per pound per day (about 165 ml/kg per day).

To ensure that the infant's needs are generously met—and to simplify the arithmetic—it is reasonable to call that 2 3/4 oz., 3 oz. and that 165 ml, 180 ml. With this slight over-allowance it is legitimate to simplify weight calculations by taking them only to the nearest 1/2 lb. or 250 g.

If a parent sets out to calculate the food requirements of any individual infant it is essential that this is done on the basis of the baby's *ideal* weight (usually referred to as his "expected weight") rather than on the basis of what the baby actually weighs *now*. If the actual weight is used there is real risk of underestimating the baby's needs and, if only the calculated amount is offered, of underfeeding him. This is because the baby may, at any moment in time, be lighter than his optimum weight for any one of a variety of reasons. If he is fed as if that lighter-than-optimum weight was his natural weight, he will be unable to catch himself up. Most babies lose some weight in the few days after birth, for example. If an individual baby regains that weight very slowly, due to illness, to breast milk being slow to come in, or due to reluctance to suck, there could be a vicious circle such that having been half-starved in his first fortnight he continued to be half-starved because he was fed as if that starved weight was his personal ideal.

Parents who wish to make calculations at all must therefore learn to calculate the expected weight of their baby. It is an easy and a rough and ready procedure, but an important one.

(a) *If the baby is less than 10 days old*
The calculation is based on the likelihood that he will lose around 1 oz. or 30 g per day up to and including day 5 and that he will put on 1 oz. or 30 g per day up to and including day 10. He is therefore "expected" to weigh the same on day 10 as he weighed at birth. Start with his birthweight.

Subtract 1 oz. or 30 g for each day up to and including day 5.

Add 1 oz. or 30 g for each subsequent day up to and including day 10.

(b) *If the baby is more than 10 days old*

The calculation is based on the likelihood that, having regained his birthweight at 10 days, he will subsequently gain around 1 oz. or 30 g per day.

Start with his birthweight which is also his expected weight for 10 days.

Ignore the vagaries of his post-natal weight loss and gain and simply add 1 oz. or 30 g to that birthweight for every day from day 10.

For example, what is the expected weight of a baby born weighing 6 lb. 14 oz. (3.1 kg) who is now aged 15 days? Assume that he weighed 6 lb. 14 oz. (3.1 kg) at 10 days; add 1 oz. (30 g) for each of the five days between day 10 and day 15 and the expected weight is 7 lb. 3 oz. or 3.3 kg.

Having done all that—which looks a great deal more complicated than it actually is—this same infant's likely food needs per 24 hours are calculated by multiplying his weight in pounds by 3 oz. or his weight in kilograms by 180 ml. Since we are working to the nearest half pound or 250 g we call that weight 7 lb. and 3.25 kg. He is therefore likely to need around 21 oz. (600 ml) of made-up milk per 24 hours.

Expected weights, expected daily weight gains, and likely food intakes *are not rules.* A particular baby may want and need twice as much as these calculations would suggest or may thrive and gain weight on much less. For personal reasons, the mother of one infant of average birthweight who was breast-fed on demand test-weighed him after every feeding in his first six weeks. Her records, summarized in Figure 3, give an unusual opportunity to demonstrate the "fit" between his demands, the milk supply which those demands evoked, and the weight gain which resulted.

UNDERFEEDING

Most parents and their advisers do now accept that the only sensible way to treat a hungry baby is to feed him. "Demand feeding" is still an unfortunate *phrase* as to many people it carries heavy connotations of screaming infants being indulged, but the ideas behind it have nevertheless largely replaced the rigid schedules which once bedeviled so many families.

Many authorities suggest that as long as a baby *is* fed "on demand" and with a suitable milk, underfeeding is extremely unlikely. Attention has shifted, perhaps too completely, to the problems of overfeeding and infant obesity (see p. 81). I believe that underfeeding remains a real factor, in some families, leading not only to sub-optimal infant growth but also to sub-optimal parent-child relations.

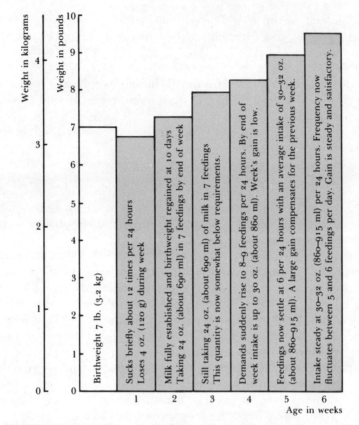

FIGURE 3. MILK INTAKE AND WEIGHT GAIN OF ONE INFANT BREAST-FED
"ON DEMAND"

During the first week his frequent demands get the milk supply established. He loses some weight meanwhile but quickly regains it and is over his birthweight in week 2.

By his fourth week the supply which he has established and kept flowing by taking 3 1/2 oz. (100 ml) 7 times each 24 hours becomes inadequate for his increasing weight. Hungry, he demands more frequent feeding which results in a 6 oz. (170 ml) increase in intake. The low-weight gain for this week reflects the days early in the week when he was not getting quite enough but by the fifth week he is getting plenty and therefore makes a large compensatory weight gain while settling to only 6 feedings in the 24 hours. During week 6 there is plenty of milk for his needs, weight gain is again good, and feeding frequency drops.

Underfed Breast-fed Babies

Many mothers believe that their babies would be underfed if they were fed exclusively from the breast. A very high proportion of breast-fed babies are given bottles of formula while they are still in the hospital. This may, in itself, reduce the efficiency with which they suck at the breast and stimulate milk production. It may also reduce mothers' confidence:

"Every time the nurse brought her to me she brought a bottle too. She seemed convinced that the baby wouldn't get enough from me."

Many mothers continue to offer bottles of formula even while they are trying to get a supply of breast milk established at home. Sucking milk from a bottle demands a different technique from taking milk from a breast. Many babies find a bottle "easier" and, always offered both, rapidly come to prefer the bottle. Once again there is a double discouragement to breast-feeding in this situation. The baby puts less effort into breast-feeding and therefore provides less stimulation to the milk supply *and* he discourages his mother by seeming to reject what she offers in favor of the formula. It is not surprising that such a high proportion of mothers find that breast-feeding has simply petered out, with the baby taking less from the breast and more from the bottle until it no longer seems worth offering the breast at all. In the British National Survey [153] "Insufficient Milk" was by far the most frequent reason given for abandoning breast-feeding in the early weeks. Neither the mothers themselves nor the researchers can really know either whether there *was* insufficient breast milk or whether there *need have been* if the attempts to breast-feed had been handled differently.

Some hospitals and advisers are careful not to introduce babies to bottles or to imply in any way to mothers that their infants might need anything other than what is provided by the breast. But breast-fed babies can be underfed, continually but to a small extent, without their mothers realizing it until the scales in the doctor's office give them a shock because the baby is failing to gain weight, or is doing so very slowly.

If the breast milk is marginally inadequate over the 24 hours, this can be enough to reduce the weight gain, without the infant's behavior alerting the mother. Often, for example, the milk is scantiest in the evening. The baby may indeed be more restless during the evening than he is during the day when supplies are better. But because he seems content by day the mother may put his evening restlessness down to colic or simply to this being his chosen period of wakefulness. Similarly if the baby continues for some weeks to demand two feedings during the night the mother may assume that this is simply his pattern—that it is a question of maturation rather than chronic underfeeding. She may be confirmed in this view by the very copiousness of her milk supply in the early morning. It is hard for a mother who wakes each day soaked in milk, with hard swollen breasts, which positively spurt as the baby starts to suck, to realize that later in the day her milk may be inadequate.

The breast-feeding mother cannot tell how much her baby has taken. This is both the beauty and the bugbear of breast-feeding. When all goes well it is beautiful. The baby sucks, thrives, and grows; the mother neither knows nor needs to know what he takes and, after a few weeks, will probably not even glance at the clock as she prepares to feed him, nor count up the number of times she has offered the breast today. But when all does not go well, following the baby's distressed and inchoate demands can be exceedingly difficult. The mother follows the approved advice to offer the breast whenever the child seems hungry; she tries to believe that, given every opportunity to stimulate those breasts, the child himself will force them to produce the amount he needs. She offers the breast again and again. Sometimes it is accepted and "a feed" is taken, but sometimes it is rejected with furious wails. Was the child not hungry after all or was there too little milk there for him to feel even momentarily satisfied? When he cries again half an hour later is it because he is now hungry—having not been so the last time—or is it because he is *still* hungry having been so all along? If day and night blur into an exhaustion of constant feeding, the mother's fatigue may, in itself, reduce the supply of milk. If, at the end of such a week, the scales show that the child has gained little, only the most convinced advocate of exclusive breast-feeding will struggle on for long because no loving parent will half-starve a baby when an easy answer is no further away than the nearest store. Many mothers sadly describe their disappointment when breast-feeding "fails," yet explain the overwhelming relief of watching three or four ounces of formula vanish down their baby's throat: "It meant that I *knew* he couldn't be hungry so I could think about other things that might be making him unhappy . . . you can't *think* when you're struggling with breast-feeding."

The mother who wants to breast-feed but is "struggling" and "can't think" will often ask advice from the nearest sympathetic and/or knowledgeable person. Support from another mother who has successfully breast-fed her own child can be invaluable. Organizations such as the La Leche League increasingly arrange for this kind of person-to-person support. Even more valuable can be reassurance from a health professional. Some health visitors take great pride in helping new mothers to establish full breast-feeding. But this kind of support is not available to every mother. In the recent British Survey many of the mothers who abandoned breast-feeding in the early weeks said that they had been advised to do so by a midwife, health visitor, or doctor. Of course they may have misinterpreted or misrepresented what was said to them, but there still are authorities who automatically suggest offering a bottle to any baby whose mother wonders whether he is hungry after breast-feedings.

I believe that such mothers badly need some objective way of assessing what their babies are getting from the breast and the extent to which they are growing and thriving. This is why I take an unfashionably positive view of baby scales in the home *for mothers who are worried*. It is argued that introducing scales simultaneously introduces anxiety. But that is invalid when anxiety is already present. It is argued that if mothers can consider a weight they will look at that rather than at their babies, but again that is invalid when the mother, looking at her baby, has been unable to decide whether all is well or not. It is argued that a mother who weighs her baby before and after every feeding, perhaps for 24 hours every three or four days, ruins the relaxed and casual bliss which ought to be intrinsic to breast-feeding. But that is invalid too when the whole reason for introducing the scales is that feeding is *not* relaxed, casual or blissful.

Although the use of baby scales in the home is frowned upon by most American authorities, such scales are found very useful and comforting by breast-feeding mothers in other countries. Of course it would be idiotic to rush for the scales every day to check on a thriving baby. His contentment and health are a far better guide to his satisfactory growth than any other measure. But where there is cause to wonder whether he is getting enough breast milk, test-weighing can give a quicker, easier, and altogether more illuminating answer. The procedure is simple. For one period of 24 hours, the baby is weighed, in his clothes, before the breast-feeding and after it. His clothing is not altered between the two weighings, and his diaper is not changed either. The difference between the before feeding and the after feeding weight is an exact measure of the breast milk he obtained at that feeding. Knowing the amount taken at one feeding is useless, because the baby's hunger and the supply of milk vary throughout the day. But the total taken at each feeding during the 24 hours tells the mother what she needs to know.

What does the resulting sum tell the mother? It tells her nothing *absolute,* but it does give her one piece of hard data to add to her observation of and thinking about her baby.

If the sum total for the 24 hours is as much as, or more than, the infant's calculated daily requirement for his expected weight, then the mother can be reassured about her ability to provide enough for him. She may not be providing enough at that moment, because he may be a hungry baby who needs more than that average or he may not be being fed according to his personal timetable (see p. 37). But if he is already getting that much from the breast, he will certainly be able to adjust the demand/supply situation if his mother persists. Equally, that quantity which is enough on paper may indeed *be* enough; there may be other reasons for his discontent. Being thus reassured about his food will probably enable both his parents to think more calmly and constructively about other aspects of his daily life.

If the sum total is less than the infant's calculated needs for his expected weight, then it is likely his discontent is due to hunger. The same scales will enable his mother to check: if there is low or no weight gain, then the infant is certainly not getting enough to eat.

Far from finding themselves made more anxious by this discovery, or more inclined to offer formula immediately, many mothers who really want to breast-feed find that factual knowledge of a milk shortage makes it far easier to cope with. As one such mother said, "If you want to be a good cow and you find that you aren't, it is really quite fun working at it. It's the not knowing that is hell." Instead of resenting and worrying over the baby's fretting, such a mother can understand it and set to work to help her baby put it right, by encouraging him to suck whenever he wishes, by expressing any milk left after feedings at which the supply is abundant, and by adapting her own life. Some mothers, who had been living in chaos and trying to get other things done against the demands of an unhappy baby, relaxed the pace, called on any family or outside help they could find, and determinedly rested. Others decided that harassment had been preventing them from eating properly or from drinking enough, and they made real efforts to take time for proper meals and to notice and drink when they were thirsty. Only half joking, one mother said, "He [her husband] realized that I couldn't cook supper for us and produce it for the baby. If he got my meal, hers was ready for her when I'd eaten it. He called it 'spoiling me' but he had to admit it was worthwhile."

If a woman is working to increase her milk, she will need hard evidence concerning her progress. Further test-weighing over the next two weeks will give it to her. If the baby's contentment, weight, and intake do not increase she will obviously have to offer a complementary bottle-feeding, but if she can see even the beginning of an increase she may find it worthwhile to persist.

If the baby's weight gain and continued discontent suggest that he really must have more food than he can get from the breast, complementary bottles—even if their introduction gradually ends breast-feeding—are certainly better for him than the only other solution—the early introduction of "solid" foods. Fashions in the timing of the introduction of mixed-feeding swing wildly but in recent years reliable opinion has set the ideal later rather than sooner. Many authorities now believe that a fully breast-fed baby is probably best on breast milk alone throughout the first half year and that bottle-fed babies need no solids before four to five months. To introduce cereals and other purées much earlier than this, simply because not enough breast milk is available, would be irresponsible. If breast milk alone is the ideal, a good formula, carefully made up, is certainly the next best thing. It is sad to hear some passionate advocates of breast-feeding boasting that their infants "never knew what a bottle was" when half their calories have been tipped into them from a teaspoon from a few weeks of age.

Underfed Bottle-fed Babies

These are usually the unfortunates whose mothers take advice from books like this one too literally. Such a mother painstakingly works out her baby's "requirements," and then makes up 21 oz. (600 ml) of formula, divides it into 6 feedings of 3 1/2 oz. (100 ml) each, and feeds that to the baby. Then she congratulates herself because he always drains his bottle. Finishing a bottle is not a virtue in small babies. It is a reproof to mothers. If he drains every drop, there is no way of knowing whether he would have liked more. Even if 21 oz. (600 ml) in 24 hours happens to be just right for him, it does not follow that he will want the same amount at each feeding, nor that he may not have extra hungry days and less hungry days. For bottle-fed babies, calculated "requirements" should only serve as data for mothers to think about if the baby fails to gain weight or seems discontented. If the mother knows roughly what he is likely to need and knows he is taking at least that much, then she can exclude hunger as a cause of discontent, and can seek advice if lack of hunger is leading to low weight gain. Knowing what he needs, she should see to it that each bottle contains at least 2 oz. (about 55 ml) more. If he drinks it, fine; if he does not, equally fine.

Extra Fluids

Small babies have a large surface area in relation to their weight and they can therefore lose a great deal of fluid in sweating. If the weather is hot or the infant has any fever—especially with an illness which also gives him diarrhea or makes him vomit—the need for extra fluid may become urgent. Many of the infants admitted to the hospital each year have deteriorated not just because of their illness but because of the dehydration associated with it.

Breast milk or formula is a baby's drink as well as his food so thirst without hunger places him in a real dilemma. This is especially acute for the bottle-fed infant because even with modern low-solute formulae, the milk contains more sodium than breast milk. If he takes a bottle because he is thirsty but not very hungry, the milk may make him even thirstier. If he cries immediately after being fed and is offered more formula, a vicious circle of discontent can be set up.

I believe that all bottle-fed babies should be offered plain boiled water once or twice a day when they are awake between feedings, and more frequently if they are unwell, taking less milk than usual, or when the weather is hot. Of course the water can contain fruit juice, but since most babies suck sweet drinks more readily than unsweetened ones (see p. 82) it may be sensible to accustom them to plain water as well.

Extra water is a more controversial topic for breast-fed babies. That food-and-drink-combined is everything the infant needs and some mothers do feel that having to introduce a bottle at all, even for water, spoils breast-feeding's simple perfection. The mother who does feel like that can safely follow her inclinations as long as her infant is well, contented, and clearly getting plenty of milk. But if there is ever a shortage of breast milk, or if the baby loses his appetite and/or runs a fever, he too will need extra water.

FREQUENCY AND TIMING

A baby's digestion is such that a full meal, taken calmly over a reasonable period—in 25 minutes, say, rather than in sips over an hour—will probably last him for between 3 and 4 hours. But that is once he is settled, once his digestion has begun to have a pattern. He has, after all, to learn to accept comfortable fullness and near emptiness, rather than the constant "topping up" of nutritional needs which went on in the womb. Further-more he has to accept our diurnal rhythm, to accept a long period unfed during the night. All this takes time. Because it takes time, the much disputed questions about whether babies should be fed "on demand" or "on schedule" make very little sense. If a pre-calculated rhythm is im-posed on the baby's feeding, he will eventually accept that rhythm, and be ready for food at roughly the pre-set hours. But during the intervening weeks he will have had periods of acute distress, when his new digestion told him different from the clock. If, on the other hand, his mother tries, in the early weeks, to follow the demands of his digestion, she will end up similarly placed. He will only want food at the 3–4 hour interval. The only difference is that the mother will have suffered some inconvenience in the intervening weeks, instead of the infant suffering hunger and frustration. The advantages of pre-set feeding times do not outweigh the advantages of a more contented baby for many mothers. The hunger cry of a very young child is extremely difficult to resist. Many who reared their children during the 1930s and 1940s can tell horror stories of sitting weeping in nursery doorways, listening to their baby, watching the clock, uterus and breasts aching with empathy as the crying got more desperate and the minute hand slower.

Few of today's mothers would put themselves and their babies through that kind of unnecessary hell but, as so often happens with shifting fashions, our escape from the extremes of scheduled feeding has led some mothers into difficulties with the extremes of demand feeding. Properly interpreted, feeding on demand means exactly what it says: the baby demands food and the mother gives it to him. He leads; she follows. Some mothers go one step further and believe that if it is good to feed a baby as soon as he demands food it must be even better to feed him when he is *about to* demand food. Infants in such families are never allowed to awaken without being offered food nor to stay awake without food being offered and re-offered, sometimes at 10-minute intervals, until they fall asleep again. The result can be an infant who is never hungry nor replete; an infant who takes his food, a few sucks at a time, all through the day and night. While I know of no evidence to suggest that this is physically harmful, it cannot be psychologically or develop-mentally helpful. True demand feeding gives the infant confidence that when he expresses a need it will be met. By preventing him from express-ing (perhaps even from experiencing) his needs for food, his mother unwittingly deprives him. True demand feeding also helps the infant, at his own personal pace, to adapt himself to the mature rhythms of eating periodically and of sleeping through the night. Continual offers of food prevent this. Worst of all, perhaps, the mother who always greets her infant's awakenings or responds to his wakeful sounds and facial expres-sions with food tends to undervalue other kinds of interaction with the baby and perhaps to misinterpret or to miss his expressions of needs other than hunger.

So, while a return to an imposed "schedule" would be extremely retrograde, it is perhaps valuable to remember that the aim of demand feeding is not to feed an infant either all the time or at random times, but to feed him when he wants food and to help him to evolve a pattern of feeding times which suit him first, and later, the whole family. There is no doubt that some infants settle into a feeding pattern far more quickly and easily than others and that a few are happy to be fed more or less at the mother's convenience where others definitely are not. If the infant always has to be woken for his feedings anyway, then there is obviously no reason why he should not be woken to suit the mother's wishes. She is having to tell his digestive system that it needs food, rather than it telling her; so she might as well tell it that it needs food at the "right" time. If, when he wakes, the baby stops crying when he is picked up, and waits calmly, then again there is no reason why his feedings should not be delayed if the mother prefers. But if, as is more usual, the hunger cry is urgent, the calming on being lifted transitory, then nothing is gained by waiting. With some babies something may actually be lost. In the early weeks, a baby whose experience and expectations are so limited can quickly cry himself into such a state that when he is finally fed he cannot calm down enough to suck properly. He may suck a little and fall into exhausted sleep before he has had enough. The whole dilemma then has to be faced again when he wakes an hour or so later. The actual feeding, sleeping, and crying times of one baby girl who was breast-fed "on demand" are shown in Figures 4 and 5. They clearly illustrate both the irregularity of her demands at 5 days of age and the regularity of the pattern which she had spontaneously adopted by the time she was one month old.

Infants vary in how long it takes them to differentiate night from day, at least in terms of sleep. At the beginning, if the baby happens to go for longest without a feeding during the night hours, it is either pure luck (in which case he may return to sleeping most of the day and waking every three hours at night, equally randomly) or it simply reflects the greater peace and darkness of the house at night.

For the first 4 or 5 weeks, almost all babies need feeding at least once during the mother's ordinary sleeping hours. If she is unlucky the mother may be woken twice. The effect of this night waking on the mother is often underestimated. She may be able to make up the *hours* of sleep she loses by napping in the afternoon, or going to bed early, but she cannot right the destruction of her sleep patterns. Maternity nurses—that rare breed of women who live in, and help to take care of the newborn baby and the mother—do not reckon that they can undertake the infant's night feedings *and* work an ordinary 8-hour day as well. Agencies supplying them will not send them to houses where this will be expected. Yet mothers have to undertake the night feedings and work what often amounts to a 12-hour day as well, *and* they are the ones who have recently given birth. Fathers can share this burden, and it is probably important that they

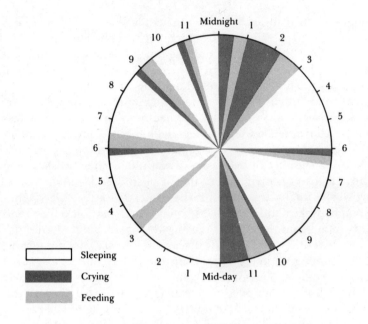

FIGURE 4. FEEDING, SLEEPING, AND CRYING TIMES OF ONE DEMAND-FED
INFANT AGED 5 DAYS

The randomness of basic behaviors in the newborn period is shown very clearly by this baby who, by 28 days had settled into a chosen pattern very similar to that which might be imposed upon a baby fed "on schedule."

On day 5 the time interval between feeds ranged from almost 5 hours (after 10:15 A.M.) down to 1 1/2 hours (after 11 P.M.). By day 28 no two feedings were closer together than four hourly.

On day 5 there is not only crying before feedings—this being the mother's cue to feed the baby—there is also crying after feeding on several occasions. The feeding given at half past midnight failed to settle her, although the episode did finally terminate with the feeding given at 2 A.M. Her crying after her 10 A.M. feeding ended without a further feeding and

should do so, both because of the actual help they can offer and because taking a full share of responsibility for what is involved in baby care at this early age is likely to help the father feel that the baby is truly his as well as his wife's, rather than an intruder on his wife's attentions to him. Private interaction between father and new baby in the middle of the night can have an effect on their relationship that is almost magical. If the baby is bottle-fed, the father can fully share the night feedings, either by taking alternate nights or perhaps by coping with the second feeding if the baby has two during the night hours. If the baby is breast-fed he obviously cannot take over completely, but even then he can be the one to go to the baby, change him, bring him to the mother in bed, sit with them to ensure that the mother does not fall asleep while feeding, and then return the infant to his crib. But these egalitarian ideals do not

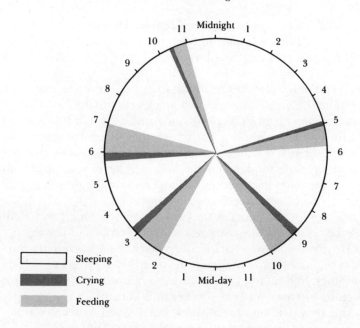

FIGURE 5. FEEDING, SLEEPING, AND CRYING TIMES OF THE SAME INFANT
NOW AGED 28 DAYS

it is clear that her distress was not due to hunger as she then slept until 3 P.M. and was awakened to eat. On day 28 crying is little more than a hunger-signal and only at 3 P.M. was there any crying at all after a feeding.

On day 5 feedings, combined with sociable time awake, seldom lasted more than half an hour at a time, but by day 28 they extend to almost an hour except for the 11 P.M. feeding at which the mother was clearly trying to convey to the baby that this was sleeptime not playtime.

It is interesting to notice that the baby spent less time asleep on day 5 than on day 28, largely because she spent more time crying and being comforted. By her fourth week pleasant social time and peaceful sleeping time have both increased.

always work out in practice. Many mothers find that they wake anyway the moment the baby cries (and perhaps have to kick their still sleeping husbands!). Once awake, many find it difficult to go to sleep again until they know the baby is settled. In these circumstances some find that having the father do most of the actual work is not sufficient compensation for having him exhausted as well as themselves. They may prefer to let him sleep, but have him cope with breakfast while they catch a last blissful hour; or cope with everything and everybody on Sundays while they lie in half the morning and nap all afternoon.

Unfortunately, before he is about 6 weeks, little can be done with the baby himself which will increase the parents' chance of a long sleep at night. If the baby is woken for a feeding just before the mother goes to bed, he *may* give her 4 or 5 hours. But equally, waking him may simply break what would have been a long sleep period. He may wake 3 hours later all the same. Persuading him to take every drop he can hold *may* keep him asleep for an extra half hour—or it may give him gas and indigestion.

But like everything else in the settling period, night feeding does eventually rationalize itself. Around 4–6 weeks the infant's pattern of night hunger becomes clear. Perhaps he is woken for a feeding at around 11 P.M. and then wakes around 5 A.M. Once this is regular it is worth seeing whether if he is fed at midnight he will last until a more civilized 6 A.M. Equally if he always wakes at 9 P.M. and then again at around both 1 and 5 A.M. it is worth seeing whether waking him at midnight will enable him to skip the small hours' feeding altogether.

But at this age inconsistency is the order of things. One good night does not predict another. Nor is there the least purpose in leaving the baby to cry. He may cry himself back to sleep because he was not urgently hungry, and crying tires him. But what is the point? His crying has already woken the mother, and he will certainly wake again within the hour with the hunger really intense. Water and other milk substitutes are similarly useless. Sucking may put him back to sleep, but if what he sucked was not food it will not satisfy his hunger, and he will wake again, probably just as the mother enters deep sleep. She would have saved precious sleeping time if she had fed him in the first place.

3

OTHER PHYSICAL FUNDAMENTALS

SLEEP

VERY FEW RELIABLE STATISTICS EXIST to tell us how many hours in the 24 babies actually sleep. This apparently simple question is very difficult to research: researchers must either observe infants themselves, continuously, over several days and nights, or they must ask the mothers. The first procedure is enormously time consuming and therefore expensive, as well as imposing a great burden on the family being studied. The second method is usually very unreliable. Most mothers do not *know* whether or not their small infants are actually asleep. They only know whether or not they are quiet and undemanding.

Books of advice on child rearing tend to imply that new infants sleep practically the whole time except when being fed or handled. By implication they suggest that there may be something wrong with the infant who wakes up before he is hungry, or who refuses to go to sleep after a feeding.

The few small-scale observational studies which have been carried out give a quite different picture. N. Kleitman and T. G. Engelmann [129], for example, studied ten infants at home. At the age of 3 weeks their average sleeping time was 15 hours, and the variation around that average was enormous. If 6 hours in the 24 are allowed for feeding, changing, cuddling, bathing, and generally caring for the infant, that average of 15 hours' sleep still leaves 3 hours in the 24 when the infant can be expected to be awake just because he is not asleep.

At one extreme, there really are babies who sleep almost continually in the first few weeks. Their mothers rightly assume that they will settle as soon as they are put in their cribs after a feeding; they expect to have to wake them up for at least one or two feedings in the day, and they take an 8-hour sleep-span at night for granted from very early on. At the other extreme, there are perfectly healthy, normal babies who never sleep for more than 10–12 hours in the 24.

A new baby cannot have "sleep problems" himself, unless he is ill, or being maltreated. Provided he is reasonably fed and moderately comfortable he will sleep when he needs to. Any problem is his mother's, not his. Often new mothers find it very difficult to relax and get on with what they want to do if they know their baby is not peacefully asleep. Obviously relaxation is, and should be, impossible if the baby is sending out distress signals. But if he is simply awake, because he is an awake kind of baby in an awake kind of mood, there is nothing the mother can do to put him to sleep. Somehow she has to re-adapt her expectations, stop feeling that the baby *ought* to be asleep, and find a companionable *modus vivendi* with him. In this respect he is behaving more like a 3–4 month infant than a newborn; reference to Chapter Fourteen may therefore be helpful.

Many mothers find it useful to help their newborns toward a complete differentiation between sleep and waking. At this stage many infants spend long periods in between the two states, as if they neither knew how to be quite awake nor how to be quite asleep. This real-life observation is supported by a growing body of research differentiating the sleep patterns of newborns from those of older people. Where an adult usually spends about 20 percent of his sleeping time in light ("random eye-movement") sleep and the remaining 80 percent in deep sleep, an infant's sleeping is divided 50-50 between the two types [176]. It is during those long periods of "light" sleep that the infant appears neither fully awake nor soundly asleep and is often kept from progressing into deep sleep by being handled as if he were wakeful.

While parents can do nothing about their infant's biological sleep mechanisms, their lives, later on, will be far easier if they know that the infant is definitely sleeping and therefore needing nothing, or awake and therefore likely to need company and care. Both the baby and his parents will come to feel this separation between the two states most quickly if, from the beginning, he is helped to associate certain places and situations with sleep, and other places and situations with being awake. If the infant is always put either into his carriage in the garden, or in a special corner of the living room, or into his crib when he is expected to sleep, he will eventually come to associate those places with sleep. If, on the other hand, he is left to drop off on his mother's lap in the middle of a cuddle, he is far more likely to drift vaguely from wakefulness to dozing to wakefulness again.

Putting the infant into special regular places to sleep does not mean that the house must be hushed, or other people's activities curtailed for him. New infants are woken up far more easily by internal stimuli, such as hunger, or passing a stool, than they are by external ones. Most will sleep in the middle of a family row, or with the television set on, or three toddlers playing soldiers around the carriage. What disturbs them is any violent *change* in the level of outside stimuli. When the row ceases, the television set is turned off, the room lights are turned on, or the telephone rings, the baby may wake.

Having to feed the infant in the night is disturbing enough for the mother; additional night waking can turn her life into a somnambulistic nightmare. Most infants in this age group only wake at night when they are hungry, but some wake very frequently indeed. Often the trouble comes from the infant sharing his parents' bedroom. Studies have shown that all babies "surface" several times during each sleep period. They open their eyes, perhaps lift their heads and move their limbs. If nothing stimulates them, they drop straight back into sleep again. They do not "want" anything; they are not hungry, or cold, or uncomfortable, so they do not cry. If the baby is in a separate room, the mother knows nothing about these small awakenings. But if the baby's crib is beside her, *she* is probably woken by his small rustlings. She gets out of bed and looks into the crib. The baby sees her, or hears her, and that moment of consciousness at once turns into a demand.

While the mother may get more sleep if she does not know about her infant's momentary surfacings during the night, the evidence shows that she gains nothing at all by ignoring his real awakenings. T. Moore and L. E. Ucko [158] found that the infants who woke most often in the night in their early months were the ones whose parents were most afraid of "spoiling" them, and therefore most reluctant to pick them up when they cried. Some mothers short-circuit the problems of night-waking and night-feeding by willingly sharing their beds with the infant from the beginning. Some eminent pediatricians now recommend this and have done a great service to parents by demonstrating, through film and other material, that even the youngest infants are at no risk of being squashed or smothered. But while keeping the infant in the parents' bed may solve some problems, it also raises others. The pros and cons are well reviewed by Martin Bax [17]. We shall return to the subject later (see p. 335).

ELIMINATION

The stools of fully breast-fed and bottle-fed babies are very different. Breast-fed babies pass from the "changing stool" described on page 15 to a stool which is an orangey-yellow liquid paste, with a slight "sour milk" smell, entirely different from the smell of the stool of those on a mixed diet.

While this is often called the "normal" stool for a breast-fed baby, there are quite alarming variations on the theme which are also entirely normal.

Many infants take as much as 3 to 4 weeks to arrive at the "normal" stool. During this period the baby may pass as many as 12 movements a day. They may be violently expelled; they are often bright green in color, and contain obvious mucus and lumps of curd. Taught about the dangers of gastroenteritis in small babies, many mothers assume that their new-borns have violent diarrhea.

Diarrhea *can* occur in a breast-fed baby, but it is extremely uncommon. If the baby is under 3–4 weeks, and is otherwise well and thriving, his extraordinary stools are no cause for alarm. If he really did have diarrhea at this age he would have other signs of illness, such as lack of appetite, listlessness, and dehydration—with eyes that looked sunken, a depressed fontanelle and very low weight gain.

By about 3 weeks the color and consistency of the stools will probably have changed to the mustard-like substance described earlier. The frequency may remain. Perfectly normal breast-fed babies sometimes have more bowel movements in a day than their mothers know about; they are always soiled whenever the diaper is changed. Research workers have followed babies who were passing twenty movements in the 24 hours, and babies have been mistakenly admitted to a hospital on this account alone. If the baby is well the mother can reassure herself by checking with the doctor and then stop counting.

Just to complicate matters further, this same breast-fed baby who has been worrying his mother with his frequent stools may, over a period of a few days, slow right down to a point where she begins to worry about constipation. Many babies on the breast have periods when they only pass a movement every 2 to 5 days. Occasionally it may be as infrequent as every 10 days. No treatment is needed, and all home treatments, such as soap sticks and enemas, are wrong. It is not known why these periods of extreme infrequency occur, but it is thought that the loose and unbulky stools of the breast-fed baby simply do not provide enough stimulus to the bowel to lead to emptying. Such phases seldom last long. Over a few weeks the baby is likely gradually to revert to having two, three or more bowel movements per day.

Often it is difficult to distinguish between the loose green stools of the breast-fed baby under a month old and the so-called "starvation stools." These are usually small, frequent and dark. They are semi-fluid, often contain mucus and usually are semi-transparent. If a baby who has been passing the yellow mustard-like stools described earlier *begins* to pass stools of this description, then it may well be a sign of underfeeding. If the baby is still having the explosive green stools of the changing period it may be difficult to tell the difference, and the mother will probably have to rely on other signs of underfeeding to give her the cue. The importance of the starvation stools is that they are sometimes taken for diarrhea. This can be tragic for the baby, since the treatment for diarrhea will almost certainly include semi-starvation, and that was what he was suffering from in the first place. It cannot be too strongly stressed that if the baby is still fully breast-fed, underfeeding is a far more likely cause for loose, frequent, dark stools than is diarrhea. Certainly the mother, with her doctor, should review the baby's weight gains and his general contentment or restlessness together with his readiness to suck more frequently if offered the breast.

Among these factors she may find indications of hunger. If she does not, or if her doctor feels that the stools indicate a true diarrhea rather than underfeeding, then she could ask for bacteriological tests to be done on the stools to make sure that there really is infection present. Apart from the discomfort for the baby of being taken off most of his milk feedings when too little milk was the original cause of his atypical stools, the mother is likely to find that by the time the baby has been semi-starved for his diarrhea she will be hard put to it to get back to breast-feeding. If the baby is not allowed his usual sucking time her milk will lessen, and it is difficult to keep it up by manual expression alone. Furthermore, if he is not to have much breast milk he will have to have fluids from a bottle so that by the end of the episode the whole natural relationship of hungry/thirsty baby to breast full of milk will have been jarred. If the child has true diarrhea, despite the protection of being breast-fed, then he is ill and must, of course, be treated. But if the mother wants to go on breast-feeding him it is worth taking a great deal of trouble to make absolutely sure that ill is what he is.

Babies fed on cow's milk have stools whose exact color and consistency depends on the type of milk preparation they are receiving. In general their stools are, from the beginning, much more formed and solid than those of the breast-fed baby, with a color that is a pale brown rather than mustard yellow. The smell is more like that of a child on a mixed diet.

Bottle-fed babies tend to produce fewer bowel movements than breast-fed ones. Because of the different chemical composition of cow's milk, particularly its relatively high casein content, the bowel contents move much more slowly through the intestines. This effect is increased if the baby is not receiving much carbohydrate content in his food, since the fermentation of carbohydrates in the intestine hurries the passage of the contents.

Unlike breast-fed babies, bottle-fed babies occasionally become genuinely constipated. Instead of a day or two without a bowel movement being followed by a perfectly normal, soft one, the movement is hard and dry and its passage causes obvious discomfort; it is the texture of the stool which matters, not the red-faced straining which may accompany defecation. Extra fluid is usually all that is required. As well as offering extra drinks of water, parents should check that the baby's formula is being made up correctly. An over-concentrated feed will always predispose to constipation as well as being bad for the baby in other respects. If extra water is not accepted or is ineffective, diluted fruit juice can be tried. Carbohydrate—in the form of sugar—has a slightly laxative effect. Now that infant formulae are manufactured so as to form a complete food, modified as far as possible to match human milk, it is a mistake to add sugar to the baby's bottles. If his constipation persists a doctor should be consulted.

Since the trace of sugar in fruit juice often rights constipation it is logical that too much sugar is a frequent cause of non-infective diarrhea. Some mothers—perhaps responding to advice from older women accustomed to now out-dated formulae—routinely add sugar to their babies' bottles. Others rely heavily on sugar-water or highly sweetened fruit juices between feedings. Infants vary widely in their carbohydrate tolerance, but many, especially in their first weeks, cannot tolerate much extra.

Intolerance for fat may also give a bottle-fed baby loose, offensive stools. Such babies used to be given "half-cream" milks in their early weeks, but it is now known that the *type* of fat in the formula is far more likely to cause problems than the *quantity* [14]. Breast-milk fat is quite different from cow's milk fat. The former is well tolerated and well absorbed where the latter may not be. Unsaturated vegetable fats are closer in composition to those in breast milk and the infant may tolerate a formula in which the butterfat is replaced by mixtures of vegetable fats and oils. A baby who cannot cope with the fat in his formula will not only have diarrhea, he will also be failing to use the fat and may therefore be deprived of nearly half the calories he is intended to receive. The diarrhea may then be associated with low weight gain and/or very frequent demands for food. The choice of the infant's formula should be discussed with his doctor.

Since infants find it difficult to digest some of the proteins in cow's milk, an insufficiently modified or diluted formula may produce bulky, grayish, greasy motions with an unpleasant smell. Once again, the baby's food should be discussed with his doctor.

Diarrhea due either to fat intolerance or too much carbohydrate usually begins slowly, developing only over several days. It can easily be differentiated from infective diarrhea, or gastroenteritis, which usually begins suddenly. Such disorders can be of any severity from mild to extreme, but in babies of this age group they should always be taken seriously. An infant who is vomiting and passing frequent liquid movements will become dehydrated very rapidly indeed. Even diarrhea without vomiting can cause a degree of fluid loss which is serious, especially if it is associated with a rise in temperature.

As a rough guide, bottle-fed babies who suddenly develop diarrhea with or without vomiting and fever should be seen by a doctor on that same day. It will help the doctor to decide what treatment, if any, is needed if, while waiting, the mother keeps all soiled diapers and makes a note of how much fluid the baby has drunk. If he is in the least reluctant to take his food he should be offered plain boiled water—as much as he will drink.

Even before the beginning of mixed feeding certain substances can produce very marked color changes in an infant's stools which sometimes alarm parents. For example if the baby is given grape juice his stools may be purple; if iron should be prescribed for him his stools may be black.

Blood in, or on, the stools (after the first day or two, when it may be due to swallowed maternal blood) must always be referred to a doctor. But if it is in the form of streaks or flecks on the outside of the movement it is likely to be due either to an anal fissure—especially in a bottle-fed baby who has been constipated—or to the careless placement of a rectal thermometer.

Unlike the stools, a baby's urine seldom concerns a mother very much. Very young infants do not concentrate their urine as much as older people, nor do they wait until the bladder is "full" before passing it. Wet diapers are therefore the rule rather than an event; some studies have shown urination to occur as often as every half an hour in the early weeks.

The only cause for concern which is at all common is sudden *infrequency* of urination. A baby at this age, if he is taking enough fluid and is not dehydrated due to fever or diarrhea or vomiting, is most unlikely to remain dry between feedings. If he is found to be dry after one 3-4 hour interval, he should be watched. If he is still dry at the end of the next couple of hours advice should be sought, in case some obstruction has occurred.

Occasionally the urine suddenly becomes extra strong smelling. It may be so concentrated that it stains the diaper yellow and reddens the baby's skin. Again, lack of fluid on a hot day, or when the baby is feverish, is the most usual cause, but if the smell is actually foul or "fishy," there is just a possibility of urinary infection, and a doctor's advice should be sought. In this case a urine specimen will almost certainly be wanted, and the mother will save everybody time and effort if she can catch one in a clean container and take it with her.

TEMPERATURE CONTROL

Newborn infants can regulate their own temperatures, so as to remain comfortable in environments of differing warmths, but the mechanism by which they do this is not nearly so efficient as in older people. If an infant is placed in circumstances which force him to use the most extreme temperature-regulating mechanisms of which he is capable, keeping his temperature stable takes so much of his "physiological energy" that he functions less than perfectly in other respects. If he is forced to keep himself warm when the outside temperature is too cool for him, he will have little energy to spare for anything else.

There is, for any infant, at any particular stage of his development, what is termed a "neutral thermal environment." This simply means the outside environmental temperature at which the infant remains at a constant temperature without expending any energy in doing so. This temperature can be established, for the individual baby, by measuring his metabolic rate in terms of his oxygen consumption. The question being asked is: "At what temperature is this infant consuming no extra oxygen —not increasing his metabolic rate—simply in order to maintain his normal temperature?"

The lower limit of the neutral temperature range is usually referred to as the "critical temperature," because cold is a far more frequent enemy to young infants than heat. An extensive study of the "critical temperature" for babies of normal birthweight was made by J. W. Scopes [198]. At birth it was found to be 88–92° F (31–4° C). It remained well over 80° F (27° C) for at least 2 weeks after birth.

Scopes's experiments were carried out with naked babies in the controlled environment of an incubator. At home, babies are usually dressed, and clothes steady the infant's temperature, helping him to stay both warm and cool by reducing conduction, convection, radiation, and evaporation. Scopes found that the temperature inside an infant's wrapping shawl may be 89° F (32° C) when the air temperature is only 77° F (25° C). Such a combination of air temperature and clothing would be ideal for a newborn, but rather too hot for a 6-week baby, who is better able to regulate his heat, and uses less energy in doing so.

Clearly, if infants are to use a minimum amount of energy on keeping warm they need higher environmental temperatures than are usually provided. The normal advice given to new parents is to keep any room used by the baby at a temperature of 68–70° F (20–21° C). Such a temperature is perfectly adequate while the baby, who was already warm, is well wrapped up, but it becomes woefully inadequate when he is undressed for a change of diaper, or—worse still—put in a bath. After such an event, the infant may have to work extremely hard to get himself warm again.

Of course it does not harm a healthy baby to have to expend a little energy on creating heat. But the baby who is exposed to actual chilling is in a very different situation. If he is mature and awake, he will respond to actual cold as efficiently as a full-grown man: his metabolic rate will shoot up; he may actually treble his oxygen consumption. But fast as he *makes* heat, he cannot conserve it; the metabolic effort must go on and on and on, until outside warmth relieves his body of the necessity.

The immature baby—usually the premature one—may be in an even worse situation. He tends to lack the deposits of "brown fat" which are important sites of heat production, and are only laid down in the last weeks before birth. Such a baby may be quite incapable of the increase in heat production the cold demands of him.

Babies who are deeply asleep when the environmental temperature begins to drop are at risk too. Infants do not appear to begin the metabolic adjustment that results in increased heat production until they are on the verge of waking up. If the temperature in the baby's room drops rapidly while he is deeply asleep, he may have lost so much body heat before he surfaces that the battle to maintain his temperature is lost before it begins. Bedrooms which cool rapidly at night are an obvious danger here. A thermostatically controlled central heating system may switch itself off at midnight, and the infant's room temperature may drop 15 degrees in an hour, especially if it is not well insulated. If a thermostat with a time switch is used for the rest of the house the infant's room must be separately heated. Covers which can easily be dislodged are also a danger, especially if plastic pants are not used, so that the infant's wet diaper cools him by evaporation. There is a good deal to be said for swaddling the infant at night, or for using a baby sleeping bag.

If an infant is having to work hard to regain lost heat, parents—thinking he seems a little chilly—often make the tragic mistake of putting extra wrappings around him. More clothing will only insulate the cold *in* and make it infinitely more difficult for the baby to regain his heat. If he has become cold, he needs to be warmed *first* and then wrapped up so that warmth is insulated in.

Babies who are allowed to become really chilled may develop the "neonatal cold syndrome." The infant gives up the battle to make heat. His respiration and pulse (which were rapid while his metabolic rate and level of oxygen consumption were high because he was trying to make heat) drop very low. He lies still. When handled, he is lethargic and cannot muster the energy to suck properly. As the syndrome develops, he may refuse to suck altogether; his hands and feet become swollen and pink and his skin feels cold to the touch. It is vital that medical help be sought urgently if this happens. The baby may have succumbed to the cold syndrome because he was predisposed to it by illness. Even if this is not the case, his re-warming has to be extremely slow and careful, and must be carried out with medical help.

High temperatures are far less of a problem for young babies. The upper limits of the "neutral thermal range" have proved difficult to measure experimentally, because infants tend to wake up and cry and kick when the temperature goes up very high. They raise their metabolic rate and their oxygen consumption in crying, so that it is impossible to tell whether they are also doing so to cool themselves. But it is clear that the vast majority of very young babies are extremely content with an environmental temperature as high as 90° F (32–3° C), provided they are not swaddled so that natural evaporation from the skin is prevented. Many parents have discovered, almost by accident, that their restless infants sleep more peacefully, and are more active when awake, if their rooms are allowed to get very warm indeed.

Radiant heat can, however, be unexpectedly dangerous to young babies. Most mothers are aware of the danger of sunburn. But even a 60-watt light bulb can burn a new baby's skin if it is too close to him, and many mothers have been horrified to find red marks on a baby who has been put on a cozy rug by the fire.

CRYING

Crying is the young infant's only sure method of communicating with his caretakers on whom his very life depends. Later, the baby's mother will recognize all kinds of other cues, which will help her to interpret cries, or may themselves be sufficiently communicative. But in the very first weeks the baby's facial expressions, physical movements and non-crying noises are often unfocused, and therefore difficult for either mothers or research workers to interpret. The baby must cry. It is the only absolutely reliable signal for assistance or care in his repertory. Many mothers feel that they would prefer it if their new infant never cried. In fact if he never cried, they would never know, certainly, that he was content. Because he cries when he is *not* all right, his not crying can be taken to mean that he is all right.

Some research workers have attempted to add up the total minutes per day that new babies cry and to give an average figure. This is not a very helpful way of looking at crying. If crying is regarded as signaling, then its duration becomes an index of the sensitivity of the receiver of the signals. In other words how long an infant cries reflects the length of time it takes his mother to attend to him and to find out what he needs. Such a measure may tell us something about the mother, but nothing about the baby. A more useful index might be the number of *times* in 24 hours that the infant uses the crying signal. As far as I know there are no figures on this.

The causes of crying have been extensively studied. One of the most straightforward reports is that by Peter H. Wolff [225]. He studied a series of newborn babies in a hospital nursery, and followed them up in their homes to several months of age. Many of the following comments are based on his fascinating paper.

Hunger

Hardly surprisingly, hunger is the most common reason for crying in the first weeks of life. At any visit to the nursery, many more babies were found to be crying in the half hour before they were due to be fed than in the half hour after they had been fed.

When a baby is feeding, many different things are happening simultaneously. They include sucking, swallowing, filling of the stomach, and absorption of food. Furthermore feeding tends rapidly to become associated by the baby with being picked up and held. Wolff was able to separate and examine these different elements, by studying a series of babies who had incompletely separated tracheas and esophagi. Otherwise healthy, the babies were at first fed by a tube into the stomach. Later they were fed by mouth in the normal way, but with the tube left in place in case it was needed.

Wolff found that if the babies were allowed to suck a pacifier for the 20 minutes a feeding would have taken, but were given no food through the stomach tube, none of them settled; sucking alone, without food, was not enough to stop them crying.

If they were fed through the stomach tube, but were given nothing to suck, all settled happily. The lack of sucking did not appear to bother them.

If they were fed normally, by mouth, but the milk was removed from the stomach through the gastrostomy tube, they did not settle. Even sucking real food was not enough if the food did not remain in the stomach.

If that same milk was returned to the stomach through the tube they did settle.

If they were fed normally by mouth, but were propped with their bottles rather than being held, they settled; being picked up and held did not seem to be relevant at this age.

Cold

As we have seen on page 50 very young babies function best, physiologically, if high ambient temperatures are maintained. This study also showed that they cry more and sleep less if their cribs are kept at around 78° F (25–6° C) (which would be a high temperature for an ordinary home) than if they are kept at 88–90° F (31–2° C). It seems that although the lower temperature may not in itself be enough to make the baby cry, it predisposes him to cry about other things. Mild discomfort, mild hunger, and noise are more likely to penetrate his sleep and disturb him if he is less warm.

Wet or Soiled Diapers

Many mothers and nurses believe that a baby will cry if his diaper is wet or soiled. Wolff tested this among babies who were crying shortly after a feeding. Nurses picked all the babies up and changed them, but in half the babies they put back the wet diaper, and in the other half they put on a dry one. All the babies settled happily. The actual wetness made no difference at all. Presumably it is being lifted and having the position changed which stops crying in these circumstances.

Spontaneous Jerks and Twitches

Almost all new babies jerk and twitch in their sleep. Very few find this disturbing when they are deeply asleep, but in the drowsy period before deep sleep takes over, some babies jerk awake and cry over and over again; they find it difficult to get *past* the jerky drowsing state *into* deep sleep.

Being Undressed

A mother often assumes that a baby's crying when he is undressed reflects her own clumsiness or inexperience. Indeed if a baby is roughly handled or feels loss of support while clothes are pulled off of him, he is likely to cry. But some cry literally for the loss of their clothes. In Wolff's sample one third of the babies objected increasingly vigorously to being undressed from their first to their third weeks. Babies who react in this way convey great pathos. They remain calm while outer garments are removed, and become increasingly tense, usually finally dissolving into crying when the mother attempts to remove the last garment next to the skin—usually the undershirt. I have seen a 3-week-old girl literally hang on to her undershirt with her fingers.

This reaction is not related to cold, as it occurs whatever the temperature. It appears rather to reflect the loss of restraint, and the loss of skin contact. It is as if the baby fears the unrestricted movement and air on his skin which will give so much pleasure in a few weeks' time.

Such babies invariably stop crying when they are redressed, and can always be pacified for the moment by being covered with a blanket or towel. It has been shown experimentally that this covering must be of textured material—plastic or silk is ineffective—and that it must cover the chest and stomach. Covering the arms and legs does not stop the crying.

Pain

From the moment of birth, babies cry if they are hurt. Their reactions to various procedures, such as heel prick to obtain blood for study, or to circumcision, make this quite clear.

Their reactions to internal pain, from gas and so forth, are more difficult to gauge. It seems likely that a great deal of crying is put down to gas when it is really of another source. Nevertheless a baby who is crying for no other reason that can be discovered does sometimes stop once he has got rid of gas from one end or the other. Fortunately a baby who does need to belch will normally do so in the course of the handling which his mother gives him while looking for other sources of discomfort.

Over-Stimulation

Too much, or too intense, stimulation of any of a baby's senses is liable to make him cry. Very loud sudden noises, sudden very bright lights, too sudden or violent a movement, too sharp or bitter a taste, too hot or cold or tickling a touch can all overstep the limits and cause distress.

Interestingly, almost any of these acute stimuli will momentarily silence a baby who is already crying. But this is merely a pause while he focuses on the sound or sight or feeling; once it is registered the crying is redoubled.

Mistiming

Stimuli which a baby appears to enjoy when he is alert and happy often cause distress if he is grumbly or tired. Rocking him, swinging him, tickling him will all give him pleasure by the end of his first month. But all of these have been shown to work in reverse if they are used to "jolly him along" when he is impatient for a feeding, or to "cheer him up" when he is crying. It seems likely that stimulations of this kind are at the upper limits of acceptability for very small infants. The baby can cope with and enjoy them when he is at his best and calmest; at other times they are just too much. It is like the older person who can enjoy being frightened by a ghost story when he is feeling well companioned and protected, but cannot cope with his own fear if he is alone in a dark house.

Other kinds of mistiming also often cause crying. They vary widely with individual infants and individual kinds of mothering, but some are fairly general.

1. The most obvious: mistiming feedings and keeping the infant waiting.
2. Offering food at the wrong rate—almost always too slowly—so that the distress of hunger breaks through the relief of feeding, thus creating a vicious circle with the infant crying because he is hungry and staying hungry because he is crying too much to suck.
3. Bathing or changing or otherwise manipulating a hungry baby who would enjoy these ministrations once fed.
4. Altering the surroundings—light, or sound, or movement—when the baby is half into sleep. If he must be pushed in the carriage, let the ride start before he settles, or once he is soundly off.

Lack of Kinesthetic or Contact Comfort

Most of the causes for crying discussed so far are simple to remedy once they have been discovered. But most parents bitterly discover that their infants sometimes cry without obvious reason. It is this apparently cause-less crying which tends to drive mothers frantic. The sadness in the noise churns them up emotionally; their inability to stop it makes them feel woefully inadequate as mothers.

Some authorities take such crying lightly. They may attribute it vaguely to "gas" or to "colic"; some even suggest that infants must cry to "exercise their lungs." The mother is advised to do everything she can to make the infant comfortable and then to leave him to cry himself out.

Working from the simple and universal observation that such infants always stop crying when they are picked up, other people suggest that they cry to *be* picked up. While close to the truth this is a risky way of looking at the problem. It suggests that the infant is capable of a kind of reasoning and planning which will be impossible for him for months to come. He cannot say to himself, "If I cry and go on crying she will come and pick me up." If the mother is encouraged to believe that he can think in this way she may be tempted to feel that she should not give in to the infant.

In these early weeks it is more likely that the infant cries simply because he feels uncomfortable. In the absence of any other obvious cause for discomfort he may be missing physical contact with his mother. He does not cry to be picked up; he cries because he has been put down.

Western civilizations are unique in the amount of physical separate-ness which they impose on infants. We have invented innumerable gadgets—from carriages and cribs to babychairs and bouncers—which make it safe for mothers to put their infants down. In other times and other parts of the world it would be dangerous to put them down for more than a moment. So infants spend their days carried by the mother or another female relative, their nights cuddled against the mother or in a huddle of bodies. Such a child seldom meets the situation of physical aloneness until he is mobile enough to travel voluntarily away from his mother.

It seems that in our preoccupation with sucking and feeding as a psychological need for infants we may have come to neglect the whole area of contact comfort. Our infants are usually cuddled while they eat, so both needs are met together during feeding times. But an increasing body of evidence (largely from animal studies) suggests that if the two are sorted out, experimentally, the infant's need for contact comfort often exceeds his psychological need for sucking. A selection of such studies is well reviewed by J. P. Scott [199]. For example, A. J. Brodbeck bottle-fed half of a batch of newborn puppies by hand. The other half sucked their milk from a machine. But Brodbeck gave all the puppies identical amounts of handling and petting. All became equally and intensely attached to him. The puppies loved the hand that petted whether it also fed or not. H. F. Harlow [102], in his famous study of baby rhesus monkeys, provided two "substitute mothers." One was a cold uncomfortable structure made of wire, which held the infants' feeding bottles. The other was a warm comfortable padded structure which provided no food or sucking. The infant monkeys would feed from the wire mother, but it was to the cloth mother that they went when they were tired or afraid.

If crying does not stop when the baby is held on the mother's lap, walking with the baby often produces miraculous silence. The actual position in which the baby is held can make a difference too. Just as the baby who hates to be naked can be comforted by having his chest and stomach covered, so the baby who is being held will usually relax most if he is held against his mother, so that he is looking over her shoulder with his chest and stomach pressed against her.

Mothers in our culture cannot carry their babies constantly. Too much else is expected of them, and too much that they do is impossible with a baby on the back. Often contact comfort of a similar kind can be given by wrapping the baby up. Again there is a way that works and a way that does not. The idea is to provide a constant, unchanging contact between the infant's body and the wrapping material. If the infant is too loosely wrapped the contact varies every time he moves, and this changing stimulation, in combination with a slight restriction of his limb movements, may have exactly the opposite of the desired effect. He becomes increasingly restless and cross. If the wrapping is sufficiently firm, the shawl or crib sheet remains in contact even as he moves, so that he moves *within* the swaddling, rather than moving *it*. Wrapped like this he is quite likely to drop off to sleep in mid-cry.

Plastic makes life very uncomfortable for babies who yearn for contact comfort. Plastic-covered mattresses, changing tables, and floor mats are desperately unwelcoming surfaces for a creature who, if he were a few million years less evolved, would be clinging to his mother's fur. He will be happier on warm, textured materials.

Other Methods of Dealing with Crying

Crying can almost always be halted by picking up and cuddling, or at least by cuddling while walking. The problem for desperate parents is where to go from there.

In the very early weeks of life a large variety of continuous, regular rhythmical stimuli predispose infants to sleep. It seems that they act by blocking out the changing, minor, internal or external stimuli which were preventing the baby relaxing into sleep. The principle is much the same as the counter irritant whereby you forget your headache when you stub your toe. P. H. Wolff [225] has demonstrated the efficacy of "white noise." J. A. Ambrose has [32] shown that rocking is universally effective, if carried out at the correct rate. He found that rocking, through an arc of about 3 inches at a rate of 60 rocks per minute or above, stopped all babies he studied from crying, and that most babies became relaxed and went to sleep within short periods. Some mothers habitually rock their infants, others have found the method useless, or do not use a rockable crib for the baby. It may be that those who do not find rocking useful do not rock fast enough; it is quite difficult to keep up a rate of 60 rocks per minute by hand. Various people are experimenting with mechanical aids to rocking, including an attachment by which a portable crib or moses basket can be hung from a ceiling hook on strong springs that supposedly maintain a rocking motion over a long period. At present such gadgets seem too cumbersome and expensive to be worthwhile, but it seems likely that such an aid will be developed in the near future. Meanwhile, the easiest way to rock a baby at the effective rate is to walk with him. Sixty steps per minute is a slow walk for an adult. A baby in a carrier or sling on the back or front of a parent, or held at the hip or shoulder, will automatically feel that soothing rate as he or she parades up and down the living room. . . . One father claims to have covered several miles in this way during his daughter's early months and to have worn a path in the carpet by doing his walking within sight of the television set. More and more parents are discovering that babies who are habitually carried, rather than confined in carriages, seldom need rocking to end crying jags. They are *being* rocked and therefore seldom cry.

Many researchers, including Wolff, together with hundreds of thousands of parents, have demonstrated that non-nutritive sucking stops crying, *provided* the baby is not hungry. Sucking a pacifier did nothing to quiet the hungry babies in Wolff's study, unless they were simultaneously fed by tube. But slipping a pacifier into the mouth of a crying baby who is *not* hungry is very often effective. Pacifiers also seem to protect sleep, so that stimuli which disturb the non-sucking infant, making him move restlessly and eventually cry, merely make him suck vigorously if there is a pacifier in his mouth. It is as if the activity engendered by the stimulus was channeled into sucking, and the infant thus lulled back into peace.

4

THIS BABY
IS A PERSON

IN THE VERY EARLIEST WEEKS of a baby's life it is easy to write about him as if he were a precious object rather than a person. There is so much to learn about him—his physical appearances, his feeding, his elimination, his sleeping, his crying, his general physiological reactions to the world, and he is so unpredictable—that "baby books" sometimes imply that parents should be, or will be, caught up in his physical care to the exclusion of all else. Professionals involved in helping parents with a new baby sometimes actually treat the infant as if he were an especially precious little animal. The brisk, kindly efficiency often displayed to mothers at early feedings, in medical consultations about the baby or during clinic checkups, can prove a powerful barrier to communication with them because mothers seldom feel objective about their infants. There are still mothers who *believe* that newborn infants are blank slates for them to write upon; who will state, if asked, that infants at birth can neither see nor hear. But the tremendous spate of research on the interaction of mother-infant pairs which took place in the seventies showed that even these mothers do not *behave* as if this were so [195]. Consciously, unconsciously, or with a mixture of the two, mothers behave *as if* their newborn infants were in active and meaningful communication with them. By acting and reacting as if the infant's movements, facial expressions, sounds, and eye-gaze were meaningful, the mother provides a framework within which they can become so.

In the first weeks of life the infant does not react to people as one person reacts to another. He does not have the capacity to recognize individuals nor even to be aware of where he ends and the person holding him begins. What he does have is an inbuilt predisposition to interact with people in ways which are both qualitatively and quantitatively differ-

59

ent from the ways in which he will interact with anything else. Many
studies have been made of the sights which interest an infant most, the
sounds which attract and hold his attention, the sensations he most
clearly seeks to repeat. All of these are most frequently and readily available in the form of an adult care-taking human being. In 1971, Bowlby
[32] put it like this:

> Newborns do not respond to people as people, nevertheless (as we have
> seen) their perceptual equipment is well designed to pick up and process
> stimuli emanating from people and their reactive equipment is biased to
> respond to such stimuli in certain typical ways.

While certainly true, that statement implies a separateness between the
infant and the stimulating adult which more recent work has explicitly
rejected. Schaffer [195] says:

> A neonate may be an essentially a-social creature, in the sense of not
> being capable as yet of truly reciprocal social relationships and of not yet
> having the concept of a person. However, the nature of his early interactive
> behaviour is such that it is increasingly difficult to avoid the conclusion that
> in some sense the infant is already prepared for social intercourse.

Subtly the emphasis has shifted from a realization that infants will
pay selective attention to human stimuli to a realization that this attention
is already in some sense "social." Schaffer, and many others, believe that
it is no longer meaningful to attempt to study the behaviors of very young
infants alone. What they call a "dyadic orientation"—viewing infant-and-
mother or infant-and-caretaker together—is essential [194]. While we
can describe some of the behaviors which most clearly demonstrate infants' readiness for social interaction with people, we cannot describe the
individual baby's behavior in relation to his particular mother or caretaker just because their behavior will be a composite which is peculiar to
the two of them.

PHYSICAL CONTACT

As we have already seen earlier, infants are usually at their most contented when they are held by the mother in one of the positions which
simulate clinging. Unlike infant monkeys and apes, human babies cannot
cling until they are several months old. Indeed the 4–5 month infant may
be very much easier for his mother to carry than is the lighter newborn,
just because he holds on so efficiently by this later stage.

There is some evidence of an instinctive tendency to cling, left over
from earlier evolution. In 1918, E. Moro, a German pediatrician, described a reflex by which newborns reacted to any sudden change of
position, and especially to any change which made them feel they were
about to be dropped, and which caused their overheavy heads to fall back
on their unsteady necks. Put down carelessly in his crib, so that he does

not feel the security of the firm mattress before his mother's hands start to release him, the infant throws out and then bends both his arms and his legs, gives the impression of being violently startled, and usually cries. This reflex—called the "Moro response"—puzzled research workers, who could not see what function it could serve in evolutionary or survival terms. In 1965 H. F. R. Prechtl [180] showed that the Moro response takes a very different and far more comprehensible form if it is evoked while the infant's hands are being gently pulled. In these circumstances his palmar grasp reflex is also brought into play, and the Moro response takes a form which clearly suggests a sudden gripping, with hands, arms, and legs. It is now thought that this response is, in fact, a leftover from a time when the infant habitually clung to his furry mother, and that it would have been evoked by any sudden movement on her part that made the infant feel he was going to be dislodged.

The instinctive desire to cling probably explains the discomfort which infants display when they are held in positions which prevent them from making full body contact with the mother. Few, for example, are happy if they are carried in a cradled position, with the mother's hands under their heads and shoulders, thighs and knees. Few like to be laid across the mother's lap, or to be held with their backs to her.

As we have already seen, being firmly wrapped in soft textured material often comforts distressed infants who cannot be carried. Similarly, physical exposure in open space usually alarms this age group. Even if the infant's clothes are not removed, he is likely to appear worried and tense if he is put down on a hard flat surface, or if he is held in space. He needs, all the time, to feel the kind of contact which he would feel if he were clinging to warm fur. Modern baby-aids are a great help to *mothers,* but many of them directly contradict the needs of infants. Weighing a baby provides a composite example. He is undressed—which he may well find frightening—and then placed in a hard plastic or wicker basket, suspended in space. The basket descends suddenly under his weight, and makes a sharp sudden sound as it reaches the bottom of its travel. To weigh a baby without tears takes real understanding, foresight, and skill.

SEEING

If the infant is predisposed to remain in close physical contact with human beings, so he is innately predisposed to look at their faces rather than at anything else. From birth an infant will focus his gaze for about 2 seconds on any new sight which is brought before his eyes. This brief focus shows that he has "noticed" the object. The length of his gaze thereafter can be taken as a measure of his actual interest in it, and some very interesting research has been carried out into the kind of object which newborns look at for the longest.

R. L. Fantz [81] found that at 48 hours of age infants looked longer at a colored pattern than at a plain block of color, and longer at a circle with eyes, nose, and mouth sketched in than at a plain circle. Most interest of all was always elicited by a face-pattern which also moved. These very new infants were therefore selecting for visual inspection objects which had the qualities of a human face.

Studying 4-week-old infants, Wolff [226] found that infants would look for much longer at an actual human face than at any other object, however garish the alternative objects were. Many mothers confirm this for their own infants, pointing out the difficulty of persuading the baby to look at a new toy which is continually disregarded as he looks back to her face. But perhaps fewer mothers realize to what extent they themselves encourage this face-watching. Papousek and Papousek [173] observed many mother-baby pairs, using sophisticated visual recording techniques. They found that mothers performed many movements designed to achieve and then to hold onto mutual visual contact with their infants, moving their heads to stay centered in the infants' visual field and to keep their eyes on the same plane as the infants', and bobbing forward to maintain the optimum distance from them (see p. 97). Some mothers explicitly deny this sort of behavior, maintaining that "he can't really see me anyway." Shown persuasive film-clips of themselves with their babies, most of these were both amazed and moved. One mother described it as "suddenly seeing how very 'us' the baby and I were."

HEARING

The human voice also seems to be innately attractive to new babies. Infants are almost always startled by loud sudden sounds, and usually seem soothed and pleased by music or by gentle, rhythmic, continuous noise. But a human voice elicits a special response from the baby. If he is crying, he is likely to stop when his mother talks to him, remain quietly alert as long as she goes on talking and cry again as soon as she stops. If he is content when she starts talking, her voice may elicit a very brief, fleeting smile, even as early as the third week of life. By the time the baby is 5 weeks old he may always smile when his mother talks to him. From this time on, he may also babble in response to her voice, although he does not yet babble in reaction to any other sound.

LANGUAGE

At the beginning a new infant has no language other than crying. Various types of cry can be distinguished by means of sound spectrographs. These do form a "language" in the sense that all infants' hunger cries have one typical pattern, all pain cries another, and so on. Mothers have to learn to interpret their infants' cries by experience. Most maintain that they would not recognize their own child's cry from those of other babies of similar age, but various experiments have shown that in fact mothers are extremely good at recognizing the cries of their own newborns. D. Formby [83] showed that of twenty-three mothers in one maternity ward, twelve successfully recognized the tape-recorded cry of their own child at 48 hours old, and all were successful during the next few days. Furthermore in the first three nights after they had given birth, fifteen mothers woke only when their own babies cried; on subsequent nights only one mother ever woke to the cry of another woman's baby. Wolff [225] found that mothers' reactions to different cries from their babies were extremely variable: they might, or might not, go at once in answer to the basic hunger cry. But the mothers in his experiment all reacted with extreme speed to their babies' pain cries—and were both furious and relieved when they found that these were tape-recorded rather than immediate.

Until about 3 weeks old, babies usually have a repertory of cries consisting of the basic hunger cry, the distinctive pain cry and what is often described as an "anger" cry, which mothers often call "trying it on." It is a grumbly, whiny cry which often lasts for some minutes, and which turns into the basic hunger cry if the mother does not intervene first.

By about 4 weeks old, the first non-crying sounds usually appear, not distinct separate sounds at this stage, but gurgly googly noises. Often they occur first of all when the infant is just beginning to feel fretful. They may give way to grumbling and thence to basic crying, in a regular sequence.

By 6 weeks there will probably be some phonetic syllables among the gurgles. Sound-making tends to become differentiated from feeling fretful at this point. The infant probably now "talks" most when he is talked to. Some babies will even "talk back" by this age, making a sound, listening to the mother make the sound back, and then making it again themselves.

SMILING

Smiling is a vital social accomplishment. It is one powerful means by which infants ensure that adults will pay them the attention they must have if they are to survive, and the very personal social attention which they must have for full development. Such a bald statement is perhaps unscientific but nevertheless justifiable because, for any normal adult, a young baby's smile is almost irresistible. The bored visitor bends only dutifully over the crib, remarking tritely to the mother on the infant's beauty. But if that infant smiles at him, he will almost certainly drop his guard and smile and talk directly and spontaneously to the baby. Such visitors have even been known to sneak back to the baby's room for an entirely hedonistic second viewing.

If smiles can entrap strangers, they can also add motivation to the work of child-care professionals and revolutionize the daily lives of parents. Nursery nurses often remark that they become very depressed when working with premature babies; although such a reaction must be partly due to the anxiety and sadness implicit in some such work, experienced nurses often mention lack of smiling, too. One experienced nurse puts it like this: "I hate to have the youngsters [trainees] in here for too long early in their training; they need to work with healthy babies and with older ones too. They need to be smiled at for getting it right."

For parents, the infant's early smiles often usher in a new era. Of the 120 mothers whom the author saw over 2 years, all but 1 made some spontaneous remark during the week in which her child began readily to smile at her, along the lines of, "Now he really knows me" or "Now she's really getting to be fun."

The actual dating of smiling varies wildly according to different authorities. No doubt this is partly because it varies wildly according to different babies. Most smile fleetingly, in response to a variety of stimuli, almost from birth. These fleeting pseudo-smiles used to be put down to gas. It is now thought that they are actual practice smiles.

By about 4 weeks these smiles tend to occur most often in response to the human voice, and they begin to have some social effect—they *look* more smiley. A little after this, the baby seems transfixed by the human face. He gazes at it, often for a minute at a time, slowly exploring its contour from hairline to chin, returning always to the eyes. By 6 weeks, about 50 percent of babies complete their detailed examination of the face by returning their gaze to the eyes, and smiling. The other half of any given group of babies will reach this stage in a diminishing scatter over the next 2 1/2 months. Only a very few—probably including those who were born prematurely—will fail to smile by 4 months.

In a way an infant's smiling, gurgling responses are the mother's reward for her devoted care while he settled himself into life. Earlier on, the baby could give his parents pleasure by his very existence, by his contentment, his growth, his obvious "all rightness." But once he begins to react to being handled in this brilliantly social, enchanting way, he gives them pleasure of quite a different sort. His smiles and his "talk" are an immediate reward to the mother who has torn herself out of deep sleep to feed him in the night, an irresistible compensation for yet another diaper needing changing in the middle of her favorite television program. Rewards are something given by one person to another and indeed most mothers do feel "grateful" to the infant for the gift of his smile. Yet it is largely the mother herself who creates that reward. As Trevarthen [215] explains, the emotions and moods of even brand-new infants are closely tied to experiences of pleasant sharing and coopera-tion with the mother or caretaker. So, in the social and emotional interac-tion between the pair of them, there is potential either for vicious circles or for benevolent ones. Infants who smile readily are likely to get more social attention from their mothers than do babies whose responses are later, slower, or less marked. But if those less responsive babies had received more affectionate social attention from birth, they might have been more responsive.

POSTURES

New babies have typical postures associated with their physical immaturity. To some extent these mediate *against* their displaying the dawning humanity of their reactions to things and to people.

Placed on his back, when he is relaxed, the middle of the back of the infant's head will seldom touch the mattress. Characteristically he turns his head toward one preferred side, extends the arm on that side, and flexes the opposite arm in toward the chest. This means that while he remains relaxed, there will be no symmetrical movements of the limbs, but merely a movement of the free ones. If his head does turn to the midline, and all four limbs thrash symmetrically, then he is either highly startled, extremely hungry, or very angry about something.

The flexed posture is important because it limits the baby's range of vision and of movement. If the mother hangs something interesting, be it a mobile, a rattle, or even her own face, directly above the crib, the infant is unlikely to see it because his head is turned. If the object is deliberately brought within his field of vision, he will, by 2 weeks of age, follow it through a very small arc by a combination of head and eye movements. By 4 weeks old he will probably follow it through a horizontal arc up to 90 degrees, and a little way vertically also. By 6 weeks he may actually search his surroundings for things to look at, turning his head to look for new objects of interest, but his visual field is still limited by his posture.

If the baby is placed on his stomach, he will turn his head toward a preferred side, and probably adopt a characteristic posture with his arms and legs flexed under him and his bottom in the air. Unwary mothers have allowed this position to convince them that they had given birth to a genius who would crawl at 1 month old. The posture vanishes in a few weeks. Meantime in active babies, unwarily placed on inadequately covered plastic mattresses, it can lead to sore elbows and knees as the infant "scrabbles" on a slippery surface.

All the postures of the newborn when he is not lying down are dominated by his gradually acquired ability to manage his own head. At the beginning his head is quite literally too heavy for the muscles of his neck and back. If his mother does not support it with a hand at his back and fingers spread between shoulder blades and neck, it simply flops, uncontrollably. The baby's own drive to acquire control is very obvious. By 1 week old, if he is comfortably held against the mother's shoulder, he will lift his head away in little intermittent jerks, so that it feels as if he were deliberately bumping his head. By 3 weeks he will be able to hold his head clear off the shoulder for several seconds at a time. By 6 weeks most will be able to support their heads for a minute or two while the mother is still; a few will be able to remain in control while they are being carried about.

Throughout this age period mothers who want their infants to prove the truth of what we have said about their interest in human faces, their preference for patterned, moving objects and so on, must allow for the typical position of their heads. Only very gradually does the infant begin to be able to turn his head at will. In these early weeks he cannot show that he is interested in looking at something unless he is put in a position from which he can see it. And that means directly in front of his eye-line, and remarkably close to the bridge of his nose (see p. 97).

USING HIS HANDS

From the earliest days, a finger inserted into the loosely closed fist of a baby will be grasped. Indeed experiments have shown that in the first 2 days of life this grasp reflex is so strong that the baby can in fact hang all his weight by his grasping hands. This ability passes quickly though, so it is not an experiment recommended for home trial.

This kind of reflex grasping has to be distinguished both from deliberately holding *on* to an object and from the very earliest signs of reaching out for an object.

By 3 to 4 weeks, many babies will hold on to a rattle or similar object once it has been put in their hands. They may indeed get some pleasure out of the movements *it* makes as their own arms randomly move. It goes without saying that the object should be light, as the baby's arm is as likely as not to land the rattle in his own eye.

By 4 to 5 weeks, although the infant still cannot voluntarily grasp an object but must have it placed in his hand, merely touching his hand with it may lead to movements of the arm, and unclenching of the hand. It is as if the infant knows that he has to use that arm and hand to get the object, but simply lacks the coordination needed to take it.

An infant's most successful holding on and early taking hold usually occur in the context of being held by the mother or some other adult. If the baby is held in a clinging posture, the adult's body supports him so that his head does not flop, and his limbs do not take up the characteristic asymmetry which they display when he is lying in his crib. Held thus he is more free to move than he is when he is lying down. Even though he must still have a rattle put into his fist before he can hold on to it, he will manage to get and to hold a handful of his mother's hair or the neckline of her sweater. Before he has ever managed to reach out and take a toy, he will have managed to get hold of his mother's nose or chin as she feeds him.

5

DIFFICULTIES IN GETTING SETTLED

EARLIER CHAPTERS HAVE ASSUMED that while the first 4–6 weeks of a baby's life may, in many ways, be hell for his parents, they are a settling period, during which one by one problems will resolve. The unpredictable waking hours that made it impossible for the mother to plan her day gradually give way to more regular intervals. The extraordinary stools give way to something more reasonable. The circulation, the skin, the hair all become more like those of an "ordinary baby," and with the advent of different types of crying, some smiling and some non-crying sounds, the mother begins to feel she is dealing with a person. And we can all manage those.

But babies vary. There are satisfactory models and less satisfactory ones; ones that are easy to operate and others that are tricky. The genetic lottery produces some mother-infant pairs which are better matched than others.

The physical care and the emotional sensitivity given to a baby interact with what he has already brought into life. As well as his genetic characteristics, including his sex, he brings a vast range of experiences in the womb and at birth. Many of these are still incompletely understood, but it is clear that factors such as the efficiency of the placenta and some aspects of the mother's health in pregnancy, together with the timing and nature of the actual birth, can all affect the "kind" of baby who emerges. Although both the existence and the importance of differences between individual newborns are now widely accepted, researching the nature and effect of such differences is fiendishly difficult [172]. Every baby is part of a dyad from the moment of birth (quite apart from having been so *in utero*). Babies can be described, compared, and contrasted at any given moment in time but at no time can observed differences be *assumed* to lie within the infants rather than within each infant-plus-caretaker combination. The research is fascinating and there is no doubt that with the current investment of expertise in the field, our knowledge will increase during the next few years. But for the moment each individual research study is subject to verification by the next and each interpretation of findings open to argument. Those of us who are primarily concerned to smooth life for babies and parents must still rely on general observations of what babies are like, almost irrespective of where their characteristics came from or of their lasting importance in development.

Obviously all parents want to give their particular infant every possible advantage, whether or not he appears to have any problems. But it is less obvious that some "types" of baby are very much easier for some mothers to handle than for others. If a mother gets the kind of baby she was expecting, the kind who needs the sort of handling which comes most naturally to her, she will have an easier job than if she gets a baby who needs handling in a way which takes positive thought and effort from her. The very wakeful baby, for example, is likely to be much more of a problem to a woman who likes her life extremely organized, with the housework completed in the morning, leisure in the afternoon, and the place spotless when her husband comes home from work, than he is to a more casual easygoing woman who does things as they need doing, and finds it easy to drop the ironing to play with the baby and to vacuum the living room at 9 P.M.

MISERABLE BABIES

Some babies are born inclined to the miseries. It is impossible to say how many, because the definition is subjective, and in any case many babies who seem inclined this way are being made so by the way they are handled. Often their discontent, their sad fretfulness, appears to center around digestive troubles. But this may be because when a very young baby is miserable, more food, or different food, is the first solution people tend to turn to. These babies do not seem to settle happily into patterns of being definitely, soundly and comfortably asleep; awake and ravenous; full, awake, and happy; and then asleep again. It is as if little bits of all these states remained jumbled up with each other. The baby is tired and fretful but he cannot relax fully into sleep. Having whined his way through a period, he is crossly hungry, but not joyous in his sucking. He may be slow and difficult to feed. Finished, he is awake but not very sociable; he quickly tires of being held but is not pleased to be put in his carriage or crib. He probably wakes often in the night. Some, but not all, of these babies gain weight slowly. They may actually look unhappy. They are the opposite of that stereotype the "bonny baby."

Anything or nothing may help, except the kind of despair which too easily strikes parents who are overtired, and who feel constantly criticized by this infant who *will not* reward their care with happiness. Food is certainly a starting point. Is he getting enough if he is breast-fed? Offering more frequent feedings or a supplementary bottle will answer that. If he is not on the breast, it is sometimes worth changing the formula. He might, for instance, actually *like* another milk better. It would certainly be worth asking the baby's doctor about trying a different formula.

Temperature is another possibility. Like the small mammals who blossom, and double their eating and their activity when they are made warm after getting too cold, some babies are kept constantly below their optimal temperature (see p. 49). It is worth trying to keep the infant's room at 75° F (24° C) and *not* putting him out in his carriage for a few days.

Sometimes extra physical contact produces a private minor miracle. The late Dr. Doyne Bell, a consultant pediatrician at the Charing Cross Hospital in London, once said that if he was faced with a very sick baby under 3 months, the first thing he did was to institute necessary treatment. The second was to assign that baby a nurse who would carry him, wherever she went, all day, every day, awake and asleep, until he started to be better. Since then I have seen mothers do the same thing with sad babies. A "snuggly" will hold the baby comfortably against the mother's chest and stomach. Alternatively a simple sling on the mother's back, made out of a small crib sheet, makes it possible for her to do simple household jobs, while a kangaroo-type sling, worn on the front, gives the baby that preferred face-to-face position (see p. 56). It is not a scientific method and nobody can say why it works when it does. But it could be that the baby is not ready to adapt and settle to extrauterine life, that he misses the constant jolting and movement of life in the womb, or the warmth or some other aspect of the symbiotic tie with his mother.

JUMPY BABIES

Another group of babies, less worrisome, less all-engulfing, but nevertheless more difficult than most to handle, are the very jumpy ones. Most small babies startle to loud noises, turn away from bright lights, throw up their arms and cry if they feel loss of balance when they are picked up or put down. But there are some who startle and cry, tremble and pale at quite minor stimuli. These babies seem happiest if outside stimulation is reduced even below the level suggested for all newborns. They may relax and sleep more calmly if they are securely wrapped up, literally rolled into a crib blanket so that they make a loose parcel. Obviously they need to be lifted with due notice, never unexpectedly, never from behind, and always very gently and slowly so that their muscles have time to adapt to each change of position as it is made. In extreme cases mothers may find that they are easiest to handle if they are carried and fed still wrapped up. Most of them will be among those who hate being naked, seeming to lose security with every garment, every touch of the air on bare skin. Baths are not, of course, strictly necessary. Every bit of a baby can be adequately washed and dried without ever fully undressing him. Carriage riding may

be a mistake too. The outside air moves; the baby sees a blur of movement, and every curbstone may make him jump and cry.

Nothing will finally right this situation except the baby's maturation.
There is no way in which this can be hurried. In the meantime, caring for
him can be even enjoyable if it is seen as a challenge. The challenge is
simply whether each day can be got through without him ever being
frightened or made to jump. It takes constant thought. It means never
being distracted so that the overhead light is suddenly switched on in a
dark room, never sitting down to feed him just where the telephone is
going to ring in his face, never hurrying downstairs with him under your
arm to answer the door, never pulling his undershirt over his head because the strings are in a knot.

SLEEPY BABIES

At the other end of the spectrum are the babies who sleep and sleep, and
who go on being sleepy and lethargic past the 4–6 weeks point. Very
occasionally babies have been known to succumb to malnutrition because
they did not demand food, and could not wake up enough to suck properly. This is extremely rare, but nevertheless a salutary warning. Exceedingly sleepy newborn babies need a little extra thought and care from the
parents because they sometimes make fewer demands than they actually
ought to make for their own sakes. Where the vast majority of babies will
be hungry when they need food, and say so, loudly, these babies sometimes demand fewer feedings than their bodies need for optimum early
growth, so that they fail to gain weight if nobody wakes them up to eat.
They may sleep for a 12-hour stretch at night right from the beginning,
and then get sore bottoms because they stayed in the same wet diaper for
so long. When they do get around to a feeding, they are likely to go back
to sleep after an ounce or two, and then sleep on, unlike most babies who
if overtaken by sleep in mid-feeding just wake up that much sooner for
the next one.

The quantities of food which are suggested as necessary for babies
of different weights (see p. 30) are only a very rough guide, but in this
sort of situation a rough guide is quite enough. If, over a period of many
days, the baby regularly takes less than two thirds of that guide amount,
and only that much because his mother wakes and reminds him, she must
make sure that his weight gain is regularly checked. If the doctor seems
to feel that she is being over-anxious she can explain that this is a baby
who is very sleepy, and that she simply wants to be sure that his unde-
mandingness over food represents contentment with what he is getting
rather than a physiological inability, due to immaturity, to know what his
body needs. Modern pediatricians, perhaps especially American ones,
have worked so hard to help parents relax about their babies' feedings
that they dislike any suggestion that weight gain *as well as* contentment
are needed in the assessment of adequate feeding. Yet a trained nurse

has, literally today, written to me to recount the sad story of her second baby's near-starvation. Her letter ends with these words: "Please tell other parents that not all babies cry when they need food. If ours had cried between feeds, even *once*, I would so happily have fed her, day *or* night, as I had done her brother. But she didn't and just those few weeks when I was too busy to get to the clinic to weigh her left me, a trained nurse, with a baby who weighed the same at three months as she had weighed at four weeks."

If he is eating enough, and gaining weight, and seems cheerful and normal on the rare occasions when he is really awake, then probably he is only reacting to extrauterine life as the sad baby did, but dealing with it more comfortably. He also is unready for it, and is going to be dozy until he is. All the same, it is important that his willingness to be shut away for hours in his crib should not lead the mother to *expect* him to behave like this. It is vital that he be offered social contact: people, things to look at, conversation. If the mother feeds him and then tries to play with him and he goes to sleep in her arms, it is fair enough to put him back in his bed, but it is a mistake to assume his sleepiness without giving him the chance to behave differently.

WAKEFUL BABIES

Many parents assume that sleep is the natural state for new babies, interrupted only by feedings and other necessary physical care. Some therefore classify their babies as "wakeful" if they are *ever* awake and contented. The assumption is false (see p. 43) and it is also unfortunate. A baby who is peacefully awake, either for "average" or for greater than "average" hours in each day, can easily be turned into a baby who is miserably awake and crying. If he is lying contentedly in his carriage looking at sunbeams, tucking him away in a darkened room for a nap he does not need is likely to make him cry, not sleep. Leaving him for nights which last longer than his sleep and steadfastly ignoring the kind of crying which says "I'm bored" rather than "I'm tired" will also tend to turn simple wakefulness into misery for everyone. Parents cannot force a baby to sleep. Attempts to do so create a no-win situation for all concerned and often lead to the parents seeing their baby as cross and over-demanding when all he is really demanding is the simple human right to be awake.

If a baby's sleep needs happen to fall within the average range, just accepting his wakeful periods and trying to enjoy them with him will prevent that kind of vicious circle. But if his sleep needs happen to be unusually low, acceptance and enjoyment are not so easy. The most wakeful baby with whom I have ever worked was a second-born girl, delivered at home. Her delighted parents cuddled her, put her to the breast, touched her head with champagne and settled her into her crib beside their bed. She lay there peacefully but she did not go to sleep and neither could they. It was 6 hours after the birth before she slept and then it was only for half an hour. That baby was contented but she was awake. Her parents were happy but they were tired. Three years later the baby is a highly active, joyous little girl who has *never* slept for more than 10 hours in any 24 or woken less than 3 times in any night. Her parents love her dearly but they are still tired.

If extreme wakefulness is not to be turned into misery, yet parents are to survive, ways have to be found to integrate the baby into adult activities from a very early age. Unlike most newborns, such a baby cannot be cared for and companioned in spurts, with pauses for adult life and recuperation in between. His positive presence has to be accepted and catered for continually. I believe that acceptance is the key because it banishes the resentment which otherwise overwhelms the parents when others talk of the bliss of long nights without feedings or the guilty relief when children settle for a Sunday afternoon nap. If there is acceptance, practical measures can help too. A baby who is human enough to require company and entertainment but too young to "play" will be most contented if he can simply be with a parent. Carrying slings, carriages which can be brought into kitchens, safe floor-corners in each room and comfortable places to prop the baby to watch his parents watching television can all help. So too can their adoption of new activities which do not exclude a baby. One father, for example, took up gardening because it kept both him and his infant son happily in contact with each other. He read far less than he had done previously but he preferred the gardening to trying to read against constant interruptions or to doing nothing but talk to the baby. Many mothers similarly find that if a wakeful baby has to mean that they cannot do concentrated, private things, alone, they are less bored and frustrated if they can find things to do which feel productive while being companionable.

Many mothers will, of course, have toddlers to cope with simultaneously. A baby who is awake most of the day certainly impinges more on the older child than a baby who is tucked away asleep much of the time. The early weeks may be very difficult. But over a few months, the wakeful baby and the toddler often come to be a comparatively easy combination. The baby will watch the toddler's activities and, with any luck, soon seem like the older child's ideal: a constantly admiring audience.

Life with a baby who is genuinely extra-wakeful is certainly exhausting; perhaps only parents who have one such baby and another with more usual sleep requirements can truly understand just how much difference the sleep factor makes. Perhaps the only real comfort lies in the fact that, if the parents can remain positive and loving, the baby who spends less time asleep will spend more time learning. Such children are often accelerated in various aspects of their development and tremendous fun to be with, as long as parents can keep their eyes open.

.   .   .

Mothers often act as if broad differences of these kinds between babies had some bearing on the personality of the child later on. They may have and they may not. Many studies have produced results in both directions. It may be that it is impossible to prove the matter one way or the other without taking a great deal more than the usual account of the *mother's* reactions to the baby's behavior, rather than merely concentrating on how he behaves. If a sleepy no-trouble baby comes to be taken for granted, during his first 6 months, as an easygoing placid type, his mother is likely to treat him as such. He may get, for example, a great deal of social attention, because the mother is not afraid of him getting too demanding or getting into bad habits. She may be happy to bring him out of his crib at night to show off to visitors and so on. At the same time she may assume that he will not mind if she leaves him with a neighbor for a few hours, or loses his pacifier. In all sorts of ways he may be steered toward growing up in a way which represents some sort of continuum with his infancy.

On the other hand a different mother may resent the newborn's sleepiness. She may work at stimulating the infant, do everything she can think of to jog him into awareness. She may expect him to be upset by things which she believes ought to upset a baby. She may subtly steer him along quite a different path.

While it is certainly not true that parents can decide what kind of person they want their infant to become, and bring him up in such a way as to produce the required model, the way they do bring him up affects his behavior from the beginning. And the way they bring him up is at least partially dictated *by* his behavior. The infant's environment and handling are therefore something which he and his parents together provide: a given type of baby and a given type of mother may interact in different ways to produce quite different results.

With all babies who have difficulty in settling into life and who have been passed as healthy and normal by their doctors, a policy of wait and see is by far the most sensible. As the infant gets a little older, most of these early problems will resolve. And as he becomes more consistent in his behavior it will get easier for the parents to see what handling he needs. In the meantime it is best if no labels are attached to him. It is a pity if a newborn's jumpiness, which was actually merely associated with immaturity of the nervous system and a stressful delivery, leads to him being known as a "nervous child," a "highly strung type," so that he has to fight his way out of over-protection when he reaches robust toddler-hood.

PART II

FROM SIX WEEKS TO THREE MONTHS

Making Patterns

6

FUNDAMENTAL
PHYSICAL PATTERNS

THE FIRST SECTION OF THIS BOOK was called "Settling into Life." An infant is "settled" once his behaviors begin to make sense. It is likely still to be extremely idiosyncratic sense, but nevertheless sufficiently clear for his mother to feel she can understand him.

Predictability is the essence of this "making sense." By around 6 weeks most infants have reached a point where their behavior on a Monday to some extent predicts their behavior on Tuesday. In earlier weeks the infant might cry himself into a lather over his bath one day, and barely bother to wake up for it on the next. Once he is settled, he is likely either to enjoy his bath or hate it; either way his feelings about the matter are likely to be consistent.

This predictability gives most mothers an enormous upsurge of confidence, even where the infant is predictably difficult! Once the mother knows what to expect of the baby—even if it is the worst—she can begin to plan her own activities around him and to make reasoned assessments about whether she is handling him in the way he needs. It is the very randomness of newborn behavior which makes it so depressingly difficult for mothers to know whether or not they are doing a good job.

Between about 6 weeks and about 3 months, all the infant's physical functions tend to become patterned along with his emotional reactions, his likes and dislikes. These patterns make up norms for that particular baby. Deviations from them therefore become cues for the mother that there may be something amiss. The more accustomed she becomes to her particular infant's patterns, the more automatically she will tend to adjust her behavior to fit in with them. If, for example, this particular infant always sleeps well and soundly between the first two feedings of the day and, equally, always remains wakeful during the afternoon, the mother

77

will probably find herself reacting quite differently to crying during these times. If the baby cries between the first two feedings, she will pick him up, perhaps change him, but put him straight down again, assuming he will go back to sleep "because he always does." If, on the other hand, he cries during the afternoon, she will probably go to him, pick him up and begin to play: she does not expect him to return to sleep.

FEEDING

Most of the problems of feeding, whether from breast or bottle, should be over by 6 weeks. The baby now has clear expectations at feeding times. He does not yet visually recognize his bottle as it is prepared, but it takes no tactful evocation of reflexes to get him sucking once the nipple is presented. His sucking is more rapid and efficient than before. Sleepy babies may still tend to suck themselves to sleep after only a couple of ounces, and having done so they may be unwakable. If this means that they wake again, hungry, in a couple of hours, it is extremely tiresome for the mother. But there is nothing that can be done except to ensure that the baby is fully awake before the feeding starts, to concentrate on him, trying to get him to watch the mother's face while he sucks, and to wait for him to mature.

In theory babies can be adequately fed on breast milk or formula alone until 3, 4, 5, or even 6 months, depending on whose theory is being propounded. In practice very few babies in the United States or indeed anywhere in the West are fed in this restrained way. In Huenemann's study [108] the average age for the introduction of solid foods was 6 weeks. The least socioeconomically privileged families introduced solid foods at 4 weeks while the most privileged families introduced them at 7 weeks. In Basedon's study of Negro and Puerto Rican infants, more than half of the 1-month infants were already being given solid foods [15]. The situation in the United Kingdom is similar. Data from the National Survey [153] and from numerous smaller-scale studies show that nearly half of all babies receive some solid foods by the time they are 8 weeks old.

In the past 2 or 3 years strenuous efforts have been made on both sides of the Atlantic to reverse this trend and persuade mothers that it is better for babies to have nothing but milk—preferably mother's milk—until they are at least 3 months old. Health professionals, supported by numerous books and articles on infant care, positively recommend waiting. Even the babyfood manufacturers have altered the slant of their advertising campaigns so that their products are not directed at such young infants. It may be that the gap between what is advised and what is actually done, in homes all over the Western world, is slowly closing. But it seems unlikely that it will close altogether until professionals achieve unanimity in their views and practicality in their advice.

What, for example, *is* the optimum age for the introduction of any food other than breast milk or formula? The most recent edition of Dr. Spock [208] suggests 2–4 months and then proceeds on the assumption that the baby is being introduced to solid foods at 3 months. In a series of authoritative articles in the *British Medical Journal* [218], Valman suggests 4–6 months. There is already enough leeway to confuse the mother who is trying to decide whether to offer her baby something extra to his milk today, next week, or next month. But opinions become even more confusing when they are expressed by people with particular interests and specialties. A recent article in the *Journal of Pediatrics,* for example [106], is concerned with the dangers to sleeping babies who regurgitate food. The author believes that this danger is increased by early cereal feeding and he therefore implies that a milk-only diet should continue for several months. Authors who are especially concerned with the avoidance of allergy (see p. 25) tend to advise exclusive breast-feeding for as long as possible [91], while those whose overall purpose is to emphasize the perfection of breast milk as baby food naturally tend to denigrate any other [136]. Many advisers from the La Leche League, or from Britain's National Childbirth Trust, suggest that 6 months is the very earliest age at which fully breast-fed babies should be offered anything else. But whatever the age range suggested, and whether a particular baby is breast-fed or given formula, all acknowledge that there can be no single age which will be optimal for all babies because the variability of individual needs and circumstances is so wide. Practical advice must be directed toward helping mothers to make decisions over feeding which are right *for their particular babies.* To do this, advisers need to know not only what mothers do at present but why they do it. When solid foods—usually, but by no means necessarily, cereals—are introduced in the first few weeks it is not because mothers believe them to be nutritionally correct but because they believe them to be problem-solvers. They are given to "help her sleep through the night" or to "keep him contented for longer between feeds." Many of these mothers may have misconceptions about normal baby behavior. We have already seen that people tend to expect small babies to sleep much more than many do (see p. 43). Caretakers may be interpreting normal (or bored) wakefulness as hunger; or they may simply be unwilling to tolerate the wakefulness and are anxious to end it with food whether it is due to hunger or not. There is an interesting difference here between mothers whose babies are breast-fed and those who are bottle-fed. Breast-feeding mothers who think that their babies are hungry, or not lasting long enough between feedings, tend to assume that their own milk supply is scarce and give supplementary bottles of formula. But bottle-feeding mothers know that their babies are already having whatever they classify as "plenty of milk" and they therefore tend to give solid foods in addition rather than even more formula. Some mothers certainly believe that the solidity of a spoonful of cereal—even when it is mixed into 6–8 oz. of milk—is somehow magically more satisfying than the equivalent number of calories in milk alone.

Adding solid foods very early is also often a means whereby a mother tries to keep her baby to an approved—or tolerable—number of feedings in each 24 hours. Feeding a baby 7, 8, or more times is extremely time-consuming. Many breast-feeding mothers accept it in this age period both because they know that their breast-milk supply depends upon the baby being allowed to suck and because the process of breast-feeding is far less inconvenient than the mixing, fetching, and warming-up of bottles for feedings. But bottle-feeding mothers tend to believe that babies only need feeding every 4 hours, and that giving up the small-hours feeding is a sign of growing up which must be maintained at almost any cost. In fact, with modern low-solute formulae, bottle-fed babies are likely to need feeding more often than they did in the old days, so every 3 hours would probably be more realistic than every 4. Furthermore, taking 5 feedings instead of 6 in the day cannot logically be called "progress" if it is achieved by giving the baby the equivalent of a sixth feeding but in a different form.

How much does an early introduction of solid foods really matter? Again reliable opinions vary. Most authorities would agree that *if* breast-feeding goes smoothly and the baby is contented and gains weight steadily he will be optimally fed and optimally protected against possible later allergic reactions if he has no other food at all during his first 4 months. If he is hungry, more frequent breast-feeding will usually be the answer. If he still seems hungry and/or his weight gain levels off, then supplementary formula will be better for him than solid foods.

A bottle-fed baby cannot manufacture extra formula for himself by more frequent sucking but, if he seems hungry, he can be offered more. But there are limits to the quantity of milk which his stomach can hold *at one time.* The usual limit is recognized by the bottle manufacturers who sell nothing larger than an 8 oz. bottle. If 7–8 oz. of formula is all that he can hold at one feeding, and 6 such bottles in the 24 hours still leaves him hungry, then he can only be given more formula by being given it more often. And this, as we have seen, is something many mothers are reluctant to offer.

The danger in this situation is that the mother attempts to make those existing feedings "more nourishing," either by putting more milk powder in proportion to water, or by adding a cereal. Various studies carried out early in the seventies [212, 69] showed that babies whose bottles were thus fortified tended to gain weight extremely fast and to become obese. The weight gain could have reflected a real need for extra food in the studied infants, but the obesity showed that they were receiving an excess over their needs for growth and energy. At that time it was thought that obesity in early infancy was related to a tendency toward obesity in later life, altering the chemistry of the body by increasing the number of fat cells and the production of insulin (which metabolizes sugars) and growth hormones.

Recent research suggests that the etiology of adult obesity is a great deal more complicated and variable than that model suggests [132]. An excellent paper by Poskitt [179] summarizes long-term studies and suggests that it is more likely that fat parents will have fat babies than that fat babies will grow up to be fat parents. In other words, there are certainly familial traits in weight, but they may be more closely related to genetic factors than to dietary ones. But while it no longer seems likely that allowing a baby to become obese in early infancy will condemn him to a struggle against obesity for the rest of his life, there is not yet any doubt that infant obesity matters. Very fat infants have been variously shown to be later than others in achieving a range of developmental milestones, to be more liable than others to upper respiratory infections, and to be at risk of atherosclerosis ("furring" of the arteries) from an even earlier age than most.

Clearly then it is important that early solid foods should not be allowed to make a baby fat, but it may be that awareness of the likelihood of this happening has led health professionals to be over-alarmist about it. At least one recent study has shown that small amounts of solid foods given before 4 months have no effect on the infants' rate of weight gain. In a review called "Infant Feeding, the Perennial Problem," Professor Brooke [38] says, "A few spoonfuls of cereal in the evening often turns a difficult baby into a contented one and there seems no reason to deny a mother this useful remedy."

But Professor Brooke refers to "spoonfuls," not to thickened bottles. If extra food is to be given to a very young baby, potential problems are probably more likely to be avoided if it is not mixed with his formula. A baby's bottle is his drink as well as his food. If he is accustomed to drinking, say, 7 oz. at a time and his mother has packed extra calories into that same amount of liquid, his accustomed drink may give him far more food than usual without his *appetite* being given a chance to refuse it. He may indeed get fat. Furthermore, if the extra calories are in the form of extra milk powder the result, even with modern low-solute formulae, will be an overdose of sodium that will place a heavy load on the infant's kidneys. If he is then thirsty and cries and is given yet another over-concentrated bottle he will be caught in a vicious circle. While a baby cereal, without added salt or sugar, mixed into the infant's normal formula would probably do no harm, it is better to treat the formula as sacrosanct and to make it up exactly according to the manufacturer's recommendations, always. A recent report [217] on some British infants admitted to the hospital with uremia due to excessive protein intake may serve to illustrate the point. Their bottles had been regularly "fortified" with a product designed and marketed as a "food drink" for convalescents and other adults unable to take a normal diet. Although the packaging carried specific warnings against its use for babies, the mothers had ignored these in favor of the equally prominent claims for its excellent nourishment.

Until or unless there is greater agreement among authorities *and* those whose job it is to advise parents coping with individual babies, I believe that it is best to assume that no food other than breast milk or formula will be needed during this age period and to try to meet the infant's demands for food simply by offering him more of it, even if this means offering it more often. A big meal every few hours is in no way better for a baby (or anyone else) than smaller, more frequent meals, it is just that the former is more convenient for parents. If as much milk as the baby will willingly drink does not seem to satisfy him, then his behavior, pattern of weight gain, and daily handling should be reviewed with the doctor or clinic. If it is decided that this really is a baby who is exceptionally hungry—perhaps because he is exceptionally energetic or needing to make a growth spurt to catch up on a low birthweight or early illness—then the solid food should be given by spoon and should not be in a high-protein form nor have added salt or sugar.

Taking food without sucking is extremely difficult for young babies. If food is placed on the tongue, the baby cannot get it far enough back in his mouth to swallow; it simply trickles out of the corners of his mouth. The trick is to use a tiny spoon, and to hold it to the baby's lips so that he can suck off the contents. If he likes the taste positive enthusiasm will develop quite quickly. The more usual technique of waiting until his mouth is open and then dumping the spoonful right at the back of his mouth often leads to gagging, and even more often to a complete rejection of spoon-feeding—sometimes for weeks.

Conventionally, a baby cereal is the first offered food, although there is no reason why a tiny quantity of a puréed root vegetable or bland fruit should not be given instead. If a cereal is offered, many authorities believe that it should be based on rice rather than wheat as the latter is rather more likely to provoke an allergic reaction. Cereals, mixed to semi-liquid texture with some of the baby's usual type of milk have the advantage of a familiar taste. Once the baby will accept such food from a spoon his need for extra nourishment can be met with fine slack purées of almost anything the parents normally eat. Our view of what is "suitable" for a very young baby is culture-bound. Finely mashed avocados, for example, might seem a peculiar choice to people in Great Britain since avocados are an expensive luxury. But they are often used for infants in California or Jerusalem.

There is a fair amount of evidence to suggest that babies have a natural preference for sweet foods and drinks. Newborns in an experimental situation, for example, suck for longer on a bottle containing sweetened water than on one containing plain water, while many somewhat older babies eat cereals enthusiastically if they are sugared but not if they are served plain. For the sake of the baby's future teeth, his later figure and his eventual dietary and health habits, it is important not to rely on sweetening food to persuade the baby to eat it. At this age especially, if he does not want the food unless it is sugared he is probably better off without it. Furthermore, habit plays a large part in everybody's eating and if he becomes accustomed to very sweet foods now, it will be far more difficult to persuade him to eat cornflakes rather than "frosted" breakfast foods when he is older. Some common sense is needed about sugar, even at this early age. It would be idiotic to expect a baby to eat stewed apple so sour that it makes an adult screw up his face. But if he is to have yoghurt, it is a pity if he is never offered it plain just because his parents prefer the sweetened fruit varieties.

If much added sugar is to be avoided, so too is added salt, including the less obvious forms of it such as the concentration in bouillon cubes, commercial soups, and the various savory spreads and yeast extracts which are said to be good for children. The baby's portion of food may taste very bland to an adult, but his palate has not yet been coarsened by life's insults and his kidneys are not yet mature enough to cope easily with added seasonings.

A certain amount of tact is often needed in the timing of the "solid" part of a meal. A very hungry baby expects to suck either breast or bottle. If he is offered solid food first, he may reject it with fury. Equally if it is offered at the end of his milk feeding he will probably not be hungry enough to bother with it. A sandwich system seems to work best, with a good suck to assuage the first hunger pangs, followed by spoon feeding, and finishing up with whatever further quantity of milk the baby wants.

Whatever system is used, it is important to remember that the solid food is an extra. It will be some weeks before the solids become the infant's principal food and the milk becomes a beverage. Unless the infant is extra hungry, he does not *need* any solid food at all at this age, and many authorities would argue that he is better off without it. Solid food should be used simply to bridge the gap between his hunger and the amount of milk his stomach can comfortably hold. There should be no question of trying to persuade the infant to take more solids, and then cutting down his milk.

SLEEPING

At this age sleeping is usually intimately bound up with eating, the baby being inclined to go to sleep immediately after a feeding. But even if he was one of the newborns who slept for 20 hours out of the 24, he is likely, by now, only to be sleeping for about 16 hours, and he will probably begin to have wakeful periods which are not entirely dependent on food.

Most babies fall into one of two groups. The first "type" tends to fall asleep after each feeding and to wake in about 3 hours, ready to be sociable for a period before hunger overtakes him and the eating-sleeping cycle repeats. The second "type" of baby tends to have one period of the day during which he is wakeful, often the second half of the afternoon.

During the morning he wakes to be fed, goes to sleep, and wakes again ravenous. But after his lunchtime feeding he naps, perhaps for an hour only, and then is awake for most of the afternoon.

By 6 weeks, almost all babies will be prepared to spend one period of about 6 hours asleep. Hopefully, this is the parents' "night." But often the baby's *preferred* long sleep period is from, say, 7 P.M. to 1 A.M., rather than the midnight to 6 A.M. which his parents would prefer.

Whatever the individual baby's pattern, once it exists, it can be tactfully manipulated. Such manipulation usually works best if it is done on the basis of feeding the baby a little *before* he demands food, rather than on the basis of making him wait a little time *after* he demands it. Adjusting the baby's long sleep period toward the parents' night, for example, can usually be accomplished painlessly by waking the baby for a feeding at midnight, rather than waiting for him to wake the parents at 1 A.M. For a few nights he may wake in the small hours all the same, but eventually he will adapt, and may even begin to wake himself for that late-night feeding, pushing his long sleep forward.

Adjustments of this kind are often bedeviled by the fact that mothers regard "giving up a feeding" as a sign of progress in their infants, and are therefore extremely loath to give an extra one. They would rather he went for 5 hours without feeding than slip in the extra feeding that will give them more sleep. This is a peculiarly old-fashioned view of child rearing, reminiscent of an era when hungry babies were labeled "demanding," and when withholding their needs and satisfactions was regarded as a parental duty and "good for their characters." It has also become increasingly inappropriate as the composition of milk formulae has altered during recent years. A baby who is bottle-fed on a highly adapted milk formula with its lowered fat and protein content is likely to experience hunger more frequently than did the infants fed on the old dried milk. If the mother can make herself feel better about extra feedings by calling them "snacks," so much the better. The need for them will occur whenever efforts are made to change the baby's eating pattern, particularly when attempts are being made to persuade him that he does not need breakfast at 6 A.M. and again when he is being persuaded to accept three family mealtimes per day rather than specially timed feedings.

Whatever the bottle-fed baby's timings, he will, at 6 weeks, probably still demand six feedings in the 24 hours, though some babies may already be down to five. Breast-fed babies will demand, and should get, just as many feedings as the current balance between hunger and milk supply suggests.

Over the next few weeks, feedings will be combined rather than abandoned. Taking the old standard timings of 6 A.M., 10 A.M., 2 P.M., 6 P.M., 10 P.M., 2 A.M. as a pattern, the 2 A.M. feeding will be the first mothers will want to abandon, and this will be accomplished by pushing the 10 P.M. feeding forward toward midnight, and pulling the 6 A.M. back probably nearer to 5 A.M. Most babies—except those who were premature or who are gaining weight very slowly or working at building up breast-milk supplies—will be ready to do without that sixth small-hours feeding by the time they are 10–12 weeks old. In the meantime there is no other way, apart from adjusting the timings of the feedings either side, of hurrying the process. Left to cry it out, the baby will, in the end, go back to sleep. But not for long. He will wake again, probably just as his mother relaxes back into sleep. He is hungry, and there is nothing to be gained by pretending that he is not.

Once he has accepted five feedings in the 24 hours, the "night" can be very gradually stretched, even though five feedings will remain neces-sary for some time. Twenty-five percent of the National Survey babies [153] were still having five or more milk feedings in each 24-hour period when they were 4 months old. If, fed at midnight, the baby begins to sleep on until 7 A.M., the mother may prefer to start waking him earlier in the evening, so that she herself can go to bed earlier. If the baby does not wake himself for that late-evening feeding, the mother can suit herself whether she prefers an early night and an early start to the day, or a later bedtime and a more leisurely start to her day.

ELIMINATION

By 6 weeks, a mother will recognize her baby's stools as normal for him, and can therefore use a marked *change* in those stools as her only cue for concern. The variation between very frequent and very infrequent stools may continue in breast-fed babies; bottle-fed ones are likely to produce a more regular 1–4 stools per day, and these are likely to be more formed than those of the breast-fed baby.

As in the very first weeks, a *sudden* attack of diarrhea, whether or not there is vomiting, is reason to seek medical advice quickly, while a gradual loosening of the stools over several days is more likely to reflect an excess of sugar or other carbohydrate in the milk, or in extra drinks.

Constipation is not constipation if, when the stool is finally pro-duced, it is of normal consistency. Many infants produce their bowel movements with much scarlet-faced straining, giving every appearance of constipation. But only if it is hard or dry, or difficult for the baby to expel, does it require dietary adjustment. As in the earlier weeks, more water, or possibly some well-diluted fruit juice, is probably all that will be needed.

Some babies, as they adopt more regular feeding times, also adopt more regular elimination times, the two functions often being linked, so that the baby passes a movement while he eats. A few mothers try to make use of this eating-elimination connection, by holding the baby on a potty in the middle of a feeding or immediately after it. Some movements can be caught in this way, but it is very doubtful whether the time the mother saves on washing those diapers equals the time she spends in potting the baby. Furthermore, if she attempts to catch the movement, she will inevitably often fail and may well be irritated. It seems a pity to introduce frustration into the feeding situation.

E. Newson and J. Newson [170], who studied the child-care practices of mothers in a large industrial city in the midlands of England, found that 20 percent of mothers had in fact "held out" their babies in this way from the first 2 weeks of life. Sixty-three percent had started training the child before he was 8 months, yet only a minute proportion had actually succeeded in training their babies by 1 year. The sum of wasted hours of mother and baby time represented by these figures is enormous (see p. 246).

CRYING AND COLIC

As in the earliest weeks of life, some babies between 6 weeks and 3 months cry more than others. Those who were miserable as newborns may still tend to the miseries at this age. Some, who were very jumpy as newborns, may still find a lot of causes for fear and unhappiness in the stimulation of a normal family environment. Yet others may cry for comparatively long periods in the day because their mothers deliberately delay fulfilling their expressed needs for fear of spoiling them. On the other hand there are babies who by 6 weeks are so readily consoled by adult handling that they rarely cry more than momentarily. Whatever the cause of the original distress, the baby stops crying when his mother picks him up, and is then easily made comfortable.

As the patterning typical of this age period takes place, some unfortunate parents recognize in their babies a particular syndrome of distress which is usually known as "three-months colic" although "evening colic" describes it better.

A baby with evening colic typically refuses to settle after his late-afternoon or early-evening feeding. If he falls asleep, he quickly wakes again with spasmodic attacks of screaming. During these attacks, he draws his knees up to his stomach, screws up his face, and gives every appearance of being in acute abdominal pain.

Evening colic, if it is going to occur at all, usually begins in the first fortnight after birth, but it is often not recognized as distinct from the disorganized behavior of the rest of the newborn baby's day, until his behavior at other times has settled and become predictable. Only when he is feeding and sleeping with some regularity do the parents realize that this particular trouble *always* occurs after this particular feeding of the day.

The facts available about evening colic are both inadequate and contradictory. Its frequency, cause, palliation, and cure are all matters of hot professional dispute. What cannot be disputed is that a baby with the true evening-colic syndrome presents a trial to his parents' marriage, their self-confidence as parents, and their sheer physical stamina.

R. S. Illingworth [111] made a detailed study of fifty cases. He found that the average time which the trouble lasted for an individual baby was 9 weeks. Half the affected babies had stopped having colic by 2 months of age, more than three quarters by 3 months of age, and all by 4 months of age.

The number of babies affected can hardly be guessed at. Some authorities put babies who tend to suffer from flatulence or other colicky pains in with those who have true evening colic. Others include all babies who show a tendency to cry in the evening, and many of these are breast-fed babies who are hungry in the evening because the mother's milk supply tends to be scantiest at this time of day.

Rather than trying to assess how many babies *do* have evening colic, it is probably more useful to describe those who do *not* have it, whatever the appearances may suggest.

A baby who cries in the evening, but in the same way and to the same extent as he does at other times of day, does not have the evening-colic syndrome. His evening crying is simply part of his normal crying pattern.

A baby who cries in the evening and will take a feeding and be comforted by it has not got colic either. He is hungry.

A baby who cries in the evening, brings up gas and then sleeps as usual has not got evening colic. He has gas.

A baby who cries in the evening until he is picked up, and is then happy until he is put to bed again has not got colic. He has probably decided to have the early evening as his wakeful period, and is simply not ready to be alone and asleep.

The baby with true evening colic cries in a different way from at any other time of day. His screams are piercing. They leave him shaky and sobbing between attacks. Everything comforts him momentarily; nothing comforts him for more than a few minutes. The trouble appears to be abdominal, and burping may relieve him long enough for him almost to drop off to sleep on his mother's shoulder, but the screaming begins again. Putting him on his tummy, rubbing his tummy, wrapping him tightly, all bring temporary relief, but just as the parents dare to hope it is over, the screaming starts again. The baby may suck ravenously, but he does so only for a minute or two, then he rejects the nipple and screams again. If the baby is left alone, with no help offered, the pattern is little different. Listening parents will live through minutes of scream-ing, blessed minutes of silence, and then screams again. Most parents feel that they have to do what they can to alleviate the attack; at the same time they have to accept that they cannot give real aid. Tired at the end of the day, needing to talk to each other and to relax, it is little wonder that evening colic is remembered with real horror by parents whose infants suffered from it.

A list of some of the causes suggested by eminent authorities may at least save some parents from shopping around from doctor to doctor, unable to believe that such an acute phenomenon can be transitory and, in the end, unimportant. Various authorities have suggested all the following causes, and more: overfeeding, underfeeding, too rich, strong or weak feedings, food given too hot or too cold, too often or too seldom, too fast or too slowly; allergies to certain foodstuffs, hernias, intestinal deformities, ulcers, appendicitis, gall bladder trouble. Pediatricians have tended to blame the mother for faulty feeding techniques, suggesting that the basic trouble is gas, and failing to explain why the mother should feed the baby wrongly at one, and only one, feeding in the day. Illingworth has demonstrated that however thoroughly a baby is burped after his early evening feeding, if he is subject to evening colic he will have it all the same.

From the psychiatric angle, explanations have tended to center around the mother. Maternal fatigue and irritation at the end of the day have often been suggested, since it neatly explains the regular timing of colic attacks. Such attacks, however, do not tend to cease when the mother is temporarily assisted by her husband or put to bed for the day by her own mother. M. Lakin [135] described the mothers of babies with colic as being less confident in their maternal role, less loving toward their infants, and having more marital conflict than the mothers of non-colicky babies. These findings could well be the *result* of having a baby with colic, rather than a cause. They are, in any case, completely contradicted by J. L. Paradise [174]. He found no psychiatric factors whatsoever in the mothers of babies with colic. The only difference of note between these mothers and the mothers of non-colicky babies was that the mothers of the evening-colic babies tended to be highly intelligent. Paradise thought that this difference probably only reflected the fact that intelligent mothers would tend to take notice of, and seek advice about, colic in their infants.

While it is clear that ordinary gastric flatulence (gas) is not the cause of colic, and while X-ray studies have shown that there is no excess of gas in the bowels of colicky babies, S. Jorup [116] did find unusually strong contractions of the colon while the baby was having attacks of pain. He believes, and Illingworth [112] agrees with him, that the probable cause is normal gas being trapped in loops of a highly mobile colon. Overall, Paradise [174] believes that the colic attacks reflect an immaturity of the central nervous system. These two suggestions may logically go together, so that one is left with immaturity of the infant's physiology leading to painful but insignificant and temporary malfunction of the colon.

Illingworth [110] studied the effects of a drug called Dicyclomine Hydrochloride. Its action reduces spasm of the colon and he has found it so effective in true evening colic that he has said that babies for whom the drug does not work must have been wrongly diagnosed in the first place. Some doctors still do not believe that any medication can much alter the evening-colic pattern and they therefore recommend even the most desperate parents simply to wait it out. But Dicyclomine Chloride is increasingly prescribed and Illingworth points out, in the latest edition of his classic work *The Normal Child* [110], that it is now sometimes given to infants whose exact symptoms do *not* fulfill the criteria for evening colic. While it would obviously be foolish to use this, or any other, drug simply as a placebo for excessive crying due to some other cause, parents can perhaps accept a prescription if one is offered and use it to carry out a brief home experiment. If the baby is given the correct dose half an hour before the feeding which is followed by the supposed colic, it may help or it may not. If it helps they can assume that they have both the correct explanation for the crying and a genuine chemical aid. If it does not help then the crying probably has some other explanation which, with their doctor's help, they can seek.

During this age period, babies will, of course, continue to cry from pain, or hunger, or from shock or fear or any over-stimulation, just as they did when they were newly born. But now they are infinitely easier to comfort. Apart from exceptional circumstances, such as evening colic or illness or continuing pain, babies of this age can *always* be stopped from crying by being picked up and talked to. They can often be prevented from starting full-fledged crying by social distraction at the right moment. For the vast majority of mothers, the era of being faced by a baby who cried and cried, while she tried every remedy she could think of in turn, and all to no avail, should be over.

The nature of the infant's crying alters too. The basic hunger cry remains, as does the distinctive pain cry. But the "angry cry" and the "grumbly cry" which began at around 3 weeks both become much more frequent. Indeed a baby who is being fed when he is hungry, and kept pleasurable company when he is awake, may seldom produce any other cries than anger and grumbles. He is angry—or so his cry indicates—when his mother terminates a conversation he was enjoying, by turning away out of sight. He grumbles when he begins to be hungry or tired. But his crying may seldom build up to full-fledged yells.

Once the individual baby's crying behavior has settled into a pattern in this way, changes in the pattern become valuable cues for the mother. If the baby always quiets when he is picked up, and never does more than grumble while his food is brought to him, then a sudden refusal to be comforted, continuing to yell while the mother cuddles him, or crying himself into such a lather that he cannot suck, may indicate illness. Of course any baby can have a particularly grumbly day. But this usually takes the form of *beginning* to cry more often than usual. It does not usually take the form of refusing to be comforted.

For breast-fed babies, a sudden excess of crying should lead the mother to consider the baby's weight gain over the past week or two (or test weight if she has access to scales). The appetite spurt of the infant of this age group has already been described. Often, a mother whose breast-milk supply was only just adequate in the first 6 weeks finds that it becomes inadequate during this period, because the baby's increase in appetite coincides with an increase in her activities as she returns to her normal life fully recovered from the birth. If the mother can find any reason to suppose that this is so, she can offer a supplementary bottle, while taking steps to increase her breast-milk supply as outlined on page 36.

BEGINNING TO MANAGE
HIS BODY

WHEN A BABY BECOMES SETTLED, in the sense of making predictable patterns in his eating, sleeping, crying, and his reactions to motherly comfort, he also tends to be sufficiently settled into his own body to start doing things with it. Of course physical and motor development are progressing daily from birth, but a sudden spurt in the beginnings of bodily control and coordination usually becomes noticeable at around 6 weeks.

POSTURE AND HEAD CONTROL

The factor which dominates an infant's physical abilities in the early weeks is the weight of his head relative to the rest of his body. At birth an infant can lift his hand, or his foot, he may even be able to lift his head a little when lying on his stomach, but he cannot *control* these muscle groups. The development of this muscular control starts at the top and moves downward. First he must get his neck muscles under control. At 4–5 weeks, he holds his head momentarily clear of his mother's shoulder, and practices doing so, so that it feels as if he is deliberately "bumping." By 6–8 weeks, the neck muscles have strengthened to a point where the infant can hold his head clear of the shoulder for minutes at a time; he may even be able to balance his head while his mother carries him gently about. But his control is still so precarious that any sudden movement on the mother's part makes his head flop again; fatigue makes him unable to hold it up at all, and he must still have his mother's hand under his neck when he is lifted or put down. By around 10 weeks his head control has developed still further; his neck is fairly steady when he is carried about. Now it is his shoulders which require support and in another 2–3 weeks they too will be steady.

The baby's posture when lying down will at least roughly parallel his development of head control. In the early weeks the infant is a scrunched-up creature. Whether the mother lays him down on his back, his side, or his tummy, he will curl inward (see p. 65).

As his head control increases, so this constantly flexed position gradually diminishes. Its departure is vitally important to what the infant can do. If, when he lies on his back, he still takes up the typical newborn flexed position, head turned to one side, the arm on that side outflung and the upper arm curled inward, he cannot use all four limbs at the same time. Only the upper arm and the upper leg are free to move. Furthermore he cannot see very much except his own mattress and underneath arm. But once he uncurls, and lies, at least when he is awake, with the back of his head on the mattress, and all four limbs free, he becomes able to do and to see all kinds of interesting things. Much the same applies to the flexed position taken up by newborns lying on their tummies. From the beginning they will turn their heads to one side to avoid smothering. But as long as their knees are pulled up beneath them and their bottoms are in the air there is not much else they *can* do. At about the same time that they uncurl when lying on their backs, they will begin to lie on their tummies with their legs straight out behind them. And as soon as they do this, new possibilities for physical activity are opened up.

By around 12 weeks, the baby kicks when he lies on his back. There is a new rhythm to his movements. He waves his arms, he bicycles with his legs. When he is awake, he is hardly ever still, and his movements flow into one another, without the jerkiness, the apparent lack of control of earlier weeks. When he lies flat on his tummy, he practices his new head control. At first he lifts his head only with extreme effort. He "bobs" up, rather as he bumped his head against his mother's shoulder 6 weeks before. Very soon he becomes able to hold this head-up position, and may even push hard enough with his forearms to lift his lower chest off the mattress too.

As early as 9 weeks most infants will have learned to roll themselves from the comparative instability of their sides onto the broader base of their backs. By 12 weeks or so, at around the same time that he learns to lift his head controlledly when lying on his tummy, the baby will accomplish the far more difficult maneuver of rolling from his back onto his side.

All these developments between about 6 and 12 weeks are vital clues to the handling the infant needs. In the newborn period his own helplessness, his obvious fear of quick movement, nakedness, or any loss of balance, made it clear that he was happiest and felt safest when he was securely wrapped, softly cushioned, totally protected. In this period his increasing physical activity, his stretching out, the smoothing out of his movements, his own control of his head, all make it clear that he no longer needs or benefits from *constant* physical padding. Once he can kick, he will kick and therefore should kick. Once he can roll, he will and should do so. Once he can move his head he must move it, and needs some payment for effort in terms of interesting things to see.

Where a hard smooth surface distressed the infant when he was younger, it now thrills him. Where earlier he would have cried if he were undressed and put on a rug on the floor, or on the center of a double bed, or on a groundsheet on the grass, now he glories in the freedom. His whole demeanor makes it clear that he is playing. It takes very little to frustrate his play, to spoil it. A rumpled rug will prevent him rolling onto his side. Too soft a mattress will prevent him getting the support to raise himself on his forearms. Restrictive clothing will stop him moving his arms and legs freely.

Very soon after the infant becomes able to balance his head while he is carried around, and to lift it when he is lying on his tummy, his muscular control will move on downward from neck and shoulders to upper back. If he is gently pulled into sitting position he will no longer droop pathetically forward so that his head almost touches his knees, his whole back bent over. Rather he will support his head and shoulders, so that he sags only at lower back and hip level. At this stage he is ready to spend some of his waking time propped up. But propping him takes some care and thought: supported by pillows or cushions, in his carriage or in a corner of the sofa, he quickly begins to slip downward—his back bends increasingly, his head is forced forward. He does not yet have an adult's ability to wriggle himself back into a comfortable position. For this reason an "infant seat" is ideal. It can be adjusted, by means of closely spaced notches, from a semi-reclined position to the almost-upright. The lowest notch will probably distress a baby who is mature enough and, at that moment, awake enough to want to be propped up. But the most upright notch has some dangers at this age. In this position the baby is beautifully supported from the base of his spine to the top of his head. But even with the vital safety straps fastened, his lack of muscular control can lead him suddenly to flop forward with a violence which will certainly frighten him. Usually it is best, at this age, to notch the seat so that the baby is supported at an angle of roughly 45 degrees. If this is done he will practice lifting his head forward from the backrest. Gradually he will lift his shoulders forward as well. When he can do this he is ready for one more notch of uprightness, and then the whole process will be repeated. The beauty of this method is that the baby himself cues the mother as to the position in which he needs to be propped.

PHYSICAL AND MANUAL PLAY

Just as the infant who still lies in scrunched-up positions is not ready for physical play, so the baby whose hands are scrunched into loose fists is not yet ready for play with objects. The hands open at just about the same time as the posture changes, so that by around 8 weeks they are open most of the time the baby is awake. And when they open, they are ready for the very beginnings of manipulative play.

The first "toy" an infant manipulates is usually his own hands. He finds one with the other, by touch alone, at around 6 weeks. He clasps them together, pulls at the fingers, opens and shuts them. But even at the 8-weeks stage the infant is probably not aware that these hands are part of himself. He uses one to play with the other as if that other was an object. At this stage he does not relate them to himself visually; he plays by touch alone, not bringing the hands up to his own eye-line.

The infant can still not reach out for a toy, nor take it if it is held out to him, but if a rattle or similar object is put into his hand, he holds on more deliberately than at 6 weeks, and he is far more likely to make it sound, because his arm movements are so much larger and freer than they were. Often it is the sound a toy makes which first leads the infant to see his own hands and what they are holding. His eye follows the sound and makes the discovery which marks the beginning of hand and eye coordination.

By about 3 months, most babies have truly discovered their hands, by eye as well as by touch. For several weeks the infant may be happy to spend minutes on end simply watching his own hands, bringing them together, spreading his arms apart until they go out of sight, bringing them back within view, pulling the fingers, opposing the thumb, as concentrated as a 5-year-old watching television.

Once the infant has got his hands under this much control, so that he can "find" them whenever he wants them, he explores them with his mouth as well as with his eyes and the other hand. He will put a finger in his mouth, take it out, look at it, put it back again. He will try putting his whole fist in his mouth, take that out for visual inspection and then replace it with both his thumbs.

Just as whole-body development gives the mother cues as to the kind of handling the infant is ready for, so this manual development gives cues too. As soon as the infant's hands are usually open, he is ready to be given light objects to hold, both for practice and against the day when he makes the connection between holding and seeing. Once he plays with his hands, watching them as he does so, he is ready for real toys as well. And once his hands go in his mouth, so will everything else. For some months the infant's mouth will be an organ of exploration. He cannot fully comprehend an object at this stage if he does *not* put it in his mouth. Mothers who are concerned over hygiene must find objects which are suitable for sucking as well as for looking and holding. Trying to stop him putting things in his mouth is wasted and misguided effort, which would be better spent on washing the toys from time to time.

Babies who have become attached to pacifiers by this point in their development are unwittingly deprived of the mouth as an organ of exploration. Very sad or fretful babies, who really need the comfort of almost constant sucking, are probably not ready for much manual play and will not therefore be missing anything. But most babies can, by this age, have their comfort sucking confined to sleep periods or times of stress, so that when they are awake and playing both their mouth and their hands are free. The close wrapping of earlier weeks is obviously inappropriate at playtimes now, too. But many babies will still settle to sleep best if they are securely wrapped, especially if they are now wrapped from the arm-pits down, so that they can still get at those precious hands. As soon as they wake up from a sleep, they are likely to fight to rid themselves of all coverings, in order to kick; indeed by 3 months a sleeping bag may be the only way of ensuring that the baby stays warm throughout the night.

All these new characteristic behaviors help to finalize the differentia-tion between sleep and waking. When the infant wants to sleep, he wants to be wrapped and warm and may need to suck. When he is awake he wants to be free and occupied. When he sleeps, it will be in crib or carriage; when he plays it may be on the floor, on a bed, in a baby chair or on an adult's lap. There is a pattern to his daily activities now, just as there is patterning in his physical demands.

8

MAKING SENSE
OF WHAT HE SEES

UNTIL ABOUT A GENERATION AGO it was widely assumed that very young infants saw little and understood less. Simple observations by scientists suggested that babies were visually attracted to lights, to large expanses of brilliant color, and to movement. The folk-teaching therefore was that they could see nothing more subtle. Parents who, experiencing the deep, meaningful gaze of their own infants, said, "I know she can't really *see* yet but it does *feel* as if she is looking at me," were told, if anyone listened to them at all, that a baby's looking at faces was either "purely instinctive" or "just your imagination." The scientific world had not yet become interested in infant vision and did not yet possess the tools for studying it. Without the tools the studies could not be made, but without the interest—and the concomitant financial investment in research—the tools could not be conceived of or designed; an interesting example of scientific curiosity and technological innovation going hand in hand.

Visual perception can loosely be defined as "meaningful seeing." The concept is different from that of simple "sight" in that what is seen must convey something which is understood, or at least noticed, to the person who is looking. There are complex degrees in noticing and understanding. Standing on the shore at night I may *see* flashes of light but fail to "notice" them in the sense of separating them out from the promenade lights, the stars, or lights from the nearby fishing fleet. Paying a little more selective attention and/or with more experience or information at my disposal, I may realize that the flashes of light come from a distant ship at sea. Now I have perceived the flashes in a meaningful way. But add yet more experience and information into that perception and I may recognize the flashes as Morse Code and therefore as constituting some kind of message. I might even be able to read the code and thus translate that original sight into a direct communication.

Techniques for finding out *what infants see* are simpler to imagine, to design, and to use than are techniques for eliciting *their degree of understanding* of what is seen. It is not surprising then that it was this aspect of work on infant vision which got off to a flying start in the fifties and sixties. Only a decade later did research into the perception of what is seen reach a comparable fever-pitch. It is continuing now, in the eighties, and there is still a great deal to be done.

Infants are born with visual equipment which is complete, anatomically, but immature in its functioning. The specific immaturity which led observers to believe that all they can see is light, movement, and so forth is an immaturity of distance accommodation. When a human being focuses on objects at different distances, the lens of the eye bends and changes shape. In the mid-sixties, researchers using a technique called dynamic retinoscopy [103] discovered that, at birth, infants' eyes operated rather like fixed-focus cameras. Their "ideal" focusing distance was approximately 8 inches from the bridge of the nose and the lens made no accommodation for objects at a greater distance. The power to accommodate for distance was said to develop rapidly and to approach adult levels by about 4 months of age. More recent work [11] using a technique called photorefraction has further refined our knowledge of infants' distance accommodation. Researchers have now found that it is not that infants *cannot* accommodate their focusing to varying distances but that they usually *do not*. The ability is there but learning to use it accurately and consistently takes time. At 9 days 80 percent of the babies they studied could focus accurately at 2 1/2 feet but only 50 percent often did so, while only 20 percent ever focused at 5 feet. By 3 months, 80 percent could focus at 5 feet and 75 percent did so consistently.

In the first weeks of life then a baby will not be able to see anything far away, and may well not see clearly anything more than 8–10 inches away.

The apparent interest which infants have in bright lights, bright colors, and movement simply reflects the fact that in normal family handling these are the only things which the infant can actually *see* during most of his waking hours. Left in a crib or carriage, in an ordinary room, the nearest object which is within the infant's eye-line will probably be a ceiling light fixture some 7–10 feet (2.10–3.05 m) above him. It will be nothing but a blur. If the light is lit, its brightness may catch his eye, as may the bright window or a blowing curtain, even though they are too distant for him to see their shapes or contours. It is easy to see how the myth grew up that these were the things babies preferred to look at. It was all they were given, except human faces, and their passion for those was assumed to be purely social.

Infants are capable of fine visual discriminations from birth. Researchers such as Robert Fantz [81] have studied both what they can see, and what they choose to look at, using a variety of techniques.

Fantz, for example, found that within 12 hours of birth infants could differentiate between a plain gray disc and an identical disc striped in black and white. But at this age they could only tell the difference if the disc was placed less than 9 inches (23 cm) from the bridge of the nose, and the stripes were at least 1/8 inch (0.32 cm) across. Given that these brand-new infants *could* see the stripes, they all preferred them to the plain gray. The actual visual acuity of the infants in this sample increased very rapidly between 2 and 4 months, so that by 3 months they could discriminate the striped disc from the gray at 15 inches' distance (38 cm) and with stripes only 1/64 inch (0.04 cm) wide. But this would still be a very marked degree of visual handicap in an adult. Janet Atkinson and her colleagues [10] also tested infant acuity and compared their results with those from their focusing investigations. They found that the babies' acuity was, at all ages studied, worse than could be explained by their immature focusing. The explanation must therefore lie within the brain itself, in the reception of visual messages.

If due allowance is made for their lack of distance accommodation, infants look more readily, and for longer, at any complex pattern or interesting shape than they do at simple objects even if they are bright or highly colored. If movement is added to the complex, interesting object, they like it even better. In Fantz's study, for example, all the babies from 5 days old to 6 months "preferred" black and white schematic face sketches to identical ovals of brightly lit brilliant colors. Furthermore the more complex the schematic face, the better they liked it; faces with shading and expression were preferred to simple eyes-nose-mouth sketches.

This kind of research work has given rise to a great deal of controversy, not over the facts of infant visual perception, but over their interpretation and the theoretical framework into which they best fit.

Some researchers believe that infants see, without understanding what they see, until such time as they are able to touch and handle objects. Supporters of this view would argue that when, and only when, the infant begins to handle things, he puts together the feeling of the object and his experiences of its behavior, with the sight of it, and then understands it. Other researchers believe that the purely visual perceptions of the very young infant, not yet old enough to handle objects, are more important than that. They believe that infants see, and understand a good deal about what they see, so that by the time they *can* reach out and handle things, they do so with a certain store of knowledge about those things.

But most authorities would probably now say that this kind of thinking about infant perception—whether visual or in any other sense

—is wrong-headed. It leads to experiments concerning isolated reactions to isolated experimental events even though babies "best" performances almost always occur when they are being asked to react to the complex of stimuli which emanate from a real person. Trevarthen [216], for example, has recently sounded a warning note to would-be experimenters:

> It is important, however, to emphasize that the responses of young babies to real persons shows that they are better able to recognize and respond to these physical features when they are combined in dynamic patterns that can only occur in the activity of a person willing to communicate. Experimental procedures generally work against recognition of this important effect.

Readers of experimental results should certainly have it always in mind that the behavior of a young infant, viewed naturalistically as he interacts with an adult caretaker, will almost always be more organized, complex, and interactive than is his behavior in an experimental situation. But if experimental procedures do not ideally explore the possible behavior of an infant, they do nevertheless allow us to consider the complex being-that-is-a-new-person bit by bit, and to obtain at least some information about different aspects of his development. On the whole the weight of the evidence from experimental procedures in this area do suggest that seeing, even without being able to handle what is seen, does teach the infant a great deal about his world.

The infant is not only capable of seeing the difference between one thing and another (provided they are brought close enough to his eyes), he actually chooses to look at just those things, and just those aspects of things, which are likely to be most useful to him if he is visually learning about the world. He likes to look at complicated, patterned, contoured objects, and movement increases his interest. Thus he is sure to study human faces—which fit that prescription so well. And it is vital that he *should* look at people, in order to interact socially with them. He is less interested in colors and in outline shapes than he is in patterning, texture, detail, and complex contours. These are just the visual cues which make for recognition of objects. If the infant were to concentrate on color and outline shape and, using these cues, learn to recognize a brown dog seen sideways on, he would be markedly confused by a Dalmatian met face to face. It is *not* color and outline shape which remain constant under different lighting conditions and viewing positions, but just those patterning, detail, complex contour variables which interest him so much.

At 6–8 weeks, infants look equally readily and for equal lengths of time at familiar things and at new ones. But by 2–3 months the infant much prefers to study things he has not seen before. By looking less at things he has already "visually learned," he gives himself more time to look at new things, still choosing the most complex and the most patterned new things available for him to see.

Until about 2 months most infants will choose to look at a pictorial representation of an object, rather than at the real thing. But just at the developmental point when the baby's hands begin to be open while he is awake, and he becomes ready to start handling things (see p. 94), he transfers his interest, and will study a doll rather than a picture, a ball rather than a disc [81].

At about this time, too, he makes it clear that he has visually learned about human faces. As we have seen, the infant has been interested in looking at people's faces since very early on. By 6 weeks he may have smiled at his mother or some other adult. And he will smile too at schematic face representations, or pictures of faces. At around 2 months his mother will get a smile most easily if she smiles and talks and moves her head all at the same time. Her talking may be more important even than her smiling. Each time the baby does smile at her, he first makes a visual examination of her whole face, going from her hairline down her face to the chin-line, and then returning his gaze to her eyes. Then, and only then, will he smile if he is going to.

At this same 2-month point, the infant becomes remarkably fussy about the "correctness" of any pictorial representations of human faces. Offered a simple but correctly arranged eyes-nose-mouth diagram, he will look at it in preference to a more interesting, well-shaded but wrongly put together face. While he may smile at a correct sketch, he will not smile if the drawn eyes and mouth have their positions reversed, or if he cannot see the nose.

During the infant's third month, the talking which made it easier for his mother to get him to smile earlier on becomes less and less important. Her face and her smile become enough to elicit his response. But the features and the feature-order that he has learned in all that careful visual scanning of faces remain vital. His mother will not get a smile if she is in profile or wearing sunglasses which hide her eyes. By 3 months, the infant has moved to yet another stage: he may still smile at pictures of faces, but real people now elicit his smiles more quickly, and when the smiles come they are bigger and smilier. He now not only knows what a face ought to look like, in terms of those vital hairline, eyes, nose, and mouth features, he also clearly knows the real from the phony.

Recent evidence suggests that there may be visual as well as social learning involved here. Carefully designed experiments [84] have shown that stereoscopic depth perception or stereopsis—the ability to see three-dimensional objects in 3-D rather than flat, like photographs of themselves—seldom develops before 3 1/2 months and goes on developing during the first half year. We do not yet know whether the early inability to see in 3-D is due to the baby having difficulty in maintaining binocular vision or to incomplete neural development in the brain, but whichever it is, until a child does see in 3-D, objects are unlikely to be more interesting to him than representations of them and the latter may actually be "easier" for him to interpret.

Once a baby does know the real from the represented, his visual sophistication about faces increases so rapidly that he quickly learns to discriminate between familiar and unfamiliar people, by sight alone. He may still be prepared to smile at anyone who smiles directly at him. But whereas a stranger in a bathing cap, which hides the hairline and alters the configuration of the whole head, may be accepted and smiled at, his mother in the same cap will be greeted with a sober stare. She is not looking as he knows she ought to look. And he does not like it.

This kind of research implies that even while infants cannot manipulate objects, handle them, experiment with them, they can learn a good deal about them by vision alone. Supportive evidence comes from some animal studies, particularly those which have been carried out with infant monkeys. If infants did *not* learn about objects just from looking at them, infants who are prevented from looking until they are ready to handle objects should be no less efficient in their object handling than infants reared normally. But infant monkeys reared in total darkness throughout the first 8 weeks of their lives, when normal monkeys would be clinging to their mother's fur and looking, remain extremely bad both at visual discrimination and at using vision to direct their own activities. They are clumsy in their first forays off their mothers' bodies, seeming unable to judge distances. They are clumsy in manipulating food, and find it difficult to pick things up accurately. They behave as if they had missed out on a whole stage of learning about the world.

If we accept that human infants do a lot of learning by looking, it seems a pity not to give them the things they are interested in to look at, in a position from which they can actually see them.

We know, for example, that infants cannot see detail across the width of even the smallest room. We know, too, that they choose to give their attention to what they have not seen before. So it seems a pity to waste nursery mobiles, pictures, brilliant wallpapers, and all the other accouterments of a really interesting room on a baby who will not see the interesting features, but will probably see just enough to get bored with it all before his distance accommodation catches up. It would seem that such a room, organized when the infant was around 4–6 months, would give infinitely greater pleasure.

We know that babies like pictures of things; that they actually choose to give them their attention. Yet many a mother would feel it ridiculous to sit a 2-month baby on her lap and show him a big, bold picture book.

We know that infants focus most easily on objects between 8 and 15 inches away from them, yet we seldom make use of this knowledge.

Interesting things hung from the hood of a carriage, for example, are usually too high up for close inspection; mothers may even be afraid that putting them closer will make the baby squint. Even grandmothers, desperate for some sign of recognition from the baby, are more likely to get him to smile if they will put their faces up to the baby's own.

9

RELATING
HAND TO EYE

As we have seen in the last two chapters, infants make enormous strides in their second and third months in controlling and beginning to *use* their bodies, and in learning about things by looking at them. At the beginning, the infant's "play" with objects is separate from his looking at them. He fingers his own hands or a rattle, or he looks at his own hands or the rattle: he does not, at first, relate his touching and his looking. His manual play and his visual exploration must eventually come together so that he can handle what he looks at—look at what he is handling. Only then can the information given him by his eyes and by his hands be put together.

As long as the baby can only look at things, he remains comparatively passive within his environment. Once he can reach out and take up things he can see, he can become an active participant.

Getting hold of things is an extremely complex procedure, involving not only visual abilities, but also physical abilities: voluntary movements of the body, arm, and hand. Furthermore it involves putting all these things together into smooth, coordinated movements. The development of "hand-eye" coordination is as dramatic and as important in this first half year as is the development of locomotion—the ability to get around unaided—in the second half year.

Earlier research workers tended to see the development of hand-eye coordination as being almost entirely dependent on the infant's own maturation. He would reach out for things, grab at them, pick them up, when, and only when, his neurology and his muscle control were sufficiently mature to allow him to do so. A. Gesell was perhaps the supreme exponent of this point of view in his early pre-war work, and he was followed by researchers like H. M. Halverson [101], whose study did not even commence until infants were 16 weeks old and—as we now see it —well advanced in the development of reaching out for objects.

While it is true that infants cannot be taught to coordinate hand and eye until their neurophysiological equipment is capable of the necessary movements and adaptations, it is equally true that without the stimuli and the experiences which come from even the most restricted environment these abilities would develop very slowly, if at all. Their development is therefore an interaction between what the baby can physiologically do, and what he is stimulated into doing.

Because infants vary in their capacities at any given point in time, and because their environments vary too, it is extremely difficult to design research projects which can give us norms for development in this field. The normal baby will accomplish, at a given stage in his development, exactly what his development and his environment combine to teach him.

It is hardly surprising then that the norms for the development of hand-eye coordination are the subject of hot professional dispute. When the first edition of this book was published, Thomas Bower [30], for example, had recently reported on postures, movements, and early reaching out behavior in babies around 2 weeks old. His studies had caused a professional flurry because what he observed would usually be described as typical of infants 2–3 *months* of age, rather than 14 *days*. Bower believed that infants are in fact born with various motor and visual abilities which atrophy during the first month after birth because they are not stimulated, and then have to be relearned. He believed, for example, that if a baby a fortnight old is fully awake, and is supported in a semi-upright position, and is then offered an object within reach of his hand, he will swipe at it in a coordinated fashion. He believed that this behavior is seldom seen in such young babies only because we do not expect it of them and do not therefore facilitate it. Such infants are seldom fully awake and alert; and in our culture they are nursed lying down, and are seldom held in the right position for reaching out.

Many attempts have been made to replicate Bower's findings. One of the most carefully designed studies, explicitly intended to demonstrate or deny this revolutionary age-dating, was published by Dodwell, Muir, and DiFranco in 1976 [63]. They found no evidence to support it. Their findings, on the contrary, were "consonant with an earlier report on the development of visually elicited reaching": the same report to which my earlier account returned and to which this new edition adheres.

The most detailed, large-scale studies of the normal sequence of the development of hand-eye coordination as most researchers would see it, and of the extent to which the sequence can be modified or speeded up by extra stimulation, were made by B. White, P. Castle, R. Held, and L. Burton [223, 44].

They carried out a careful study of infants being raised in an institution. The babies were receiving good physical care, but they were given a minimum of handling or attention by adults. They were kept in a visually boring environment, with very little to see within their likely focusing range. In this setting, White and his collaborators were able to study both the normal development of coordinated hand-eye behavior, and the extent to which it could be speeded up if more and/or different stimuli were offered to different groups of infants.

Where newborn infants spent much time in gazing unfocusedly into space, it was found that by 6 weeks most of them spent some of their waking time in voluntary visual exploration. Their visual range was, of course, still limited by their flexed posture and their inability to move themselves around. But they would focus on the hand toward which their heads were flexed, or on the edge of the crib blanket, or the crib bars.

Offered a bright, complicated party favor to look at, all the infants would focus readily on it, provided it was shown to them within their best visual range—8–9 inches (20–22 cm)—and provided it was offered on the side to which the infant preferred to keep his head turned. The infant's interest in this object was usually shown not only by his ready focusing on it, but also by a marked change in the level of his physical activity. If he had been moving his free arm and leg when he caught sight of the object, he would typically "freeze to attention." If he had been still when he first saw it he was likely to become physically excited, and begin to wriggle.

At this age the infants would try to keep the object in view, by "tracking it" with their eyes if it was moved in a small arc. But they lost interest immediately if the arc took it beyond their best focusing distance. They had not yet got sufficient visual distance accommodation to enable them to keep it in sharp focus as it moved away.

By 2–2 1/2 months, the infant's typical posture had changed, so that much of the time he lay with the back of his head on the mattress, and his head, arms and legs all free to move. Some of the infants in White's sample already had their hands open for some of their waking time.

At this stage the babies were usually looking at *something* when they were awake, and there was far more visual searching than before, with the infants swiveling both their heads and their eyes to find something to look at. Often they chose to watch their own hands waving in the air. But they appeared to have little idea that those hands were within their own control; they would simply look at a waving hand if it happened to appear in their view.

The experimenter came in for a good deal of interest at this stage, and the infant's attention was even more easily caught by the party favor, which he would track visually by moving his head as well as his eyes. Changes in level of activity were more marked than at the earlier age. For the first time this whole-body change in level of activity was sometimes translated into action directed *at* the object, so that if it was presented in exactly the right place, exactly within the ideal focusing distance, and toward the infant's favored side, he would occasionally swipe at it with his hand, instead of just wriggling with excitement at the sight of it.

By around 3 months the infant's range of visual adaptation had increased to a point where he could keep the party favor in focus when it was as close as 3 inches (8 cm) to the bridge of the nose, or as far away as 20 inches (51 cm). Visual tracking through quite a wide arc was efficient, and the infants would follow the object through a vertical movement as well as horizontally. By this age the infants were watching their hands *as* they played with them. Offered the party favor, they might swipe at it as they did earlier, or they might display a very clear stage in learning how to get hold of it. If the object was presented to the baby's preferred side, he might focus on it, raise the hand on that side toward it, and then glance repeatedly from hand to object, as if measuring, visually, the distance between the two. If the stimulus was presented centrally, so that it was equidistant between the child's hands, he might raise both arms toward it, and then clasp them together across his chest.

By this stage the infants were clearly aware of a connection between what they could see, and their own arms and hands; they had grasped the idea of looking and reaching, but could not yet carry the look-reach sequence to a coordinated conclusion.

These age-norms, which will be carried through into the stage of fully efficient reaching out for objects, in Chapter Sixteen, were found to be surprisingly open to environmental adaptation. As we have seen, these infants were being reared in an environment which can best be described as "bland," containing the minimum of visual, physical, or emotional stimulation for any baby. Various changes were made, by the experimenters, to the environment experienced by different groups of infants. An increase in the daily "ration" of handling by the nurses, with all the stimulation that such handling provides, was found to produce a dramatic increase in the babies' visual interest in the world around them. The more they were taken out of their cribs, moved around, talked to, handled, allowed to see different things from different angles, the more interested they became and the more they looked around for something to look at when they were returned to their cribs.

The provision of numbers of suitable things to look at, within the infant's visual range, and designed to suit his interest in complex pattern and contour, appeared to *delay* the infants' discovery of their own hands. Infants with very little else to look at typically began to finger their hands at 6–8 weeks, while the experimental group, whose cribs were festooned with mobiles, stabiles, and pictures, did not start concentrated hand play until around 9 weeks.

But the experimental group of infants used the stabiles and hanging objects around their cribs. And they learned from them. On average the babies in this group were reaching out and grasping for objects efficiently by 14 weeks, nearly 5 weeks earlier than the control group.

Such an acceleration is remarkable. But at present there is no evidence to suggest that it is of lasting benefit to the baby. In our society, we tend to be so achievement oriented that we feel that it must be good for a baby to learn anything ahead of time. It must be a sign that he is extra bright, or extra well-handled or extra something-desirable.

But faint notes of warning can be detected in this research, and in other work within the same area. The extremes of stimulation offered to the experimental group did not produce *any* acceleration of hand-eye coordination before 2 months of age. Until that time, the experimental infants lay in their jazzy cribs, covered with bright patterned sheets, hung around with carefully chosen toys, and they cried. They cried more and were generally less contented than the control group, who lay peacefully in their white institutional cribs, playing with their fingers.

The difference between the two groups, with the stimulated babies forging ahead in their learning, came at or after 2 months. It came, therefore, at just the time when the infants were uncurling their bodies; opening their hands; getting control of their necks; beginning to kick; and starting to look around to see what they could see.

It may be that these developments are signals of the infant's readiness for stimulation; that they herald the beginning of what is often called a "critical period" for manual-visual learning. If so, infants may actually be better off if they are allowed to come to terms with their own bodies, find their own hands in peace, before they are bombarded with outside stimuli. After all, we know that in these early weeks extremes of noise and light and movement are obnoxious to infants; perhaps extremes of visual stimulation are disturbing too.

If the third month is indeed a critical period for this kind of stimulation, it is probably worthwhile to offer it in full measure once the infant *has* shown that he is ready to make use of it. Learning to get hold of objects early does not mean the infant is a genius, but it will serve both infant and mother well when they reach the stage where boredom becomes a problem (see Chapter Eighteen). Once the infant can hold and manipulate objects, he can play. And once he can play, he becomes very much easier to entertain. Besides, once he is *ready* for lots of things to look at, and swipe at, and reach for, he will enjoy having them. It seems that he may not enjoy them if they are forced on him too soon.

10

HEARING AND
MAKING SOUNDS

INFANTS DISCRIMINATE between different levels of sound from birth. Sudden, loud noises will almost always make a new baby jump, and will make many of them cry. Equally, sudden *changes* in the level of sound tend to have the same effect, so that if the infant has become used to the noise of the vacuum cleaner working around his crib, he may cry when it is turned off.

It is obvious that babies react differently to different kinds of sound. But it is not obvious, nor easy to discover, to what extent they discriminate in detail between one sound and the next. Crying when an ultrasonic boom occurs and relaxing to sweet music only suggest a very coarse degree of discrimination. We need to know all we can possibly find out about the detailed auditory discriminations of young infants, because those discriminations between sounds must at least partly explain how, and indeed why, human infants, as opposed to the young of any other species, eventually learn to speak.

Various researchers have examined the actual hearing apparatus of the human infant and compared it with that of higher animals. Very few important differences in the structure of the ear or inner hearing mechanism have been found. G. Von Békésy and W. Rosenblith [219] said: "Our measurements demonstrate that the auditory systems of man and higher animals function in many respects as if they were governed by the same principles . . ." but these, and other, researchers have found differences in the way in which the auditory apparatus is *used* in man and in animals. It looks as if the human animal is not born with unique equipment which will enable him to understand and use speech, but is unique in the use to which he puts that equipment.

Although far more research is needed, it does seem as if human infants' auditory perception may be innately programmed to distinguish between human speech and other sounds from a very early age. As we saw in Chapter Eight, a baby's visual preferences lead him inescapably toward looking at human faces. In the same way it seems that his auditory preferences lead him toward listening to human voices. In a long and careful series of studies of 700 very young babies, Rita Eisenberg [71–74] exposed infants to a variety of sounds of varied frequency. Their reactions to each sound were assessed in terms of their motor movements, their eye movements, the extent to which they were generally aroused or quieted, changes in their respiration and heart rate, and in their vocalizations. Eisenberg found that any individual infant's response to a particular sound was largely dependent on his own state at the time he was exposed to it. Hence the same sound might excite a baby who was already happily awake but produce crying in one who was already fretful. It might awaken a baby who had been dozing, but merely interest one who was quietly alert.

Eisenberg's findings about the nature of the sound, as opposed to the state of the baby, are less obvious. Sounds within the same frequency range as the normal human voice were usually reacted to positively. Such sounds led calm infants to exhibit interest, and distressed infants to stop crying. Sounds at even slightly higher frequencies than the human voice had quite a different effect. Calm infants tended to "freeze" in apparent alarm or displeasure. Many cried, and any who were already fretful or distressed became much more so.

The clearest and most favorable responses of all were seen when infants were exposed to sound within the human-voice frequency range, *and* intonated to follow roughly the patterns of rise and fall in ordinary adult speech. They reacted far more positively to this intonated sound than they did to sound in the same frequency range presented flat and uninflected. Some infants even turned their heads in apparent search for the source of sound.

No wonder mothers find that their own voices are among the best of all calming devices for infants who are upset. No wonder, too, that very young infants, incapable of seeing the picture, nevertheless often take an interest in television programs.

Further research will undoubtedly reveal other detailed auditory discriminations which infants can make. But the *reason* for their particular reactions to different sounds cannot be seen on a sound spectrograph; such reasons have to be deduced. For example Marvin Simner [203] has already shown that, even in the newborn period, infants are far more likely to begin to cry if they are exposed to the sound of another baby crying than if they are exposed to a band of "white noise" of exactly the same frequency range and volume. Nurses in hospital nurseries amply confirm this finding, dreading the infant who cries a lot because "he sets the others off." Mothers of twins complain that they are seldom given the chance to deal with *one* crying infant, because as soon as one starts to cry, the other joins him. The implication of studies such as these must be that very young infants detect distressed sounds—which they discriminate from other voice-sounds—and react to them by uttering distressed sounds of their own. Trevarthen [216] has studied babies with their mothers, from birth, and has recorded a complex of interactions between each pair which he has labeled "pre-speech." The babies he studied responded with small, but accurately coordinated sounds to the musical, lilting questioning of their mothers and coupled their "talk" with speech-like movements of their mouths and expressive facial changes. It seems, then, that even the youngest infant can discriminate and respond appropriately to social sounds too.

But this work, part of a large body of research devoted to considering infants as part of infant-mother pairs interacting with each other, is as new as it is exciting. There are still many scientists who believe that early infant sounds are the spontaneous result of changing physiological states, and nothing to do with the infant's hearing of, or discrimination between, sounds. They point out, for example, that the contented gurgles of a recently fed infant result directly from his physical relaxation, half open mouth, and slack vocal cords, and that the tiny whimpery sounds which often precede crying come from his increased breathing rate and tense vocal cords. While such explanations seem disappointingly mundane, they do gain some credence from work with deaf babies. It has been found that even the totally deaf child, one who cannot hear his own sounds let alone anyone else's, makes the same sounds, the same range of sounds, and the same number of sounds as a normally hearing child, at least during the first 2 or 3 months. Similarly, if it is experimentally arranged so a normally hearing baby is temporarily unable to hear his own sounds, he will nevertheless continue to make them. An adult who is prevented from hearing the sounds he makes finds it almost impossible to go on talking, as anyone who has experienced transatlantic telephones on a bad night for satellites will know. So perhaps these early infant sounds are not related to the baby's hearing at all, or perhaps some sounds are reactive while others are spontaneous. When enough research work has been done, some kind of consensus will emerge. For the present the question can remain academic because whether or not the sounds of the first few weeks are reactive and social, they certainly rapidly become so.

By 2 months in some babies, and by 3 months in almost all, hearing spoken sounds becomes a very definite stimulus to the infant to make sounds of his own. When he is spoken to, he looks for the source of the sound, watches the face of the talking adult, changes his level of activity (either "freezing to attention" or beginning to kick excitedly), and he usually smiles. As he smiles, he "talks back," producing small explosions of liquid sound. Every bit of the baby seems, to an observer, to go into this delightful social exchange, and every bit of him exudes dejection if his mother terminates it by turning away.

This voluntary talking usually has a close association with social smiling. The infant smiles and talks when his mother smiles and talks to him. By 3 months the specific stimuli and responses have sorted themselves out. The infant smiles when his mother smiles at him—whether she also talks or not—and he talks when she talks to him, even if she is not also smiling.

Almost all infants under about 3 months do most of their talking when they are being talked to, but there is very wide variation in the amount which individual babies also talk when they are alone. S. Nakazima [168], whose work in comparing American and Japanese infants will be referred to at length in Chapters Seventeen and Twenty-three, felt that his subjects could be divided into two quite distinct groups during this age period: those who talked most when they were being talked to, and those who talked most when they were alone. While some babies certainly do vocalize extensively to themselves when they are in their cribs or carriages, it seems surprising that Nakazima's sample babies were not also willing to talk extensively to adults. Further research might show that if they had been talked to more, or differently, they might in fact have done so, in which case the two groupings would comprise highly vocal and less vocal infants, rather than vocal and socially vocal ones.

Most researchers in this field have demonstrated a very clear relationship between the amount an infant is spoken to, directly, face to face, rather than casually as the mother moves around, and the amount he talks himself. H. L. Rheingold's studies [184] demonstrated clearly that mothers who did talk a great deal in this direct face-to-face way with their infants, tended to be able to carry on "conversations" with them, even as early as 6 weeks. The mother would talk to the baby; the baby would make a sound back, and then pause; the mother would reply, and the child would make a further sound. Conversations of this kind have been recorded lasting as much as 15 minutes, and containing a wide range of inflection and tone from the infant.

The baby who will "converse" in this way will also probably "practice" his sound-making when he is alone. Instead of a burble of sound, the listening adult hears the baby make a noise, pause, as if listening to that noise, and then make it again. This sound-practicing, together with playing with his own hands, is often the infant's best method of self-entertainment. Babies who do it are more likely than others to remain happily in their cribs after waking, or to be content if put down for a nap before they are quite ready for sleep.

But some mothers find it more difficult than others to talk to a very young baby. Where some instinctively chat whenever they are handling the infant, others feel self-conscious, and find it more natural to handle the baby silently. There is no alternative to the genuine human voice for stimulating the baby's speech. Various researchers have experimented to see whether arranging for some other sound to follow closely on the infant's own noises would stimulate him to go on and "converse." P.

Weisberg [221], for example, arranged for a pleasant-sounding bell to ring every time his sample infants uttered. This response did not stimulate further sound from the babies. The infant "talks" because he is being talked to, not just because he hears a sound. He talks when he is talked to because he is in some way innately programmed to respond to human speech.

THREE MONTHS' SUMMARY

BY 3 MONTHS babies are already complex human beings; the more complex they become, the more difficult it is to generalize about what they will (or "should") be doing at a given age. The range of ages at which they do certain things is enormous, without the babies at either end of the range being in any way abnormal. Furthermore there is no convincing evidence that a baby who is slow in certain areas of development will continue to be slow, or conversely, that the advanced 3-month infant will go on being ahead of his peers.

Generalizations of the kind given in this summary are therefore of interest in respect to the individual baby only if they are read with full knowledge of that particular baby's past development. The *rate* at which he moves from stage to stage may vary, but the *sequence* in which he does so is almost invariable. A specific example may clarify this. Later in this section will be found the statement that by 3 months most babies will be able to roll themselves from their backs to their sides. To say that an individual baby is slow to accomplish this, without knowledge of his prior development, is meaningless, because he will not learn to roll from his back to his side until after he has learned to roll from his side to his back. The latter will always precede the former. On the other hand if the baby begins to roll from side to back just around three months, he may learn the opposite maneuver almost immediately afterward, so that he ends up equal in "rolling ability" with the baby who learned the first direction at 8 weeks.

Summaries such as this one serve two purposes. They give a rough guide to what "most" babies do at a given age, and they tell people who are involved with individual babies roughly what to expect the next development to be. They do not enable anyone to make spot checks on the advanced or retarded behavior of the infant.

One further note of caution is necessary. At this age, babies who were in any way disadvantaged at birth, due to prematurity, low birth-weight, illness, acute feeding difficulties, changes of caretaker, or just to being very miserable or sleepy babies, have not had nearly enough time to catch up with infants who had a better start. Such babies are likely to be well behind. It may take them several months more to catch up to the "norm."

Behavior	Likely stage reached at 3 months	Comments
Feeding	Five feedings per 24 hours from breast or bottle.	Sixth feeding will not be dropped until baby can go for one period of 6–7 hours without feeding.
Quantity of food	6–8 oz. (170–230 ml) milk per feeding. Possibly some solids.	Not as much if birthweight was low; solids certainly not needed if milk intake is still below about 35 oz. (1000 ml) per 24 hours.
Weight	Is likely to have gained about 7 oz. (200 g) per week from birthweight except for first week; i.e., baby born weighing 7 lb. will now weigh roughly 7 lb. + 12 × 7 oz. = 12 lb. 4 oz. (3.2 kg now 3.2 kg + 12 × 200 g = 5.6 kg).	Low birthweight babies will gain at similar rates, and will therefore be roughly the same amount lighter than their peers at this age as they were at birth.
Sleeping	Very approximately 16 hours out of 24.	Actual hours of sleep will depend on how much the baby has slept in earlier weeks: the total hours will have dropped, but to what level depends on the individual starting point.
Crying	Probably no frequent, "purposeless" crying. Causes of crying are usually clear and comprehensible.	Babies who have always been "miserable" may still appear to be so. They will not become readily comfortable until their social development reaches the norm for their age group.

Behavior	*Likely stage reached at 3 months*	*Comments*
Colic	Over. Continued evening screaming is now much more likely to be due to hunger or frustration of social inclinations.	Colic, once established, usually lasts 9 weeks. Babies who started it late may continue to about 4 months. Colic after 4 months is extremely rare.
Posture	On the back, the baby now usually lies straight, with back of head on mattress and all limbs free. On face, he raises upper chest on forearms; legs straight out behind him.	All these developments go together. Baby who still lies in "scrunched-up" neonatal position on back will only turn head when placed on face.
Posture	Held sitting, he supports his own head and upper back, sagging only from the hips. Carried, he supports his head unless mother bends down or moves very suddenly.	Similarly baby who cannot support own head when carried will not support it when held sitting.
Motor activities	Provided he has reached the postural stage described above, he will now wave arms and legs smoothly, rhythmically and almost constantly when awake. Will be able to roll from his side onto his back. Once having done this, will learn about now to roll from back to side. Will enjoy being gently rocked, swung, held sitting or standing.	None of these developments will take place until head control is almost perfect. Until this stage, arm and leg movements remain jerky and unplayful. Rolling over is unlikely and being rocked and swung may actually distress him. Will *not* enjoy these things until he *has* begun playful motor activity himself.
Grasping	Hands will now be open most of the time when awake. Will grasp an object put in the hand. Will clasp one hand	Baby whose hands are still habitually loosely fisted is unlikely to be ready for manual play. Hands will open when baby is ready to use them.

Behavior	Likely stage reached at 3 months	Comments
Grasping (cont'd)	with the other, finger and play with clothing at chest level. Put fingers or objects in the mouth. May finger breast or bottle.	
Seeing	Can now readily adapt focus to objects as close as 3 inches (8 cm), as far as 20 inches (50 cm). Clarity of distance vision is much improved; adult acuity will be reached by about 4 months. Visual interest is now great. Looks at something whenever awake; swivels head and eyes to follow object. Watches mother as she moves around room.	Baby who still lies in the neonatal posture is not free to move his head in the same way, and will therefore see and follow objects very much less. Just as postural growing up is needed to free limbs for motor activity, so it is needed to free head and eyes for increased visual activity.
Coordinating seeing and grasping	By 3 months, the baby has "found" his own hands with his eyes as well as by touch. He spends much time looking at his hands, watching them as they move; putting them to his mouth and then bringing them back into his line of vision. Presented with an object within range he will swipe at it, and often hit it. A hanging ball will be swiped, watched as it swings, swiped again. Once swiping is accurate, the baby may raise his hand toward an object, glancing from hand to object to hand, as if visually measuring the distance between.	Baby will not "find" his hands with his eyes until he has begun to play with them by touch. He is unlikely to "swipe" at other objects until he *has* begun to watch his own hands moving.

Behavior	Likely stage reached at 3 months	Comments
Social responses	Now smiles readily at a smiling face, even if it is not also talking. Will still smile at masks or drawings of faces, but smiles to real people come faster and look "smilier."	*Early* social smiles are slow in coming, and usually are a response to the adult smiling *and* talking. Smiling to a *silently* smiling face follows this phase.
Smiling	Still needs to see all features, full face. Will not smile to profile. While smiling strangers still get a smiling response, familiar adults who look strange—with new hairdo, sunglasses or hats—may get an adverse reaction.	
Talking	Baby will "talk back" when he is talked to. Practices sounds when alone—often in the early morning.	Will not "talk back" until he has started to smile to a silent smiling face. This marks the separation of smiling and talking responses.
Pleasure and anticipation	When extremely pleased, the baby tends to put all his new abilities together, so that he smiles, burbles, kicks, and waves simultaneously. Such behavior is often seen as a "greeting" to the mother when she comes in to the baby in the morning. It may also be seen when the baby is presented with his bottle, or put in his carriage for an outing. At this stage, the baby may also react with this sort of pleasure to his own motor play.	"Greeting" behavior and other spontaneous expressions of delight will not be seen until the baby smiles readily at people and talks back.

PART III

FROM THREE TO SIX MONTHS

Discovering People

11

SINGLING OUT MOTHER

IN MANY FAMILIES a baby's second 3 months are seen and remembered as the period during which he stopped being "the baby" and became a distinct individual and a noticing person. He will become a full member of whatever kind of family is available to him because his signals become so clear that anyone who lives with him will come to understand them while he in his turn will interact with anyone who is available. Those available people and the environment he shares with them become acutely important to the baby as this age period progresses.

For ease of reference a book of this kind has to try to present separately the infant's different accomplishments and the shifts and changes which take place in various areas of his being. In reality, however, such separation is false. The baby is all of a piece. His eating is not separate from his mood; his "talking" is not separate from his relationships with people; his physical play is not separate from any of these things. He is probably more completely a whole than older people are. He has not yet learned to assume roles: to be one child at school, another on the street, and yet another at home. He has not learned to empty his mind of domestic responsibilities while at work nor to stop thinking about that work because it is Sunday. So even as we dissect the developing baby's characteristics, behaviors, moods, and abilities, it is important to remember that each minute fragment has a context and that the context is the-whole-child-and-the-people-who-are-important-to-him.

I believe that the infant's relationships with people who are important to him are the foundation stone for the structure of his personality. I further believe that it is during this age period, when the baby learns to tell one person from another, that we can first clearly see the structure beginning to grow. The baby is both increasingly sociable and increasingly fussy about whom he socializes with. Basic to most of the other kinds of discrimination which he will learn to make appears to be his singling out of his mother or mother-figure from all other adult people.

I phrase all this as a personal credo because, as we shall see, recent research developments have made it necessary to accept that we do not, scientifically, *know* that this one-to-one relationship with mother or substitute is vital to babies. If readers are to interpret my necessarily brief presentation of the evidence on both sides, they need to know my bias. But first we have to dispose of one misapprehension which has bedeviled discussion of mothering ever since its importance was thrown into tragic relief by the plight of orphaned children after the Second World War. This misapprehension is that when one talks of mothering or of a mother-child unit one is necessarily talking of the child's blood-mother. Infants do not know who gave birth to them. As far as we know there is no magic whatsoever in the blood tie between mother and baby any more than there is magic in the genetic tie between father and baby. What matters to the infant is that someone—some individual person—should care for him, practically and emotionally, and should therefore be available to him for his first love-relationship. If more than one person should thus be available, the infant is the richer for it. There is some evidence that he will still choose to make his most important relationship with one of them, but if one is the natural mother, he may still attach himself primarily to the other.

This issue raises many difficulties. In our society it is still usually the natural mother who does care for a baby, and therefore this relationship is most often seen between a natural mother-baby pair. To refer to them thus is therefore rational, but, however often one reiterates the point that it *need not* be the mother, it is still assumed that in some moralistic way one is saying that it *ought* to be. There are other difficulties: relationships are two-way. Mothers carry fetuses and give birth to them. Physiologically (and usually emotionally too) they are more ready than anyone else to mother the person who is born, and to start doing so immediately. We simply do not know whether the baby who is thus mothered immediately after birth and continues to be mothered consistently from that time has an advantage over others. To the mother who does this, obviously it seems so. To the mother who does not, it naturally seems important that it should not be so. Fathers who are ready, willing, and able to care for their infants need to believe that they can do so as well as their partners while fathers who wish to pursue a more conventional division of family labor have a vested interest in believing that those partners are the "right" people to undertake most of the baby care. Substitute mothers, paid or unpaid, family members or outsiders, would lose much of their motivation if they had to believe that the best they could offer an infant had to be second best.

The many groups all over the world—from the established kibbutzim of Israel to the mushrooming communes of the United States—who are experimenting with various forms of group living, have a highly charged

interest in the subject too. In some such groups—certainly in the kibbutzim—the primary emotional tie between mother and child is accepted but
is separated from the daily care of the infant which is carried out, often
rather impersonally, by trained staff working with fairly large groups of
babies. In other groups deliberate attempts are made to avoid even a
primary emotional tie, the principles and the ideals of the group being
that all infants should equally "belong" to all member-adults. Finally,
there are many people who believe that the whole institution of the
nuclear family is inappropriate to modern life (if indeed it ever was
appropriate) and therefore that infant care, the necessary activity which
forces us to maintain some concept of family, would be better undertaken
as a professional responsibility. I believe that this view is strengthened by
the appalling conditions in which our society allows, indeed expects,
women to carry out a mothering role [138]. Ours is a society where paid
work gives people not only their means to live but also their status, their
identity, and much of their social contact. We have drained people and
most of their meaningful activities out of our "homes" and into our work
places. Yet child care is left as something to be carried out by women
alone in those homes. We have thus swung away from inquiry into what
is best for babies toward descriptions of what is not tolerable for their
mothers. Whether or not each baby needs an individual mother-person,
each individual adult certainly needs other adults with whom to work and
play. Child care as a solitary and full-time activity is a new phenomenon
related to, and no more acceptable than, the phenomenon of the com-
muter. No wonder, then, that any attempt to look at a baby's first important relationships is beset by so much pain and anger.

The question "How much do mothers matter to babies?" first came
to the close attention of the general public with John Bowlby's [34] report
to the World Health Organization designed to suggest ways of improving
the care of motherless children emerging from the horrors of war. That
report and book stimulated an enormous and timely amount of discussion, and has probably done more than any other single work to improve
the lot of children who must, for whatever reason, temporarily or permanently, live in institutions. But due to the amount of popular interest it
evoked, that report, together with many of Bowlby's subsequent papers,
has been widely misinterpreted. It has been suggested that nothing less
than the 24-hours-a-day, 7-days-a-week, 52-weeks-a-year care of a baby
by its own mother would suffice to fulfill its emotional needs. Bowlby did
not say this. He said that it was essential for a baby to experience a warm,
intimate, and continuous relationship with its mother or permanent
mother-figure. But he also said, even in this first early report, that it was
important to accustom the baby, from the beginning, to being cared for
occasionally and for short periods by other familiar figures. He has never
suggested maternal chains.

The attitudes of research workers to the question of the infant's need
for a close exclusive tie with his mother inevitably depend on their atti-

tudes to infant development as a whole. In the past, students of infant development tended to subscribe to one of two radically opposed points of view.

J. B. Watson [220], often described as the father of behaviorism, saw the new infant as a blank slate on which parents could draw almost at will. For him, psychological development was a one-sided process, something that arose from what was done *to* the child. The characteristics found in that child as he grew up were seen therefore as almost entirely the result of parental handling, or, more often, their mishandling.

A. Gesell [93, 94] took an equally one-sided although opposite view. He believed that development was primarily a matter of maturation, of the child unfolding as he got older along largely predetermined lines. He believed that the child's environment could make only minimal differences to his development. It is interesting to notice that in a 1980 publication from the still highly influential Gesell Institute [7] this position is barely revised. Gesell's successors acknowledge that the environment works on the child but a child's inherent developmental patterns are still seen as primary. Indeed, where a special interest in environmental influences is expressed, it is in *physical* environmental influences—such as pollution—rather than in emotional influences stemming from people.

In recent years, a Skinnerian model, suggesting that infant learning and development takes place almost entirely through conditioning effects, has gained many advocates. This approach, perhaps epitomized by the work of J. L. Gewirtz [98], suggests that for learning to take place, the environment must provide stimuli which the child can discriminate, and reinforcers for his behavior in reaction to those stimuli. While this is undoubtedly true, it is inadequate as a theory. The fact that the infant smiles more if his smiles are pleasantly responded to is a statement of fact; it is not an explanation. Why does the infant react in this way? Why can he discriminate a smile? Why does he smile? Why does an answering smile make him smile again?

All these theories stay outside the baby's skin. More recent work has concentrated on looking not merely at what is done to the baby from the outside, nor at his inherent rate of maturation, nor even at the cause-and-effect links which are forged between the two. Rather it concentrates on looking at the cognitive structures within the baby, which mediate between information coming in to him and his own behavior. Something within the baby makes him likely to smile when his mother smiles, and *unlikely* to cry when she smiles. The baby takes an active part in shaping his own environment, in dictating what stimuli he will receive. And he takes a particularly active part in shaping the way in which his mother—and other caretakers—behave toward him. The organism which is the baby interacts with his environment; the results of that interaction change his behavior, but they also change the environment. The two are totally intermixed.

This point of view was most cogently put forward by J. Piaget [177,

178]. He saw the infant, from birth, as being possessed of certain "schemata," which are initially organized around innate reflexes such as sucking and visual orientation. These schemata dictate the newborn baby's first interactions with the environment. The sucking schema, for example, ensures that the infant will attempt to suck any object which his mouth encounters. But experience of the variable "suckability" of objects leads to changes in the original schema—for instance a thumb requires a different type of sucking from a nipple; the baby therefore accommodates his original schema by adapting it to different stimuli.

Adaptation to the environment is a constant balancing by the baby of assimilation and accommodation. Where a stimulus fits into an existing schema it is assimilated. Where it does not fit, the schema is adapted to accommodate it. Events are always selected, interpreted, and fitted into the existing pattern of cognitive structures. The flexibility of the human being is such that the inborn schemata can become adapted to an ever-increasing range of external circumstances. Finally such a complex and diversified cognitive structure is reached that the child can handle not only all external events, but their internal representations, in terms of symbols and abstractions. Piagetian ideas have become accepted as basic to the study of child development, yet many of the original papers as well as the innumerable critiques, confirmations, and extensions to which they have given rise, are difficult to find and highly technical. A 1980 account of important aspects of his thinking, written for lay people and related to the actual development of real infants, may be useful [202].

This view of development finds a parallel in systems engineering with its principles of self-organization and feedback. L. K. Frank [86] discusses this parallel, and sees the infant as "a self-organizing, self-stabilizing, self-directing, largely self-repairing open system which becomes progressively patterned, oriented, and coupled to the culturally established dimensions of his environment, natural and human." This creature is no blank slate for parents to draw on, nor a Pavlovian dog who will automatically respond to a predetermined stimulus.

As we have seen in earlier chapters, infants appear to have schemata toward other human beings. They are visually interested in the human face (see p. 99), they are interested in the human voice (see p. 109), and they respond soothedly to being held and cuddled. But at the beginning, these responses are not specifically social. When he starts to smile, the infant will do so as readily to a mask face as to his mother. When he cries, he is comforted as readily by being swaddled in a soft blanket as by being held in his mother's arms. Often mothers assume an importance for themselves, as individuals, which in the *early* weeks they do not yet have. When such a young baby cries, his mother is likely to pick him up and cuddle him and be gratified when he is comforted. Why should she experiment by putting him, instead, into a soft, warm, holding-gadget making tape-recorded, voice-sounds? Or by handing him to a friendly stranger? She assumes that she *as herself* is the comforter, whereas at this stage she is merely the readily available and concerned human being who, by her humanity, provides the sum of comforting elements.

For many years it was assumed that the baby learned to associate people with being fed; that it was the hunger drive which acted as a stimulus, and feeding as the reward, and that a child's attachment to his caretaker could therefore be simply explained. Freud placed heavy emphasis on the feeding relationship as the context within which the baby learned dependence on his mother. J. Dollard and N. E. Miller [64] made the theory even more explicit:

> In general there is a correlation between the absence of people and the prolongation of suffering from hunger, cold, pain and other drives; the appearance of a person is associated with a reinforcing reduction in the drive. Therefore the proper conditions are present for the infant to learn to attach strong reinforcement value to a variety of cues from the nearness of the mother and other adults . . .

This is a tempting idea, and one which a superficial look at real life tends to confirm. The mother is usually the person who deals with an infant's hunger or cold, fear or pain. And it is usually the mother to whom the baby becomes most attached. It all seems simple and "natural." But the theory does not fit the facts.

Mothering behavior does not appear to be necessary in any species before attachment can take place. Mothering behavior *takes place* in human infants before attachment manifests itself, because human infants are relatively so slow in their development. But in other species attachment often precedes any form of mother care. In birds, for example, chicks emerge from the shell with an inbuilt and determined desire to follow the mother bird. No contact need be made at all between mother bird and chick before this following behavior (known as "imprinting") occurs. Furthermore chicks can be experimentally "imprinted" onto almost any other moving object, if that object (even a human being) is the first thing the chick sees on hatching. The imprinted following is an instinctive attachment behavior in no way dependent on prior satisfaction of any infant need.

Moving closer to the human species, extensive research with rhesus monkeys [102] has shown that feeding is by no means the strongest drive in the development of attachment behavior. H. F. Harlow has shown that if infant monkeys are deprived of their real mothers at birth, and are offered two "surrogates," one made of wire and holding the feeding bottle, and the other made of comfortably padded cloth, they develop a passionate attachment to the "cloth mother," clinging to it, sleeping on it, returning to it in times of stress. They use the "wire mother" purely as a bottle holder.

In human infants there is a considerable amount of evidence, touched upon in Chapter Three, that not even feeding, together with all other aspects of infant care, necessarily dictate the direction of an infant's attachments. In the Israeli kibbutzim, for example, the complete physical care of infants used to be taken over by nurses from the earliest weeks of life. Contact with the natural mother was confined to a couple of hours in the day. But it was nevertheless with the mother, who offered emotional gratification but no physical care, that the infants formed their close attachments. H. R. Schaffer and P. E. Emerson [196] similarly found that infants often formed close attachments to fathers, siblings, or other relatives, even when they took no part in routine physical care or feeding.

The infant does not need reduction of hunger or other unpleasant sensations to provide him with motivation for becoming attached to people. His motivation is inbuilt, part of his cognitive structure. He has certain schemata, in Piaget's phrase, and these direct his attention to certain aspects of his environment. People are uniquely able to provide all that interests the baby, rolled into one stimulus. They are interesting to look at, to listen to, to touch and feel, to be held and moved around by. They are warm, soft, brightly colored, and so forth. The infant is made so that people will interest him more than anything else around him. The more he sees of them, the more he wants. The more he sees, the more he becomes able to tell one from another. And the more he discriminates *between* people the more he comes to want particular people, not just any people.

In what our culture regards as "normal families," the object of the baby's first real attachment is likely to be the mother, but research has made it abundantly clear that this is a matter of environmental chance. If the mother is mothering her own baby, more or less full time, she is the obvious, the most available candidate for his first intense attachment. But it is availability, not magic. If someone else is mothering the baby, that someone else will get his attachment, provided that their interaction began *before* the baby began to differentiate his natural mother from other people. Allowing for the wide age variation within which such discrimination can begin to occur, 6 weeks is probably late for an ideal adoption; and the baby's formation of attachments will almost certainly be disturbed if he is moved from one caretaker to another later than about 3 months.

Bowlby [34] believed that whether or not the infant had his natural mother to attach himself to, this first or primary attachment would be to one person only—that the infant had, as it were, an inbuilt monotropy. Other researchers have shed some doubt on this proposition. Schaffer and Emerson [196] made repeated studies of the same babies over several months, in what is termed a longitudinal investigation. They found that 29 percent of their sample of 58 babies formed their first attachments to several people at the same time. Schaffer refers to various animal studies, which showed similar findings. For example, dogs often form primary attachments to littermates as well as to their mothers, because the mother tends to begin to leave the nest just at the time the puppies are ready to attach. Similarly, Bonnet macaque monkeys have a polyma-tric rearing system, which leads to the formation of multiple attachments. It seems likely that the number of attachments made by the infant does vary with the number of relationships offered to him. But it is possible that the relationship with the mother-figure is always primary, and that the formation of the additional relationships is contingent upon the ma-ternal one, even if their formation is separated only by a few days. Mea-sures of attachment are not yet sophisticated enough for anyone to be sure exactly who, in this situation, the infant attached to first, nor which attachment is the most meaningful for the child. Bowlby [32], the last volume of whose great trilogy *Attachment and Loss* was published in 1980, certainly does not believe that the natural mother is the only possible candidate for the infant's attachment. But, by repeatedly stressing that the infant will *select* an attachment-figure out of the range of people available to him, he does imply that that chosen relationship will be the one which is of primary importance in the infant's early life.

Unfortunately it is difficult to find naturally occurring situations in which it would be possible to study an infant's attachment behavior if he was offered two adults, both equally available to him all the time. It is not known whether the infant would select one of them as his primary person, or whether he would interact equally with them both. There are plenty of highly participant fathers, but few of them are at home with the baby as much as their wives. There are plenty of mothers who share their babies with nannies—but few families where both women hold them-selves constantly available to the child. The essence of such a situation is that when one is "on duty" the other is not.

So for practical purposes it is reasonable to assume that the baby will attach himself primarily to his mother or her substitute. But her central role does not remain for long unless she earns it, and she cannot earn it simply by feeding and physically caring for the baby. In Schaffer and Emerson's sample nearly one third of the babies had shifted their primary allegiance by the age of 18 months, usually in favor of the father, even if he participated little in baby care, and could spend comparatively little time with the infant. As age increases, the choice of person to whom the baby is attached seems to be dictated firstly by the object-person's re-sponsiveness to the infant's cues and social advances, and secondly by the amount of interaction which he is prepared to *initiate* with the infant. As Schaffer and Emerson put it:

> When . . . the most available person (generally the mother) does not show a great deal of responsiveness and is not prepared to interact much with the infant, the latter is more likely to search for another object toward whom he can direct his most intense attachment behavior. . . . Thus when a relatively unstimulating mother is found in conjunction with, say, an ex-tremely attentive father, the latter is more likely to head the infant's hierar-chy of attachment objects, despite the mother's greater availability.

But that is in the future. At 3 months infants have not reached the point where they will abandon one attachment because it seems less satisfactory than another. They are only just beginning to make that first, primary one. L. J. Yarrow [227] studied a large sample of infants to see how many showed definite pleasure and excitement at seeing their mothers rather than the unknown experimenter, and at what ages they reached this stage. At 1 month, only 20 percent of the infants showed any behavior which even might have demonstrated a discrimination of mother from stranger. By 3 months 80 percent clearly differentiated between the two, while by 5 months every single infant not only clearly knew mother from stranger, but infinitely preferred her.

The development of the infant's attachment to his mother as a particular and special individual can be seen in subtle behaviors, which are not always clear unless the infant is watched when he is with mother *and* somebody else. Alone with mother, he behaves as infants behave when they are in pleasant social contact with an adult; when another person is added into the situation it can be seen that he increasingly treats his mother differently. M. D. S. Ainsworth [2] found, for example, that where most babies would smile at a mask or photograph of a face at 14 weeks, they already smiled faster and more fully to a human face. By 16 weeks the mother's face got the widest and fastest smiles of all, and being picked up by mother when he was distressed always stopped a baby's crying, where being picked up by a stranger might not. By around 4 months the babies in this sample showed quite different behaviors when they were happily seated on their mother's or the stranger's lap. On the mother's knee, they behaved as if the mother's body belonged to them, exploring her face, her clothes, her hair with their hands and mouths. But on the stranger's knee they were far more restrained, often barely touching her. By 5–6 months, most of the infants would bury their faces in the mother's shoulder or lap if they were shy or upset; they never did this to the stranger.

So the signs of an infant's discrimination of and attachment to his mother are, during this age period, positive ones. It is not that he is calm with his mother and distressed with strangers, but rather that he is free, confident, and joyous with his mother and more restrained with strangers. Few mothers can fail to be pleased when their infant, having sat calmly in a visitor's arms, comes to hers with grins and crows of delight. The more the baby singles his mother out for these charming attentions, the more she is likely to respond to them in kind. He makes her feel marvelous; mother and baby reinforce each other.

It has been repeatedly demonstrated that infants *will* make an intense relationship with their mothers or permanent caretakers if this is offered to them. It has further been demonstrated that when such a relationship has been formed, during this age period, it will have more significance for the infant than his relationship with any other adult. But the question remains: is such a relationship *necessary* to babies? Do infants only develop optimally in all fields if they are offered such an intense one-to-one experience over a long period? Do we even know, objectively, what "optimal development" is or does the user of such a phrase merely reflect the current values of his or her own culture or sub-group?

Many eminent workers in the field of infant development are trying to elucidate facts, uncontaminated by emotion or special interest. The difficulty (and fascination) of the task is best illustrated by two large volumes of recent research reporting by giants in the field. *Studies in Mother-Infant Interaction* is a large collection of papers edited by H. R. Schaffer and published in 1977 following a most exciting conference [195]. The papers report wide-ranging research projects which have in common the view that infant and mother are, from birth, a dyad. They are seen as acting upon one another; interacting with each other, and creating between them both the environment they share and maturation and development in them both. The very beginnings of every human characteristic are minutely observed and recorded, with imaginative and sometimes novel technological methods being used to enable the authors to objectify findings which might otherwise be dismissed as chance observation or even as wishful thinking. Perhaps the strongest overall impression left by this formidable collection is of the richness of communication between these babies and their mothers. Whether a particular research worker is reporting on studies of newborns reacting rhythmically to human speech or another is reporting on a small sample of 3-month babies "just playing" with their mothers, a clear impression of the vitality and centrality of the relationship, to adult as well as to infant, remains. I do not believe that any of the contributors to this volume would make blood-mothering a necessary (let alone a sufficient) condition for being one half of the whole which is the infant-adult pair. But I do believe that most of them would consider it useless to study infants in isolation from an adult other-half. The many and various infants discussed in this book come across not just as *needing* an adult caretaker in special relationship to them but as being creatures who are only complete within such a relationship.

Infancy: Its Place in Human Development [120] is not a collection of reports on research by many individuals but an account of a large-scale American study carried out by the authors, J. Kagan, R. Kearsley, and P. Zelazo. This superb study was based on the opposing view: namely that the significance of the mother-child dyad was unproven and must be examined, in detail and without prejudice. A day-care nursery was specially designed, set up and staffed, and the development of babies and toddlers within the facility compared with the development of matched controls being reared at home by their mothers. Overall, the day-care children showed no disadvantage whatsoever.

None of the research reported in these volumes can be faulted in any significant way for the care or inventiveness of its methodology. Nor is the honesty or integrity of their intentions or findings open to question. This is excellent research. Clearly both groups of workers cannot be "right" yet equally clearly neither can be "wrong."

Does this mean that the two sets of findings are contradictory? I do not believe so and I think it would be a pity if they were used to increase the polarity between those, professionals and parents alike, who believe that mothers matter and those who believe that their role is not only culturally determined but also psychologically overstressed. I believe that these two vast collections of data can both fit comfortably into a single approach to exploring the infant-mother relationship if we can rid ourselves of the emotional connotations of that word "mother" and of the unthinking assumption that if a one-to-one relationship is to be meaningful, it must be exclusive.

The babies in the work reported by Schaffer were relating to their natural mothers but it is the relating which is demonstrably important, not necessarily the blood relationship. There is little in this volume to suggest that the infants would have related differently or less richly to equally loving and attentive caretakers who were not their natural mothers. Common sense—and a little preliminary data—suggest that a blood-mother may have some advantages in starting a close relationship with her own child. Pregnancy and delivery ensure that she is physiologically "ready" to mother somebody. The fact that the infant is her own child may be an important motivating force and, of course, she is automatically in at the start: at the moment of birth. But even if natural mothers do start out with an advantage in being their own infants' "special" people, it may be an advantage which is readily outweighed by other factors. A report by Britain's National Children's Bureau called *Growing Up Adopted* [200] reported detailed assessments of adopted children aged 7 years as compared both with the rest of a national sample of 7-year-olds and as compared with those members of the sample who, usually because they were illegitimate, might have been placed for adoption but instead had remained with their natural mothers. The adopted children showed no disadvantage, on any of the many measures employed, when they were compared with the might-have-been-adopted group. While no legitimate direct comparison can be made between the detailed developmental data in Schaffer's book and the statistical survey data from the National Children's Bureau, the latter's findings do suggest that, in the longer term, the relationships offered to the infant and their social and economic context may be more important than the actual identity of the relating adult.

The infants in Kagan's study were not totally deprived of their natural mothers. They spent the first few weeks of their lives with their parents, at home, just as the home-reared babies did. When they were admitted to the nursery it was to the individual, consistent care of skilled and highly motivated mother-substitutes in a specially designed and infant-centered environment which kept in continual personal contact with the

parents, day by day. The babies were not in the constant and *exclusive* care
of their mothers but their experience of relationships with adults could
be seen as actually enriching rather than as likely to deprive. They had
mother and home *plus* another individual caretaker who, like a once-
upon-a-time Granny or nanny or a first-class child-minder of today, was
always available to them when mother was not. They also had, in the rest
of the group, aunt/cousin figures, adults and children, forming a consistent, warm group into which they could gradually emerge as a baby of this
age gradually emerges into a natural large family. Accustomed as we are
in Britain to day-care facilities so scarce that they must limit admission
to the most troubled families and so limited in budget that they cannot
offer truly personalized and consistent care in a rich and stable environment, we tend to assume that a young baby in such care is experiencing
that vital one-to-one relationship only during his hours at home. Kagan's
study shows that this need not be so.

So where do we now stand in the real world of the eighties? In
possession of a little knowledge yet still needing a great deal more. I
believe that it is amply confirmed that young infants use known and loved
adults as their completing and maturing other-halves and that this relationship has little to do with physical care and everything to do with social
interaction. Where a natural mother is her child's principal caretaker she
will find herself in this role from the beginning but if someone else takes
the full care of the child she will find herself in the role. We do not know
whether, if two people made themselves equally available to the infant
from the start, he would "choose," at this early age, nor do we know
whether a substitute mother's relationship with the infant is more difficult
to establish (for either or both of them) or qualitatively different. We do
not even know whether the infant's relationship with the completing
adult will be different if the adult is male. Lone fathers in sole charge of
new babies are still rare enough to have escaped study while full "role-
swapping" within a partnership seldom begins so soon after birth.

I think we also know that the need for one intimately relating adult
does not mean that she must be, or even ought to be, the one and only
adult who is meaningful to the baby. In these very early months, one adult
can certainly fulfill the baby's needs, but if she does so in solitude she may
risk her own happiness (and therefore the baby's) and the baby risks
losing his only completing-half if some disaster should strike her. In most
societies, even today, additional and alternative adult relationships are
unselfconsciously made available to the infant-caretaker pair because
they live within a family, clan, tribe, and community. Even in the urban
West this is more often the case than some sociological studies imply.
Often the mother must share herself among many people. She needs
private time to be herself—rather than one half of a symbiosis with the
baby—time to spend with her partner, other children, her own parents,
friends. The baby takes his place in the family, and, while remaining safely

within his mother's completing orbit, gets much of his stimulation from other people.

A simple listing of the possible combinations and permutations of "family" which the baby may meet would take a whole book in itself. The baby may be a first child, and within that position, he may be male or female. Whichever he is, he may be closely, distantly, or never followed by a sibling either of the same or of the opposite sex. Again he may be a second, third, or fourth child of either sex, in which case he may have one, two, or three siblings older than himself, each of which may be a girl or a boy, and each of which may be anywhere from 10 months to 20 years older than he is; other siblings may, or may not, be born after him. When one adds to this all the possibilities of grandparents living in the house, of cousins next door, of aunts in residence, not to mention step- or half-siblings, it becomes clear that it is impossible to define the possible people in a baby's immediate environment.

Yet from this age period onward all such relationships are important to the baby: all can be expected to affect his development to some degree. The baby is busy learning to discriminate people. Therefore he is learning to relate to people. The experience of the baby who has many people of all ages and both sexes to relate to will obviously be different from the experience of the baby who spends most of his time alone with his mother, sees his father on weekends, and smiles at the milkman.

12

STIMULATION
AND ATTENTION

As we saw in the last chapter, between 3 and 6 months people become the most vital factor in an infant's environment and therefore in his development as a person. He learns to know one person from another; he chooses the person or people to whom he becomes most closely attached, and he learns about the world through them. He needs them to mediate the world for him, to show him things, to help him to do what he cannot yet do alone and to comfort and reassure him when things are strange or difficult.

We still know very little about the differences which various kinds of family structure and family experience make to an infant's development. But we know a little about some extreme situations, about infants who are isolated with their mothers in high apartment blocks, for example, or the relative progress of infants in large families as compared with only children. It appears that the critical factor which differentiates one family environment from another, for a young baby, is the amount of social stimulation which he receives. Later chapters will touch on the evidence that such stimulation tends to speed up, or at least to optimize, development in many areas, especially in speech and in manual abilities. But our knowledge is still scattered and scanty. Social stimulation is not a clearly definable *thing*. It has partly to do with how much time adults spend in direct interaction with the baby—and this can be measured. But it has also to do with how much they *enjoy* being with the baby—the whole atmosphere of their interactions—and that is not measurable. Researchers repeatedly try to define these "atmospheric variables," trying to find ways of measuring "warmth" or "love" or "pleasure in the child." But often the definitions arrived at by one group of researchers are slightly different from the definitions of another group, and we rarely have the knowledge to judge whether those slight differences are likely to be important.

It is impossible to lay down the amount of social stimulation which an infant needs. In some areas it can be shown that particular kinds of stimulation improve his performance in specific ways. We have already seen that being talked to a great deal improves his vocal performance (see p. 111). But even this does not mean that the more the infant is talked to the better off he will be. If he were talked to *all* the time, he might, in theory, lack the peaceful times he needs for practicing his new motor skills or learning about his hands with his eyes.

In Western societies, understimulation is more usual than over-stimulation. Most mothers, because of other calls on their time and attention, have to ration the time they spend interacting directly with their infants. Babies tend to be left to "amuse themselves" whenever they will tolerate this, whether they are in the same room as other members of the family or actually alone in their own rooms or on the porch. It is a rare mother, in most communities, who would actually like to play with her baby more than that baby appears to want to play with her.

As a result most research work in this area has concentrated on demonstrating the beneficial effects of extra stimulation to infants. One group of studies—such as those by Burton, Castle, White, and Held [44, 223] and Yarrow [227]—has been conducted in institutions. In studies such as these, the level of overall stimulation offered to the infants has tended to be extremely low: the infants' lives have been so bland, uninteresting, and lonely that the extra individual attention provided by the experimenters still did not bring their experiences up to any kind of "norm" for children in families. In circumstances like these it is hardly surprising that the experimental groups showed a great increase in happiness, in interest in the world, and in performance.

Another group of studies has tended to use infants in ordinary families, and to manipulate the amount of stimulation they received in very specific areas, so as to demonstrate accelerated progress in those areas. For example, studies have been carried out to show that concentrated walking practice may lead to earlier independent walking, or that concentrated and regular periods of story telling may lead to earlier speech. In studies of this kind the interpretation of the results tends to be confused by an almost unanswerable question: is the extra *specific* stimulation responsible for the infant's improved performance, or is it the extra general stimulation of attention from the mother? From the infant's point of view, his mother's attempts to give him daily practice in using his limbs means that at least once a day she plays an intensive physical game with him. The stimulation of the game, of her attention, her physical handling, may be as important, or more important, to his development than what she is trying to teach him.

In the present state of knowledge, it is probably most valuable to look at stimulation for infants in a more general way. To avoid talking of stimulation as if it were a clearly definable thing, which can be measured, divided into "kinds," and whose effects can be separated out in the baby, but rather to consider what stimulation is, in terms of how it can be *used by* the individual baby.

Many of the things which are done for babies, with the intention of stimulating, amusing, or interesting them, are often done with so little understanding of the baby himself that they fail completely. Just as food on a plate does not nourish a child until it has been eaten, so stimulation offered to a child does not stimulate him until he has noticed and *used* it. Often parents will buy and lovingly hang a complicated colorful mobile in their infant's room—and then continue to lay him on his tummy. A stimulating sight cannot stimulate unless it is seen. Often, too, an adult will begin a stimulating interaction with a baby, smiling and speaking to him and then not have the patience to wait for his slow response. By the time the baby has begun to smile back, the adult has turned away to do something else. An interaction that is merely one-sided is not interactive nor truly stimulating.

The child has to be ready to receive the stimulus if it is to mean anything to him. At the simplest level it is no use trying to play with a baby who is trying to be asleep, nor trying to love and cuddle one who is furious with hunger. At a slightly more subtle level, new and exciting experiences will mean most to the baby when their degree of novelty is just exactly right for his particular developmental stage. Between 3 and 6 months, apart from known faces which, as we have seen, retain their fascination for the baby, the objects and events which will interest him most will be those which are just slightly different from what he has met before. Totally new events or objects, which he cannot relate at all to his existing schemata, are likely to be ignored. He will *not* enjoy a panto-mime. On the other hand things he has seen many times before are boringly familiar. In between these extremes, a ball just like his old one except that it has a different colored pattern, a piece of paper which is like yesterday's but more crumply, a music box which works like the old one but plays a different tune will all fascinate him. And then of course there are all the infinite variations in people: his father, whose hands are bigger than his mother's, whose voice is deeper, whose chin is bristly, but who stills bathes the baby in his usual bath; the aunt who pushes him in the same carriage, but not in the same way; the new food that comes in the same bowl, from the same hand, but has a different taste. J. Kagan [119] put it neatly when he said that the baby is likely to be most genu-inely stimulated by those things or events which "require tiny, quiet, cognitive discoveries—a miniaturized version of Archimedes' Eureka."

Even when careful thought is given to the kind of stimulus which is being offered to the baby, and to the use which he can make of it at one particular stage in his development or moment in his day, each baby has many individual characteristics which will affect the way *any* offered stimulus strikes him.

There is abundant evidence that some infants are born with a greater degree of perceptual and tactile sensitivity than others, and that some are more physically active than others. No authority would, I think, quarrel with this, but quarrel they do about the origins and the significance of such differences. Some of these characteristics have been described as newborn phenomena and some may, indeed, be related to the processes of birth itself. There are numbers of studies which show, for example, increased irritability in babies following difficult deliveries, or a variety of effects, including sleepiness and slowness in feeding, following heavy sedation of the mother. But if mother and baby are viewed as a pair who emerge together from the business of birth, it is exceedingly difficult to assign simple cause-and-effect directions to their behaviors. These difficulties are well described by Dunn and Richards in a paper called "Observations in the Neonatal Period" [67]. They could find no evidence that differences between babies and/or between styles of mothering which seemed related to those babies' characteristics, lasted after the newborn period. But other workers report different viewpoints. Thomas and Chess [214], for example, believe that temperamental differences in early infancy are good indicators for later personality differences, while Escalona [77] believes that differences in overall sensitivity to stimulation are vitally important in that they effect the individual infant's experiences of every aspect of his environment. She believes that there are discernible differences between infants in their sensitivity to all kinds of stimulation. She points out that infants of differing sensitivity receive quite different experiences from identical handling. For example, a highly sensitive infant may receive the same amount of stimulation from a relatively quiet unstimulating mother as the insensitive infant receives from a relatively boisterous highly stimulating one. The handling the two infants receive is quite different, but the effect may be the same. Equally, if those two infants were swapped the sensitive infant might be overwhelmed by the highly stimulating mother, while the less sensitive infant was bored and understimulated by the quiet one. In recent years there has been a resurgence of interest in the idea that too high a level of stimulation tends to lead the infant to withdraw, where a milder stimulation makes him want to explore [147].

Sometimes parents have to learn this lesson the hard way, if they have two children who vary along this dimension. The rough-and-tumble games which delighted the first baby on father's nightly return from work may drive the second into a frenzy of fear. Or the gentle lullabies which mother sang to the first baby may quite fail to catch the attention of the second.

Just as the novelty of a stimulus has to be adjusted to suit the baby —the familiar being boring and the totally new incomprehensible—so the intensity has to be adjusted too. The infant likes objects which are just slightly novel. He likes other stimulation to be strong enough to be noticeable, but not too strong.

Differences in levels of physical activity from birth have been demonstrated by many researchers, and they have also been shown to remain consistent over long periods of time [48, 124]. The newborn who is always on the move and sleeps little tends to be the wakeful 6-week baby who acquires a powerful kick very early on. Later in his first year he may crawl and walk early; even if he does not, he is likely to need endless exercise and to be furious if he is physically restricted. On the other hand, the sleepy newborn, who moves very little, may be content to be rolled in a bundle for much longer; he may never take the extreme delight in motor play that the active baby does, and he may be content to be a "sitter" until much later in the first year.

These differences appear to be innate, and independent either of the mother's behavior, or of any other factors in the child's environment [192]. And they are important. A baby's own physical activity provides him with entertainment, but it also provides him with other kinds of stimulation. As he kicks, he brings his feet into view and out again; he alters the feeling of the blankets over him; he makes a draft which tickles his nose. When he learns to roll over, earlier than most babies, he can provide himself with a new view of the world as well as with a change of physical position. A very active baby may therefore provide himself with so much stimulation that he needs less from the adults around him than does the inactive baby who depends on them for every new experience. Schaffer [193] put this point of view to experimental test. He measured the "developmental quotient" (see p. 362) of active and inactive babies before they underwent similar brief periods in an institution. At the end of the period, the developmental quotients of the inactive babies had dropped far more than the quotients of the active babies. It seemed that, even when they were deprived of much of their accustomed stimulation from handling and play, the active babies were able to make the very most of any stimulation which *was* offered to them, and to keep themselves alert by the feedback, and the changes of position and view which came from their own physical activities. The inactive babies, on the other hand, suffered far more from not being given much stimulation, because they were not able to compensate by providing it for themselves.

The infant's sex may also affect the amount and the kind of stimulation he receives within his family. Of course parents are aware, from the moment of birth, whether they have produced a boy or a girl. In some families the awareness may be overwhelming: a boy may end a one-sex run of three girls, thus delighting his parents; or he may make yet another boy to add to the other three boys, and make his parents painfully aware that they did not actually *want* a fourth child if it was not to be a girl. But where the parents were comparatively neutral about the baby's sex before his birth, the actual sex tends to impinge increasingly after 3 months, as the infant ceases to be "our new baby" and becomes "Johnny" or "Jane."

Everybody who has handled children knows that boys and girls are different. But whether they are genetically different, or whether we make them different in their behavior by expecting differences and therefore handling them differently, remains a matter of hot dispute. The dispute has been heated further by the current determination of many parents not to *impose* differences on their children, but to give both boys and girls equal opportunities to experience 100 percent of what their world can offer them, rather than 50 percent each. There is some evidence of inherent sex differences in sensitivity to some forms of stimulation, from a fascinating longitudinal study by R. Q. Bell [20]. There is also evidence of differences in behavior between the sexes in the early months from an observational study by H. A. Moss [161]. The boys in Moss's sample were more likely to be irritable than the girls, they tended to cry more, and their mothers found the causes of their crying more obscure. The boys also responded less readily, and less rewardingly, to their mothers' attempts to comfort and cheer them.

If the boys and girls in this study behaved differently from each other, they also received very different handling from their mothers. The mothers of girls tended to pick them up whenever they cried, and to be willing to pick them up and cuddle them more than usual if they had an extra fussy day. The mothers of boys on the other hand rapidly stopped adjusting their handling to fit in with their sons' crying. They picked the boys up as much as they thought proper and no more. When the boys cried at other times the mothers labeled them "fussy," and left them to get on with it.

Few studies produce such clear-cut differences in behavior between the sexes in the early months, nor such clear-cut differences in maternal handling, but other studies do suggest such differences. For example, a body of further work by Moss [162–164] suggests that at 3 months boys get more cuddling and rough-and-tumble physical play from their mothers than do girls of the same age. The girls tend to get more direct talking, smiling, and looking contact from their mothers instead. We do not know how general these differences in handling the two sexes are. But they are certainly not general or intense enough to override wider cultural differences in infant handling. In a comparison of Japanese and American families, for example, W. Caudill and H. Weinstein [47] showed that Japanese mothers concentrated more on quieting and soothing 3-month babies of both sexes than on stimulating them. The babies appeared extremely quiet and passive beside their American counterparts. The differences between the nationalities far outweighed differences between the sexes within the national groups.

It does seem likely, however, that there are neurological differences between the sexes. This is a difficult field and one which has developed rapidly since the first edition of this book. Then, two papers published in 1967 and 1970 [125, 131] had suggested that the left hemisphere of the brain (the part which normally contains the "speech processing area") developed more slowly in boys than in girls. The authors speculated that, if their findings were confirmed, they would suggest that the right hemisphere of the brain (where visuo-spatial information is normally processed) would be preponderant in baby boys as compared with girls.

In 1975 anatomical support for this speculation was produced at the Third Child Language Symposium in London. It had been found that when the temporal cortexes of girls were compared with those of boys an actual lengthening and thickening of one tiny area on the left could be observed.

Does this suggest that the differences in the way parents are reported to handle boys and girls in early infancy are appropriate neurophysiologically even if they are not socioculturally approved? Will a baby girl actually make better use of listening and talking play while a boy of the same age and stage makes better use of more physical play? It might be tempting to say: "Their brains develop differently and therefore it is only sensible to handle them differently." But there is other work, with animals, which suggests that handling in infancy may actually be able to create neurophysiological changes in brain structure. For the past ten years a group of psychologists and biologists have been working together in California on the effects of various kinds and degrees of stimulation on the brains of rats [186, 187]. Over the years they have discovered a very wide range of neurological, physiological, and structural effects arising from enriching the experiences of their experimental rats. They are rightly cautious about extrapolating their findings to human beings. But it is by no means impossible that we shall eventually find that stimulation affects not only performance but the very size and structure of the parts of the brain that control performance. So we may come full circle. Boys and girls behave differently. We handle them differently. By doing so we may be prolonging or intensifying a difference which, with identical handling for both sexes, might have been minimized or eradicated. This is a fascinating area for research and speculation but not yet for parental action.

Clearly a large number of each baby's characteristics, as well as his particular moment in development, affect the amount and the kind of stimulation he receives and can use. But this baby-oriented view of stimulation cannot be accepted alone, any more than the old views which saw the infant as a blank slate on which the parents wrote.

A sensitive response by the parents to cues from the baby is vital if they are to provide the "right" kinds and levels of stimulation for him. Maternal sensitivity is often described, in research literature, as if it were a supreme virtue. But it is made up of innumerable factors, only a few of which are under the mother's control. Much "maternal sensitivity" is the result of fortunate chance. The mother finds herself with an infant whose personal characteristics meld with her own, to provide a smoothly functioning unit. The baby is somewhat jumpy; she is characteristically calm and gentle; they do well together. The baby is very active—so is she. She asks nothing better than to have a reason for lots of walks, lots of physical play. The baby is very active in seeking social contact; she is a highly vocal, sociable person, who is delighted to find that a young baby can be "good company." In all these circumstances, and hundreds more, the mother's ability to take her cues from the baby, and provide him with the kind of stimulation he needs, comes at least as much from his demanding what comes naturally to her as from her skill.

Less fortunate mothers can be faced with an infant who demands from them a kind of handling and of stimulation which they actually find it difficult to provide. For example, some babies are more "cuddly" than others [197]. Some definitely resist being held, cuddled, tucked up, or restrained for dressing. Such a baby may be soothed by being talked to, may delight in looking at his mother and in smiling at her, but may very definitely reject her if she tries to pick him up and hold him. Yet many mothers have a permanent baby-shaped space at their left hip and shoulder; many instinctively pick up a baby if he cries, cuddle and rock him to convey their love, and carry him about when he is miserable. Handling a non-cuddly baby in the way he needs to be handled may require such a mother to make a real intellectual effort and to tolerate what she feels as emotional rejection.

Practical circumstances, too, may vitally affect that "maternal sensitivity." A mother with her first baby is often alone with him for much of the time, able to expend as much attention on him as she wishes, free to interact with him just as she pleases. Such a mother may watch the baby, be alert for his cues, and respond to them freely. That same mother with a new baby and a furiously jealous 2-year-old is quite differently placed. She has to steer constantly between the two children, making an unending series of choices, compromises, and diversions. If she is happy, and well-supported by her husband, and the new baby is a "good fit" with her, she may manage. But if her other circumstances are depressing, her husband makes it clear that he is getting fed up with his child-oriented household and the baby is difficult for her, she is likely to go quietly frantic. In these circumstances even the most "sensitive mother" is likely to take a "let quiet babies lie" attitude and ignore the newcomer unless he insists on her attention.

Fortunately those who are concerned with individual babies never know what their infant *might* have been like had he been differently handled. There is no temptation to expend hours and agony on adjusting his daily life in infancy, because there is no prescription for infant handling that will produce a given kind of child or adult. We do not have to know that we did not stimulate our infants in exactly the right way, at exactly the right time. On the whole, stimulation or handling which gives the baby pleasure is right for him. And contrariwise very few kinds of handling or stimulation which distress him are right. If he is happy and contented, his handling is good enough. If he is happier still with more of it, then he can use more if his parents feel able to give it to him. In the end the only guide to the right amount and kind of stimulation is the baby himself.

13

FEEDING AND GROWING

FOOD FOR INFANTS is not a rational subject in the Western world. Everybody is taught that correct feeding is vital to optimal development, so every mother worries—often endlessly and frantically—about what her infant does or does not eat. Yet because the vast majority of infants in our culture are more than adequately fed, the subject of their eating is seldom discussed, outside textbooks of biochemistry or dietetics, in the kind of detail which would show mothers that their worries are unnecessary and destructive. The few infants who are not adequately fed would benefit from detailed discussion too. If their mothers cannot afford to feed them lavishly, or they will not eat the wide choice of foods available to them, their restricted diet is often inadequate simply because the mother does not have the information which she needs, or worse, has misinformation.

Unfortunately feeding is tied up in our society with socialization. Eating is linked with meals; getting adequate nourishment is linked with acceptable behavior, with table manners, with emptying the plate, not being greedy, not wasting good food, and so on. Nutritional and social-moral statements are mixed together. For example, many mothers would agree that an infant should eat green vegetables. But often the mother herself does not know whether she means that it is *nutritionally* important that he should eat them, or socially and morally right that he should eat them. Is making a child eat cabbage a way of giving him sufficient vitamin C or a way of disciplining him? It is vital that issues of this kind should be sorted out. In terms of the child's development they are totally different matters. Both issues are important, but neither can be sensibly handled while they are muddled together.

The kind of general dietary advice which is given in most books on child rearing tends to reinforce this kind of muddle. After detailed advice about breast-feeding, about choosing a formula for bottle-feeding and about introducing the first solids, they tend to leap to the stock phrase "a good mixed diet." This diet, at which everybody is supposed to aim, is an ideal. If any human being is given three good meals a day, with a variety of meats, fish, eggs, cheese, vegetables, fruits, and so forth, he will, without doubt, get everything he needs to eat. The trouble is that few infants will really eat that diet and few mothers have the money or the time to prepare it. It is an ideal far removed from the realities of mother and infant at home.

This chapter, and Chapter Twenty which covers feeding in the second half of this first year, attempt to show what infants actually do eat, and to consider what they need to eat and why. It is about food, not about socialization—about food for health, not food for virtue.

Finding out what infants actually eat is more difficult than it sounds. We know (see Chapter Two) that only a very small proportion of infants are being breast-fed by the time they are 3 months, and we know that those who are will probably be receiving other foods as well as breast milk. But there our certain knowledge almost stops. The only way to find out what infants are being fed is to ask their mothers, and their replies are likely to be inaccurate. Food is an emotionally laden subject and mothers will therefore tend to answer researchers in what they think of as a socially acceptable way. In an industrial city in England John and Elizabeth Newson [170] found that mothers interviewed by a health visitor reported far more breast-feeding, giving of vitamin drops, and attendances at welfare clinics than did mothers interviewed by a university worker, who was not a representative of the health authorities.

Even where mothers truly strive to be accurate they may not be able to be. Some personal experiments carried out in an ordinary kitchen may illustrate this difficulty. A jar of a famous brand of strained babyfood, available all over the U.K. and the U.S.A., contains 3 1/2 oz. (100 g) of food. This statement, printed on the jar, is accurate if that jar is scraped out so thoroughly that it is left almost clean. But the scraping process takes at least 25 seconds. Emptied more carelessly, as a busy mother might empty the jar when getting an infant's lunch, it yields nearly 1/2 oz. (15 g) less. Such a difference probably does not matter to the well-fed baby; but it makes a great deal of difference to the poor researcher who is trying to find out exactly what the baby ate.

Feeding the same food to a 3-month baby, wearing the type of bib which catches the drips in a pocket at the bottom, I have given meals which yielded 1/4 oz. or 1 1/2 oz. (7 g or 45 g) of what would technically be called "plate waste." Mothers are unlikely to know how much food dribbled down the infant's chin.

Similar problems apply to baby cereals and instant powdered meals. Different brands require different quantities of added fluid to arrive at the same texture. If the added fluid is water, the addition does not affect the food value and need not bother the researcher. But usually it is milk. Does the mother know how many ounces of milk went into that cereal? Usually she will simply have gone on stirring in more milk until the food reached the baby's preferred texture.

Even bottles of formula do not escape these problems. Mothers will know how many bottles the baby has had. Usually they will know how much was in each bottle and whether the baby finished it. But the food value of those bottles is a vexing question—and one we shall return to when we discuss what babies ought to eat. The dangers of mixing formulas too strong have long been recognized (and have been mitigated with the modern formulae). But some mothers do seem to work on a sort of "one for the pot" principle as they add the scoops of milk powder. Leaving aside those mothers who make the bottles extra-concentrated on purpose, there is still wide variation in the concentration arrived at by mothers who are trying to follow the instructions on the container. Using a popular brand similar to America's Similac, I found that eight of the manufacturer's scoops, gently filled, and accurately leveled off with a palette knife, weighed just over 1 oz. (30 g)—exactly what the manufacturer intended. But putting a little pressure on the palette knife during leveling, so that the scoops were very slightly packed, led to a yield of 1 1/4 oz. (37 g). Worse still, hurrying, and using the edge of the jar as a leveler instead of a palette knife, I ended up with slightly rounded scoops, eight of which yielded 1 1/2 oz. (45 g). A bottle made up with my last method would have given the infant 50 percent more nourishment than his mother would report to the researcher.

So we know that only a few infants of this age are receiving breast milk. We know that most are receiving bottles of formula made more or less to the manufacturer's specification. We also know that with rare exceptions they will be receiving solid foods in addition, but we do not really know exactly how much of what.

A study published in the *Journal of the American Dietary Association* [108] showed that all social groups introduced cereals as the first "solid food," with babies in the lowest socioeconomic groups usually starting these in the fourth week while the highest socioeconomic groups waited until the sixth week. Vegetables were introduced next, between 8 and 12 weeks, while meats and fruits came later at 12–16 weeks. Almost all these solid foods were commercially prepared. Only 17 percent of the babies were ever given home-prepared food at 6 months, and only 4 percent were given no commercially prepared foods at all at this age.

As we have seen (see p. 22) infant feeding practices vary widely with geographical area as well as with the parents' years of education, but it may nevertheless be interesting to compare these figures with those of the British National Survey [153]. Solid foods were given to 1 percent of infants in the first week of life, to 3 percent by the second week, to 18 percent by the fourth week. Those percentages rose to 40 percent by the time the babies were 6 weeks old, 85 percent at 3 months and 97 percent by 4 months.

A further British study [20] attempted to find out not only what was fed and at what age, but how much of each food was given to the babies. The mothers of 300 normal infants under 1 year making routine visits to an Infant Welfare Clinic were asked, without warning, to recall the exact food intake of their infants during the previous 24 hours. Four hundred and ninety-eight different types of food had been given to the babies, almost all of them being commercially prepared. The only fresh food used at all regularly was eggs. The variation in nutritional value of the reported diets was enormous. Some 3-month infants had taken a day's diet suitable for a year-old baby while some 9-month infants had received little more than milk and jars of fruit. Few of the mothers seemed to have much idea of the varying nutritional values of the jars they were offering, and many seemed quite oblivious of the fact that they were feeding large quantities of cereal to babies who were extremely fat.

This picture, scanty though it is, is very different from a picture of what an infant between 3 and 6 months actually needs to eat. Any discussion of "requirements" or "recommended" intakes must, of course, be extremely generalized. The authorities who compile nutritional tables are careful to warn readers that they are averages worked out for large groups of people of a given age, not for individuals. Infants vary, as do all people, in their food needs, their hunger, their general enthusiasm for the business of eating, and in the speed and completeness with which they use up, or metabolize, food. *No individual baby's needs can be worked out from nutritional tables.* Such tables are intended to provide guidance for people catering for *groups,* whether in nurseries, cafeterias, or residential institutions. They are the best average guide we have but to apply that guidance to an individual's eating is to misuse them. What, then, is the point of giving the data at all in a book such as this one? I have been pointedly asked this question by many authorities who would prefer that they be deleted. They do not believe that readers can be trusted to understand the difference between a best-guess at the average requirements for all the members of a group and the actual needs of their individual child. But I do have this trust and I also believe that many parents have a very different view of "good nutrition" from that of nutritionists and that this is partly due to some common misconceptions which can only be corrected by telling parents some of the nutritionists' facts.

People are made up primarily of water, and they lose water continually through the skin, the breath, and the urine. Infants therefore need water, and will die far more quickly for lack of it than for lack of food in general or any one food in particular. A curious reluctance to give infants plain water to drink can be responsible for many feeding difficulties.

People also have to have the foods which are incorporated into the body, the proteins. Proteins are made up of twenty amino acids which are strung together in varying orders and numbers in different foods. All twenty amino acids are needed by human bodies, but all but eight in adults and ten in growing children can be made by the body out of the others.

Protein foods are usually described as either "first class" or "second class." First-class protein is so named simply because it already contains the vital amino acids in complete form, as well as all the others. Eating meat, fish, eggs, and dairy products therefore ensures that the body receives the amino acids it needs. But second-class proteins can do an equally good job by human bodies if they are eaten in a mixture. They are proteins which are eaten in plant form, rather than in the form of plants which have already been converted by an animal. They usually contain large proportions of the commoner amino acids, and have some of the rarer ones missing. A mixture of these proteins will almost always compensate for the deficiencies of any one of them, thus giving the body all the amino acids it needs.

First-class proteins tend to be expensive; indeed the eating of meat is, in many societies, regarded as an index of rising prosperity. The Western world reads of the developing nations suffering from lack of protein and, perhaps as a result, increasingly glorifies protein foods. It is often the protein foods which mothers press upon their children and the possibility of too little protein which worries them when they face a fussy eater. Anything which has liver, or egg, beef or cheese in it is "bound to be good for him." And of course the babyfood manufacturers play up to this myth: "High-protein cereal with egg," "Full of the protein your baby needs," "Full of beef for extra bounce," they say.

A certain quantity of complete (or completed) protein is an absolute requirement for growth and for continuing good health. Because of the horrors of protein-deficiency diseases, and the work which is being done on their prevention and cure in other parts of the world, we do know *approximately* the minimum quantities which are required by people of differing ages and weights. To people accustomed to eating the privileged meals of the Western world, these quantities are remarkably small. There is no benefit in a much *higher* intake. The *"recommended* intakes" given by the U.S. Department of Health and Human Services, and referred to in more detail later, already make a substantial extra allowance to cover the possibility of some infants needing more than others. And they are already set at higher levels than the *minimum* requirement figures used by organizations such as the Food and Agriculture Organization. So while controversy rages as to how much is *just* enough it can be assumed that these recommendations are generous ones.

Once proteins have entered the digestive process they are used by the body immediately, if the body requires protein for tissue repair or for growth. But if it already has enough protein, it cannot store the extra nor can it "hold" surplus incomplete proteins against their completion at a later meal. The surplus amino acids are taken to the liver, where they are converted into glucose, and released to the bloodstream for energy. Feeding an infant too much protein may be actually harmful. If protein is thus converted into glucose, there is a heavy load of nitrogen left, which may stress the kidneys which have to excrete it. Overfeeding of proteins is also inefficient. The conversion of the surplus to glucose actually uses more energy than it releases to the body. Since protein foods are vastly more expensive than the carbohydrates which the body can easily turn into glucose, using roast beef for energy instead of bread is roughly equivalent to fueling a car with cognac instead of gasoline.

Energy, for keeping the infant alive, and for his physical activities, comes from carbohydrates and from fats, both of which are converted by the body into sugars. If the protein foods have come to be overvalued in our society, the carbohydrate foods are undervalued. Efficient feeding requires some carbohydrates. An infant's need for energy takes biological precedence over his growth. Energy is the first demand which will be fulfilled out of the nutrients available to the body. Therefore if the infant is fed too little carbohydrate, those precious proteins will be inefficiently burned to give him energy, instead of being used for his growth. Carbohydrates therefore act as "protein conservers," ensuring that the infant has all the fuel he needs, so that his body can retain all the protein it needs for optimum growth. Unfortunately for a fat society, *surplus* carbohydrates are not burned and excreted as surplus proteins are. They are stored in the form of body fat.

Fats are made up of fatty acids, just as proteins are made up of amino acids. Like the carbohydrates they are used by the body for energy, and they are useful in that, weight for weight, they provide far more concentrated calories than do carbohydrates. Some special groups, such as Eskimos, who require high-calorie intakes because of intense cold, or athletes, who expend large amounts of energy, would be hard put to eat enough calories if a proportion were not in the concentrated form of fats. But in less extreme circumstances there seems to be no absolute dietary requirement for fat, other than a need for minute quantities of certain specific fatty acids. Since these fatty acids are widely distributed in both animal fats and vegetable oils, deficiencies are extremely rare. Many authorities believe that a high intake of animal fats (which of course includes dairy products and egg yolk) predisposes people to later heart disease. They urge the use of polyunsaturated fats and oils instead. While heart disease is still thought of as a problem of the later years of life, its foundations and therefore its prevention may lie in infancy. A considerable amount of research work is in progress [23] concerning infants who are breast-fed by mothers whose diets were high or low in animal fats and infants bottle-fed on formula containing varying amounts of butterfat.

In addition to these main food groups, which give the body its growth, repair, and energy needs, minute quantities of vitamins and of mineral substances are also required. Many of these are so widely distributed that it would be impossible to eat at all without getting enough of them. Many more are being discovered but are not yet fully understood. The more important ones, and those which an infant could lack, are set out in Table 1.

TABLE 1. SOME ESSENTIAL VITAMINS AND MINERALS

	Technical details	*Required for*	*Comment*
Vitamin A	Technical name is retinol. Measured in retinol equivalents because body can use a substance called carotene to make retinol, but absorbs the result less well than pure retinol. Our vitamin A is roughly 2/3 retinol and 1/3 carotene, and the measure is therefore μg (micrograms) of "retinol equivalents."	Growth. Perception of light. Protection of surface tissue and mucous membranes.	Not soluble in water. Can be stored in the liver. Excess can be harmful.
Vitamin B group	A group usually, but not always, found together in some foods. Most important are thiamine (B_1), riboflavin (B_2), nicotinic acid or niacin. Also known are folic acid (B_{12}), pyridoxine (B_6), pantothenic acid, biotin. Measured in mg (milligrams).	Control and facilitate the process by which the body gets a smooth continuous release of energy from carbohydrates. Part of enzyme system. Protects nerve cells. Prevents certain anemias.	Soluble in water. Unstable at high temperatures. Body cannot store. In the absence of information about infant requirements, recommendations are based on the amounts secreted in breast milk.
Vitamin C	Technical name is ascorbic acid. Measured in mg (milligrams).	Concerned with the structure of connective tissue. Wound healing.	Soluble in water. Unstable at high temperatures and in sunlight. Body cannot store.
Vitamin D	Dietary requirement variable, as can be manufactured by the body following exposure of skin to sunlight. Measured in μg (micrograms) or iu (international units; 1 μg = 40 iu).	Absorption and laying down of calcium and phosphorus in bones and teeth.	Not soluble in water. Body can store. In extreme cases storage leads to hypercalcemia.

	Technical details	*Required for*	*Comment*
Calcium	The calcium in certain foods is more easily absorbed than that found in other foods. Furthermore it can only be absorbed in the presence of adequate vitamin D. Much more is present in hard water than in soft. Exact dietary requirements are therefore difficult to assess. Measured in mg (milligrams).	Development of bones and teeth. Blood clotting. Muscle function.	Stored in the bones and released into the blood by the parathyroid gland.
Phosphorus	Found with calcium. Needs for phosphorus can therefore be ignored in normal diets.		
Iron	Individual ability to absorb iron is very variable, and different forms of iron are differently available to the body. Varying quantities are derived from water, from the use of iron cooking pots, and from such culturally variable adjuncts to food preparation as curry powder and red wine. Measured in mg (milligrams).	Vital component of the hemoglobin which transports oxygen all over the body in the blood.	Once absorbed, iron is used and re-used, as well as being stored in the liver. A little is lost in general wear of the body, some in the digestive juices in the feces, a great deal in bleeding.

Before this kind of information can be related to real live babies eating real kitchen-type food, a hard look at the question of growth is needed. Traditionally an infant is said to be "growing well" if his weight gain is adequate. But a baby who gained weight without gaining height to match would be getting fat rather than growing big. It is essential that the infant should gain both weight and length; it is highly desirable that he should gain them in strict relationship to each other. An "average" girl might be born weighing just over 7 lb. and measuring just over 21 inches. If at 6 months that girl weighs 15 lb. and measures 25 inches, her growth is proper. But if she weighs 19 lb. and measures 25 inches she is definitely fat. Such a weight at 6 months would only be appropriate if she were a very large baby, measuring 26 or 27 inches in length.

Infant growth is remarkably steady. It is rare to find a child who puts on either weight or height by fits and starts, except where acute or long-drawn-out illness, or extreme emotional upset, has temporarily retarded his growth. After such a period of deprivation infants commonly have a period of "catch-up growth," during which they put on weight and height at a much faster *rate* than before the illness until they are back on their old trajectory. Then, almost magically, the accelerated growth slows down again, and the child settles into his old pattern.

His own pattern is the vital point. If he starts below or above the average for height or weight, he is likely to remain at a similar position relative to that average throughout infancy; like a rocket, he has a preselected growth trajectory, fueled by his environment. Given normally adequate feeding and other care, he will grow his predetermined amount, and at his predetermined rate. While we commonly talk of the first year as being the most rapid period of growth, he will, in fact, never grow as fast or as much as he did in the womb. In 9 months he grew from microscopic to around 7 lb. and 20 inches (3.2 kg and 51 cm); if he continued to grow that much, or that fast, he would be a giant indeed.

But fortunately he does not carry on at this rate. In the first 3 months he is likely to gain somewhere around 6–8 oz. each week. By the second 3 months this has slowed up to gains of around 4–5 oz., while in the second half of his first year his weekly gain will be only about 2–3 oz. weekly.

These gains will be similar for any infant who is healthy and appropriately fed. So the actual *weight* of any individual baby at any particular age point will depend on his own starting point: his birthweight. This means that any attempt to relate individual babies to "norms" can be misleading. Norms are based on averages. If your baby was of average birthweight, then he will be near the norm for his age. If he was not near the average, the norm will not apply to him. Rules of thumb about "normal babies" can be positively dangerous. In child-welfare clinics all over the U.K. one such rubric is quoted over and over again: "A baby should double his birthweight by 6 months and treble it by 1 year." A premature baby who followed this rubric would be half starved; an average birthweight baby will probably follow it more or less; a heavy baby who followed it would be obese. See Table 2.

All babies tend to gain roughly the same *amount* of weight whatever their birthweight. That gained weight is a very different *proportion* of the bodyweight in heavy and light infants.

C. M. Drillien [66], who followed up a large group of Scottish babies from birth into school, illustrated this dramatically. She showed that

TABLE 2. RELATIONSHIP OF BIRTHWEIGHT TO ABSOLUTE AND PROPORTIONAL
WEIGHT GAINS

Expected gain in first 13 weeks = 7 oz. (200 g) per week after the first
fortnight
= 77 oz. or 4 lb. 13 oz. (2.2 kg)
Expected gain in second 13 weeks = 5 oz. (150 g) per week
= 65 oz. or 4 lb. 1 oz. (1.95 kg)

Birthweight	Weight at 3 months	Weight at 6 months	Comment
5 lb./2.3 kg	9 lb. 13 oz./ 4.5 kg	13 lb. 14 oz./ 5.45 kg	Weight virtually doubled at 3 months; approaching *treble* at 6 months.
8 lb./3.6 kg	12 lb. 13 oz./ 5.8 kg	16 lb. 14 oz./ 7.75 kg	Closely follows the rubric.
11 lb./5.0 kg	15 lb. 13 oz./ 7.2 kg	19 lb. 14 oz./ 9.15 kg	Weight not nearly double at 6 months.

premature babies followed the *rate* of growth of average- and above-average-weight infants so closely that at 5 years the *actual* difference in their weights had remained constant, although its significance had diminished. Thus the baby who was born weighing 5 lb. (2.3 kg) tended at 5 years still to weigh 4 lb. (1.8 kg) less than the child who was born weighing 9 lb. (4.1 kg). The low birthweight babies did, however, grow in length at a rather faster rate than the others, although they never grew quite as tall. They were therefore always rather taller for their weight than the heavier babies, and tended to be thinner.

Infants need to be fed according to their expected weight (see p. 30). This means the weight to be expected of the individual baby, if he was gaining at the expected rate. It does not mean feeding the premature baby, who at 3 months weighs less than 10 lb. (4.54 kg), as if he were the average baby who at the same age weighs 3 lb. (1.3 kg) more.

Turning now to the daily food intakes of babies during this quarter, we have to return to those same average figures which have just been disparaged. No other figures are available to us because figures relating *individual* food intakes to *individual* needs can only be obtained by highly complex medical, biochemical, and anthropometric measurements. It cannot be too strongly emphasized that, without such lengthy procedures, it is impossible for anyone to design the ideal diet for a given person or, in the absence of clinical indications, to diagnose undernutrition.

The figures given here—and at intervals throughout this book—are derived from the *Manual of Nutrition* [158], published by the Ministry of

Agriculture, Fisheries and Food in 1970, and the "Recommended Daily Amounts of Food Energy and Nutrients for Groups of People in the United Kingdom" [53], published by Britain's Department of Health and Social Security in 1979. The ministries concerned are at pains to point out that these figures, based on the best available information, are designed to assist in the planning of food supplies for various groups of people, the assessment of information from nutritional surveys, some of them from the U.S., and the comparison of one group with another. They are not, therefore, recommendations as to what each individual member of a group *should eat,* but recommendations as to what should be *made available* to each individual member. The figures are given here simply to provide an authoritative idea as to the kinds of amounts of foodstuffs babies of various ages and weights might use. Safety margins are, so far as present knowledge allows, built in so that an individual who does eat the average "recommended" amount is most unlikely to be getting less than he needs; he may well be getting more. In general, then, anyone looking at the figures with an individual infant in mind should regard the quantities rather as we regard those in a cook book. If a recipe says "enough for four persons," we assume that it will, indeed, provide four reasonable servings. We do not panic if the four consumers fail to eat one quarter each.

In Table 3, the quantities recommended for each infant are given in terms of calories, protein, and the essential minerals and vitamins already discussed (see Table 1). The calorie count is the sum total of the energy value of all the food taken, irrespective of the source (protein, fats, or carbohydrates) of that energy. Within that total, carbohydrate and fat are not specified. Calories not coming from proteins must come from one of these two sources, and in terms of the body's fuel requirements it does not matter which. Protein is always specified separately, as a requirement *within* the total energy of the food, because, as we have seen, the protein is an essential for its building, rather than its energy-giving qualities.

The scientific measures for nutrients are somewhat confusing. Readers who do not wish to labor with them will find that they can be accepted simply as "measures" and that in all subsequent food tables, one food can be compared with another on the basis of its *relative* richness in the given substance. But for those who are interested, the basic measures can be very approximately defined as follows:

kilocalorie (kcal)   often loosely abbreviated to "calorie" in nutritional discussion; this is the amount of energy required to heat 1 pint of water 3° F (1 litre of water 1° C). Theoretically (making no allowance for cooling) 47 kcal would heat 1 pint of water to boiling point from a room temperature of 70° F.

kilojoule (kJ)   is the modern unit of energy. There are approximately 4.2 kcal in a kJ and kilojoules are grouped in thousands so that 1000 kJ = 1 megajoule or MJ. 1 MJ = 240 kcal. Although joules are now the standard units in nutrition, most tables still give both measures and this book adheres to the more familiar kcal.

gram (g)   = 1/28 oz.

milligram (mg)   = 1/1000 gram

microgram (μg)   = 1/1000 milligram

The major part of the infant's diet at the beginning of this quarter will still be milk. Most infants will be bottle-fed. The few who are breast-fed can be assumed to be as well (if not better) off in all dietary respects, as long as the quantity of milk they are getting is adequate.

Although in America it is common practice among many families to make the switch to whole milk at 3–4 months, most doctors would agree that it is better to continue to use a formula until at least 6 months. Most of the dried milks which are marketed for general consumption are totally unsuitable for babies. They tend to lack fat—which makes them low in calories—and they almost always lack vitamins and minerals. Most canned evaporated milks are also unsuitable, especially those which contain a lot of sugar. Fresh cow's milk is, of course, the basis of infant

TABLE 3. RECOMMENDED DAILY NUTRIENTS FOR INFANTS FROM BIRTH TO 5 MONTHS

Total Calories kcal	Protein g	Minerals		Vitamins					
		Calcium mg	Iron mg	A μg	D μg	Thiamine mg	Riboflavin mg	Niacin mg	C mg
700	18	360	10	420	7.5	0.3	0.4	5	20

Infants will require approximately:
1. 52 kcal per day for every 1 lb. of their weight; and 1 g of protein.
    117 kcal per day for every 1 kg of their weight; and 2.2 g of protein.
2. Both the energy (kcal) requirement and the protein requirement are set lower by these authorities than by those of many other countries. The lower energy requirement is designed to offset the fact that American babies have been found less active than those in other cultures. The level of protein requirement is that which other authorities estimate to be necessary to prevent actual protein deficiency; many therefore recommend a level which is one third higher, in order to provide a safety margin.
3. The mineral requirements are those needed by a baby fed on formula. A breast-fed baby receives far less calcium, for example, than this, but he absorbs what he does receive much more efficiently.
4. The vitamin requirements are similar to those given by the authorities of other countries except that few recommend such a high intake of vitamin C.
5. The very variability of recommendations emphasizes the inexactness of our nutritional knowledge. The figures given by any authority can be regarded as no more than a very rough guide.

formulas. But fed to the infant fresh, it tends to make heavy casein curds in the stomach. The protein which it contains is suitable for calves, not for infants. The spray-drying processes which are used in the preparation of formulas modify these curds, making them far more digestible. Furthermore the fat, vitamin, and mineral content of fresh cow's milk is variable. Different cows, different cattle feeds, different seasons, and different methods of storage all affect milk. And a mother cannot hope to know about these variables, let alone control them.

Given that a formula specially prepared for infants is used, it probably does not matter which one is chosen unless a doctor or health visitor advises a special one. Some are slightly easier to mix than others. The few which are sold in the form of a liquid concentrate are particularly easy both to mix and measure, but they are comparatively expensive and very heavy to carry home. A formula which is stocked by a local shop is obviously preferable to one which involves a special journey, but if the baby is soon to be taken on a holiday or other trip abroad, it may be worthwhile to accustom him to a formula which will be easily available there.

At 3 months, most bottle-fed babies will be taking five feedings in the 24 hours—one at his parents' bedtime, one in the very early morning, and three during the day. Most will drink somewhere around 6–7 oz. (170–200 ml) per feeding. A baby who takes somewhere around that quantity of formula may already be getting everything he needs. If he is strictly "average" in every way, he will probably need about 200 more calories and he may just be beginning to need a little iron to replenish the stores in his liver with which he was born. An infant's need for a few more calories can, of course, be met in a variety of ways. He does not lack protein, so there is no point in giving him his extra food in a high-protein form—indeed it may be better for his kidneys if he is *not* given extra protein at this age. A few mothers may unwittingly be already supplying more than the needed extra calories by adding sugar to the formula. Every teaspoonful adds an extra 17 calories of energy value. But it adds nothing else whatever except for a sweet taste which some authorities believe can inculcate an unfortunate preference for sweet food that lasts into later life.

Baby cereals are usually the first solids added to an infant's diet. In many ways they are ideal, but as long as the baby drinks this much of a formula, the quantities which he needs will be minute. A typical infant cereal (not necessarily one advertised as "high protein") yields around 110 calories if one tablespoon of the dry powder is mixed with 3 oz. (90 ml) of milk to produce 3 tablespoons the texture of thick cream. Most of them will contain around 3 mg of iron. Added sugar will put up the calorie count by 17 per teaspoonful. Such a feeding may be just about right for our postulated baby. Some mothers add egg yolk to the diet at this early stage, rightly valuing it for its iron and its fat-soluble vitamins. An egg yolk will yield around 50 calories. Furthermore most infants will be receiving orange juice; most varieties contain a good deal of sugar as well as the vitamin C.

At this age many mothers are using jars of strained babyfood. As a source of calories there is nothing against these except that there are unexpected variations in the calorie value of different varieties. For example, while one would expect a strained fruit variety to be lower in calories than a cheese variety, one would not necessarily expect Gerber's "beef liver" to contain half the calories of their "egg yolks with ham": 92 calories per jar as compared with 182.

It should be clear that while there is no need or purpose in counting the calories one feeds to a baby, there is a very marked tendency to overfeed, and to feed a great deal of unnecessary protein. Many babies of 3 months regularly drink the quantity of formula we have discussed, *and* receive egg yolk, perhaps with infant cereal, at breakfast time, a jar of a baby dinner in the middle of the day, and more cereal perhaps with a jar of baby fruit at suppertime. Even allowing for individual variations, it is not surprising that some of these babies become obese.

Obesity in infants is too often regarded as a matter for congratulation. People tend to think that fat babies look sweet. The dimples in the plump knees make other mothers coo. The baby's "adequate" weight gain is on display for all to see. Unfairly, we react quite differently to fat *children*. Adults assume them to be greedy; their mothers are thought to ply them with sweets and other "unsuitable foods"; their schoolmates deride them. And of course the Western world is full of adults who are dieting to try to lose weight.

We do not know how general overfeeding is in this age quarter, but all the available evidence points toward its being very general indeed. A. Shukla *et al.* [201] showed that the average weekly weight gains for the 300 babies in their study were way above the expected weight gains used here, and by most authorities. In the first 3 months, for example, where one would expect a weekly gain of around 7 oz. (200 g), following initial weight loss, they found gains of 8.4 oz. (240 g) for boys and 6.7 oz. (190 g) for girls—and this without any loss during the days after birth. For the second quarter, where gains of around 5 oz. (150 g) would be expected, the average weekly gain for boys was 7.5 oz. (214 g) and for girls was 6.7 oz. (190 g). To make the picture blacker, these infants were not particularly tall. Their ratio of weight to height was higher than would be expected.

Taitz [212] studied the birthweights and weights at 6 weeks of 260 normal babies born in a region of England. More than 50 percent of them became overweight even in this short period.

When the first edition of this book appeared it was widely believed that the body of a baby who was made fat in his early months actually produced extra fat cells which, while they could be emptied of fat by a change in diet, would remain in his body so that he was, so to speak, threatened with obesity for life. Current views are more sophisticated and perhaps less alarming for parents. But it is still clearly as bad as it is common for babies to be obese.

Obesity is, at least to some extent, familial. There is evidence which suggests that a child with two fat parents is very likely to be fat himself although if one parent is fat and the other thin, obesity in the child is less likely. There is a suggestion here of a genetic component, but there may also be a far simpler explanation which is also the direct responsibility of the parents. Parents who are fat may sometimes be people who, for a wide variety of reasons, use food themselves for something other than adequate nutrition. There are people who eat for comfort and this may, in the long run, provide a pleasantly followed example to their children. Perhaps more important still are the people—often mothers—who invest a great deal of emotion in feeding others. Often such women are excellent cooks whose pride in the food they provide is justifiable but whose desire for other people to eat large quantities of it at frequent intervals is neither physically nor psychologically healthy. A child whose mother sees his rejection of her food as a rejection of her love and care does not have a fair chance to regulate his eating according to his physical needs and appetite alone.

But at this early age, even the slimmest parents with the healthiest attitudes to their own food can inadvertently make their infant obese. Early mixed-feedings are certainly partly responsible but so is the relationship of mixed-feedings to bottle-feedings. The minority of mothers who breast-feed their infants fully for a number of months tend to believe that the food they give is perfect. While a few may start mixed-feedings early as a way of avoiding supplementary bottles, most are happy to continue with breast milk alone until the baby clearly shows that he needs more food rather than the same food more often. When such a mother does start to give foods other than milk, she must give them as an entirely separate item of diet. She cannot tamper with the composition of the breast milk and the quantity is regulated by the baby himself. She therefore introduces food from a spoon and if the baby really does not want it, he can refuse. The bottle-feeding mother on the other hand may be far less sure that the formula is perfect for her baby and far more ready (as well as able) to "improve" it for him. As we have seen, some mothers routinely add sugar to complete formulae. It is but a short step from there to adding just a little extra milk powder "to make it more satisfying" and then just a little bit of cereal "so that it sticks to her ribs for the night." A baby whose bottles are tampered with in this way may be fooled into taking more calories than he needs or wants because they are hidden in the amount of milk to which he is accustomed. Furthermore, although recent modifications to formula have reduced the risks of the baby's receiving an overload of protein and sodium from over-concentrated bottles, such bottles can still make him thirsty. If he cries for a drink and the drink that he is offered is yet more food he may be cross and uncomfortable today and fat next week.

Natural appetite is the best guide to the quantity of milk to give an infant, but the workings of that appetite as a guide do depend upon the milk being consistent and plain water being readily offered.

Natural appetite is also the best guide to quantities of solid foods but, at the start of spoon-feeding, it can be difficult to follow.

Very young babies take quite a long time to associate the spoon with food: their instinctive way to satisfy hunger is by sucking, and they have to learn that it can also be quelled by spoonfuls. If you watch a hungry baby during his first spoon-feedings, spoonfuls of food are often dumped into his mouth between angry yells of hunger, the yells only gradually diminishing as the infant finds himself less urgently hungry. Furthermore such young infants are extremely inefficient with a spoon. Food which is placed in the front of the mouth is usually pushed out again with the questing tongue. It is extremely difficult to tell whether the infant has spat out the mouthful because he did not want it, or because he failed to get it far enough back in his mouth to swallow.

All in all it does seem that infants might be better off if solid foods were left alone entirely until around 3 months, and were then introduced in *minute* quantities as learning experiences rather than as foods. As we shall see in a later chapter, that "good mixed diet" is not even appropriate as a goal until the second half of the first year.

14

PHYSICAL FUNDAMENTALS
AGAIN

EATING AND SLEEPING PATTERNS

THREE TO 6 MONTHS MARKS, in many babies, a changeover from "feedings" to meals, and from almost always sleeping between meals to discrete "naps."

At 3 months, eating is still intimately tied up with sleeping, so that the infant tends to wake up when he is hungry, and go to sleep when he is full. But already there is likely to be one particular period in the day when he is usually wakeful, even though well fed. For the majority of babies this seems to be the mid-afternoon. The baby goes to sleep after his lunch and wakes again an hour or two later, staying awake until his 5 P.M. or 6 P.M. meal. Whether this pattern is a genuinely inbuilt one, or whether it merely reflects the comparative willingness of most mothers to play in the afternoon, and their reluctance to play during the morning —the conventional time for household chores—we do not know. Certainly one can find babies of this age whose chosen period for wakefulness is the morning, or the evening.

While eating and sleeping are still so closely related, the amount of manipulation of the infant's day which the mother can easily carry out is very limited. He wakes ferociously hungry, and almost all mothers, willingly or unwillingly, will feed him within a few minutes. Having eaten, he needs to sleep, and may, if the mother tries to keep him up, drop off to sleep on her lap or on the floor.

But gradually eating and sleeping become disassociated. The infant eats, and probably sleeps soon afterward. However he begins to wake up because he has had a long enough nap, not because he is hungry again. A little later still, a full stomach does not necessarily send him to sleep. If interesting things are going on around him, he may eat and then play.

He still needs his meals, and he will still take a rough average of five hours' sleep between 6 A.M. and 6 P.M., but both the meals and the naps become more adjustable.

During these months the infant becomes able to suck his fingers whenever he likes, and to get some fun—and increasing amounts of nutrition—out of mouthing hard foods clutched in his hand. Both these abilities help in disassociating eating from sleeping. When the infant wakes, the mother can feed him if it suits her—he has no objection to eating before he is acutely hungry—but if it does not suit her, his fingers or a zwieback may keep him happy for anywhere from two minutes to half an hour.

During this same period the frequency with which the baby demands to be fed drops. At 3 months a few will still be demanding a night feeding, between say 10 P.M. and 6 A.M. These will probably be having a variable five *or* six feedings in the 24 hours. They do not quite need six and cannot quite manage with five. But most are already only having five feedings by 3 months; and by 4 or 5 months many will only be having four. Once four feedings are the infant's settled pattern, his food ceases to be a matter of "feedings" and becomes instead a matter of three meals a day and an additional bottle- or breast-feeding.

How these meals are organized depends partly upon the infant's sleep pattern and partly on the mother's convenience, and the routine of the rest of the household. The infant is probably going to have breakfast, lunch and supper. In addition he is going to need a bottle or the breast *either* last thing at night, before the mother goes to bed, *or* first thing in the morning. Three common eating/sleeping patterns are outlined below:

Wakes at 5–6 A.M.   Cannot wait for family's normal breakfast time. Given bottle- or breast-feeding; sleeps again until 9–10 A.M. when given breakfast. Sleeps again until around 1 P.M., but after lunch takes only a discrete nap, being otherwise awake until after his supper at around 6 P.M.

Wakes at 8–9 A.M.   Has breakfast, and stays awake until around midday, when he is given lunch, and then sleeps at once for most of the afternoon. May not wake until around 5 P.M. Probably then wishes to be sociable, so that bedtime becomes later, after supper—around 7–7:30 P.M. He may wake, or be woken, for his late-night feeding.

Wakes around 7 A.M.   Can wait until breakfast time, then takes a nap of 1 to 2 hours between breakfast and lunch, and a similar nap between lunch and supper. His day is more evenly divided than either of the other two between sleep and wakefulness.

Obviously any combination or permutation of these patterns is possible. Their interest lies in how they can be adapted to the household. The first pattern might suit the mother who has a husband and other children to get off to work and school, and who is therefore pleased to have the infant out of the way during their breakfast time. She may be happy to play with him, or take him out in the afternoon, and glad to have him in bed early, leaving her free to give her attention to the others during the evening. She can therefore encourage him to go on with the early-morning bottle- or breast-feeding, giving it to him even on mornings when he happens to wake a little later.

The second pattern might suit a mother whose husband wanted to see as much as possible of the baby, and who, perhaps because it is a first child, does not find herself too loaded with work to cope with a baby who is wakeful all morning. She can continue to wake him for his late-night feeding.

The third pattern is, perhaps, the easiest of all, because it shows a more complete separation between eating and sleeping than either of the other two, and spaces the hours of sleep more evenly through the day. Such a baby is not likely to be as tired and cross at 6 P.M. as babies in the first group, nor as determinedly wakeful as babies in the second group. His final bedtime can therefore be adjusted, even from day to day. And the mother can choose whether she continues his early-morning or his late-night bottle- or breast-feeding; with this pattern he may soon make it clear that he needs neither.

The actual hours of sleep and the pattern of "naps" are not likely to change very much during these 3 months. As he gets older the infant may sleep slightly less at each nap, but since he is also likely to be happy for somewhat longer periods in his carriage or crib alone, the mother is unlikely to notice, or even to know this.

Sleep difficulties are unusual during this age period. Where they do exist, the problem is still the mother's, not the infant's. As we have seen, dropping off to sleep cannot be voluntarily inhibited at this age. Given reasonable conditions the baby will go to sleep when he needs to. Problems only arise if he does not need to sleep when the mother thinks he should. Sometimes she is unable to fathom the infant's preferred pattern of sleep and wakefulness; she may fail to follow his cues and try to put him to sleep when he is wakeful and perhaps to play with him when he is sleepy. Probably the most common error is to allow the infant to nap through most of the afternoon, and then expect him to be ready to sleep again by 6 P.M., as soon as he has been washed and fed.

Occasionally the pattern of concerned care which evening colic (see p. 87) has set up leads to difficulties. The baby's sleep rhythm may have become adjusted to a long period of evening wakefulness and its attendant social attention. When the cause of the wakefulness (the colic pain) ceases, the baby still wakes every evening. Unless the parents allow themselves to be trapped into taking an angry and moralistic attitude to this behavior it is usually easy to deal with. The baby wakes and is given the attention he is accustomed to, but because the pain is no longer there to keep him awake, he rapidly drops off to sleep again. A shorter and shorter period of cuddling each evening will usually suffice, so that within two or three weeks of the colic's end the baby no longer wakes at all.

TEETHING

Many sleep difficulties are put down to teething. Often an acute concern with teething will follow directly from parents' worrying about colic, or much incomprehensible crying in the early weeks. Many parents prefer to have something positive to which they can attribute their baby's misery. It is easier to remain patient with a constantly crying baby if you can believe he has a physical reason for his misery. Teething is an accepted cause, and far easier for most people to understand than more probable but nebulous causes such as loneliness.

Authorities have been concerned with teething since Hippocrates, who said: "Teething children suffer from itching of the gums, fever, convulsions, diarrhea. . . ." All the early authorities are well reviewed by L. Guthrie [100], and some of the more hair-raising suggested cures such as gum-lancing, leeches behind the jaw or wolves-teeth necklaces are described by Illingworth [112]. He has reviewed the modern evidence on

TABLE 4. ORDER AND AVERAGE AGES FOR THE ERUPTION OF FIRST TEETH

Teeth	*Average age for first appearance*
Lower incisors—the two middle teeth of the lower jaw	First at 6 months Second at 7 months
Upper incisors—the two middle teeth of the upper jaw	First at 7 1/2 months Second at 9 months
Lower first molars—the grinding teeth farthest forward in the lower jaw	12 months
Upper first molars—the grinding teeth farthest forward in the upper jaw	14 months
Lower canines, or cuspids—the pointed teeth between incisors and molars in the lower jaw	16 months
Upper canines, or cuspids—the pointed teeth between incisors and molars in the upper jaw	18 months
Lower second molars—the grinding teeth at the back of the bottom jaw	20 months
Upper second molars—the grinding teeth at the back of the top jaw	24 months

the symptoms of teething and believes that while it is not quite true that "teething produces nothing but teeth," it certainly does not produce more than a little irritability from time to time, a lot of dribble, and occasional frantic sucking or biting.

A baby of 3 months or more who cries excessively, or frequently wakes in the night, is most unlikely to be behaving in this way because he is teething. In the first place he probably is not teething, since most children do not cut their first tooth before 5–6 months (see Table 4). In the second place, if he is teething, the process is most unlikely to be uncomfortable enough to cause more than very occasional misery. If such a baby also has diarrhea, fever, convulsions, vomiting, or loss of appetite, he may or may not be teething. But if he is, it is totally irrelevant. He needs to see a doctor as his symptoms are those of *illness,* not of *teething.* In 1839, the Registrar General's report on mortality in the first year of life attributed more than 5000 infant deaths in England and Wales directly to teething. We now know that these deaths must have been due to illnesses which were missed because parents, nurses, and doctors were prepared to believe that teething could cause almost any physical symptom.

CRYING

The prime causes of crying at 3 months are still similar to those of earlier weeks (see p. 51). Crying is likely whenever the baby is physically uncomfortable; his discomforts may range from hunger through cold to physical pain. On the other hand, most babies by this age give other cues to their discomfort, before they begin to cry. The attentive mother can tell, from her baby's expression, from restless movements, from the little noises which presage full-throated crying, that something is wrong. Very often she can abort what would have been an episode of crying before it really gets under way. M. David and G. Appell [54] have described some mother-infant pairs where the mother is so attuned to the distress signals of her baby that crying point is very seldom reached. They have observed others where the mother, albeit with the best intentions, cannot spot the baby's distress until it is voiced in a full-throated roar. It may be that some of these infants do not, in fact, give the full range of subtle distress signals; or it may be that they move through the stages of growing distress very rapidly, so that the mother has barely time to see the downcast face before it crumples into howls.

Causes and cures for crying that have nothing to do with physical discomfort or its alleviation appear with increasing frequency during these months. Both are directly related to the attachment to people, and especially to the mother, which was discussed in Chapter Eleven.

In many infants a new "type" of crying also emerges at this stage. Bruner [40] differentiates it from the insistent, continuous "demand crying" which goes on at full pitch until somebody does something, by terming it a "request mode." This kind of crying is gentler and less insistent than "demand crying." But it is most clearly characterized by a built-in pause-pattern. The infant utters a series of cry-tones, tails them off and waits and then, if nobody comes, cries again. These pauses are thought to be literally an anticipation of adult response: the infant equivalent of a child's "Mom?"; "Mommy?"; "Mo–o–om." If this is the correct interpretation—and personal observation certainly suggests that it is— then Ainsworth [5], Sander [190], and the other researchers who have studied this type of cry, are probably right to regard its development as a favorable sign. They believe that an infant who develops the "request mode" is one with whom an adult has interacted sensitively and who has therefore come to expect a friendly response to his communications. It is obviously a pity if an infant who does have these comfortable assumptions about his caretakers finds them contradicted as he grows older. If "request mode" crying is ignored, it will, of course, usually give way to "demand crying." The parent who regularly waits for this to happen, saying, so to speak, "he's not *really* unhappy yet, I'll leave him for a bit . . ." may imply to the baby that polite requests are useless and that only yells and screams can be relied upon to evoke response.

As soon as the infant's social development has advanced far enough for him to discriminate between friends and strangers, mother and others, it becomes extremely rare for his crying, whatever its cause, not to be halted by being held and talked to by familiar people. At the same time much of his crying can be seen to be caused by his need for social interaction with people.

Whatever the infant is crying about, he is likely to stop when his mother picks him up, unless he is in severe pain, or sedated, or ill. If the original cause of his distress was some form of mild discomfort, he will probably put up with it as long as his mother holds him, remaining calm and cheerful while she fetches his bottle or sorts out his rumpled bed. If the original discomfort was severe, and is ongoing, he may start to cry again even as his mother holds him. But even then it is likely to be a different kind of crying, much calmer and gentler than when he was alone.

Very often, the mother can discover no cause for the crying. If she then returns him to his crib or carriage, alone, away from company, he is likely to begin to cry again immediately. He was crying for people, crying for her.

Many mothers, health visitors, and doctors believe that such crying for company is in some way illegitimate. They believe that infants have a right to cry if there is "something wrong"; and that it is the mother's job to find out what is wrong and put it right. But something wrong means hunger, or a chafing diaper, or sun in the eyes; it does not mean loneliness or boredom. If there is nothing *physically* wrong, mothers are advised to put the baby down again, and let him cry it out. It is a curious attitude.

Without his desire for human company, without his need for his mother, the baby could not develop as a normal human being. Furthermore we do not treat social demands in this way in any of our other relationships. We do not reckon that a husband who has been given his supper "should not" require anything more of us until morning. Nor do we greet friends on the telephone by saying, "Do you actually need me to do anything for you? Because if not I am going to hang up." A chat is a valid reason for the telephone call.

Usually it is the specter of spoiling which leads to this irrational behavior toward infants. Many mothers fear, perhaps only partly consciously, that if the baby is allowed to make all the emotional demands he wishes on them, they will be engulfed, drained, left with no individuality, nothing to offer husbands, friends, or older children. The relationship which the infant wants with the mother is so intense that mothers tend to want to keep it under their own control; ration it, in case it gets out of hand.

Yet only Western cultures tend to take this attitude toward young babies. It is only we to whom it ever occurs to leave a baby alone for long periods. Elsewhere the baby is automatically with the mother or grandmother or older sister all the time; carried by her during the day, cuddled up with her during the night. In many cultures the implicit recognition of this need is so strong that it is embodied in sexual taboos on the relationship between husband and wife. It is the baby who shares the mother's bed, not the husband. In Western cultures a baby in the bed instead of a husband (or indeed as well as him) is not considered either normal or desirable. Meeting the needs of a small baby places heavy demands on the relationship between husband and wife anyway; their privacy and peace together at night are vital. So we have to try and provide security and warmth by means other than a huddle of bodies.

The fear of spoiling a baby of this age is a tragic one. Implicit in it is the view that babies are demanding monsters who given an inch will take a mile. But why should they? They only want as much as they need. Given what they need, they will not demand more and more. Indeed given what they need when they show they need it, they will tend to demand less and less. It is the baby who is firmly left alone in his carriage, awake, and crying for an hour at a time, who tends to become demanding and difficult. He is the one who begins to fear his carriage or crib, because they spell isolation. The baby who is always picked up, talked to, played with, included in the household, whenever he indicates his need, has no reason to cry when he has not the need. He is confident.

Fear of spoiling often leads to a different but related kind of crying. As the baby develops new accomplishments, he has a very strong desire to exercise and practice them. Most of them, as we shall see in later chapters, directly involve the mother, either as a partner, or as a facilitator. The baby who is determinedly left alone for long periods when he is awake may be not only lonely, but also frustrated and bored. He is being prevented from doing all the things he wants to do, needs to do, is developmentally programmed to do. Play is not an indulgence, it is a developmental necessity: the child's job. It may not earn him money, but it earns him growth.

15

GETTING CONTROL
OF HIS BODY

WHERE THE FIRST 3 MONTHS of the infant's life saw him fighting and winning a battle for control over his own heavy head, these 3 months see him getting to know his own body, and finding out what he can do with it.

In the early weeks of life, it is thought that infants do not "know" their own bodies even in the sense of being aware that they are all of one piece, and a separate piece from anything else. Their awareness of where they stop and other things begin is probably extremely blurred. Their pleasure when their own waving hands move across their field of vision is just the same as their pleasure when the mother's hand is seen. When they catch sight of their own hand lying on the blanket, they do not at once move it; rather they consider it, interestedly, as if it were an object. The mother's body is often used by the infant as if it were his own—without apparent awareness that she may react, for example, to having *his* fingers in *her* mouth. The infant's own body can often be offered him in place of the mother's—by gently disengaging his clutching hand, for example, and giving him his other hand to hold instead. So the infant makes an exceedingly exciting discovery during these 3 months: he discovers that all the bits of his body are attached and part of *him,* and as a corollary, he discovers that they are all more or less under his own control. A great deal of his drive, his energy, his concentration during this period goes into making his body obey him.

In gross terms, the motor developments which take place are very small. The infant does not learn to walk during this period; he does not learn to crawl, or even to sit up properly. To a casual observer he still seems very immobile, very incompetent physically at 6 months. And compared with the young of any other species he is indeed incompetent.

Nevertheless the consequences of each small development are immense, if they are considered in scale with the small scope of the infant's world.

For several weeks he was totally dependent on his mother for the very position in which he lay. Once she had put him down, apart from turning his head, he could do nothing to change his position. Now, soon after 3 months, he learns to roll himself over, first from his side to his back (see Chapter Seven) and then from his back to his side—a small achievement, perhaps, but one with far-reaching consequences for the infant. By rolling over, he may make himself more physically comfortable, or less so. He may hurt himself, by banging his head on the crib bars or rolling off the sofa; he can change his view of the world, see new things, perhaps even catch sight of his mother. He may increase his own freedom to move around, by releasing his legs from a blanket; he may trap himself into immobility by catching his arm underneath his body. The list of possibilities is endless. The important point is that the baby is greatly increasing the stimulation he gets throughout his waking hours by providing stimulation for himself. And the stimulation is giving him innumerable lessons in cause and effect, in what is him and what is outside him, and in visual accommodation to different objects at different distances. The change in his environment which being able to roll brings about is equivalent to the change which uncurling from the neonatal position brought about at the 6-weeks stage.

As with most aspects of development, once a baby *can* roll, he *will* roll. His ability to do so will increase by fits and starts so sharp that they may catch his mother out. It takes only one extra-frenzied effort on the baby's part to turn the diaper-changing table from an acceptable convenience to a hazard that is banned too late. The baby's efforts are dedicated to rolling right over, from his back to his stomach. The earlier he has managed to roll from side to back the earlier he will roll from back to side. And the earlier he accomplishes both these maneuvers, the earlier he can be expected to manage to get all the way over. In the meantime he will try and try, and he needs to be helped over, placed on his tummy so that he can practice the preliminaries to crawling which will become so important soon after 6 months (see p. 251).

By 3 months most infants placed on their tummies lie with their legs straight out behind them, and can take the weight of their upper bodies on their forearms so as to lift their heads well clear of the floor. By around 15 weeks, the infant will probably be able to lift his whole chest clear of the floor as well as his head, and he may hold this position for several minutes at a time. A few infants, by 4 months, even learn to transfer their weight from forearms to hands, thus raising themselves even higher.

At around 4 months, while he is lying flat on the floor, resting from the head-up posture, the infant begins to pull his legs under him, rather as he did when he was newborn, so that his bottom is in the air. As with forearms and hands, some infants quickly learn that they can get even more purchase if they push up with their feet rather than with their knees.

By 5 months many babies have both the head-up and the bottom-up position perfected, but cannot put the two together so as to be on hands and knees. They therefore alternate the two, and look rather as if they were seesawing—first one end up and the other down, then the first end down and the other up. By this stage, while a true crawl with the tummy clear of the floor is very unusual, quite a lot of babies will make some progress across the floor, as they seesaw. It is not deliberate locomotion, but it is quite enough movement to take them over the top of a flight of stairs, or into an unguarded fire.

Some babies do not progress in their pre-crawling maneuvers as fast as this, because they strenuously object to being put to lie on their tummies at all. Often these are the babies who seem to be most alert to people, and to things around them. It may well be that they object to the reduction in their field of vision which being put face down brings with it. There is no evidence to suggest that such a baby is likely to be late in crawling. He may, however, be early in learning to sit up. Probably he will simply cut out some of the preliminaries of learning to crawl, refusing to be put on his tummy until he is very nearly ready to move off.

As we saw in Chapter Seven, most infants take a great pleasure in free kicking and other physical play by the time they are 3 months. From 3–6 months such play becomes much more obviously purposeful. Where at 3 months the infant enjoyed having his hands held while he was gently pulled up to sitting position, by 4 months the mother has only to take his hands for him to try and pull *himself* to sitting. By 6 months he may indeed provide all the power for this maneuver himself, using the adult's hands purely as balancing handles. Even without adult hands the baby will try to sit up. By 4 months, lying flat on his back, often during a short rest-pause following an energetic bout of kicking, the infant will lift his head clear of the floor. A month later he will be able to lift both his head and shoulders clear, and may get an amazing glimpse of his own feet as he does so. Propped up in sitting position, he cranes his head forward from the backrest, as if he yearned for a more and more upright posture. By 6 months the infant's control of his back has moved downward, so that only the base of his spine, at hip level, still tends to sag when he sits. He can sit in his carriage with only a single pillow wedged behind his bottom; and he may be able to sit alone for a few seconds, often leaning forward to put his hands on the floor for extra balance. But even the best 6-month sitters cannot really *use* the independent sitting position. Even if they can balance while their full concentration is on the sheer business of sitting, distraction by a person, or the sight of a toy, or any attempt to turn their heads or use their hands will still topple them.

A 3-month infant held in standing position tends to sag pathetically at the knees. But over the next few weeks, most babies begin to take a fractional amount of their own bodyweight on their feet, pushing down with their toes while they intermittently straighten their knees. By 4–5 months, the knee-straightening has become rhythmical, so that the infant feels as if he were "jumping" on the mother's lap. At this stage some babies acquire such a passion for the standing position that it is exceedingly difficult to persuade them to *sit* on a lap at all. They turn themselves inward, fasten their fists in the nearest portion of their mother's body or hair, and fight to get themselves upright against her shoulder. Once in position they have a delightful view of the world over her shoulder, and a view, moreover, which moves around as they jump; they are in warm contact with the mother's body, face to face, and they can exercise their legs to their heart's content. By the time the infant reaches 6 months, the mother may feel that she is nothing but a convenient trampoline for a budding gymnast!

Most of these physical activities require the mother's participation, or at least her preliminary help. The infant cannot practice his rolling over unless she puts him on a suitable firm surface, and frees him from hampering wrappings. He cannot sit himself up unless she helps him, nor stay sitting unless she arranges a suitable seat. He cannot practice taking his weight standing up unless she enters the game. Babies who are left, alone and awake, for long periods therefore have good reason to be bored as well as lonely. They need their mothers to play, not only for emotional reasons, but also as partners who provide the muscle power and the balance for these new physical adventures.

Yet placed on a mat on the floor, or even in his carriage with the blankets removed, a baby of this age period can make some entertainment for himself. Many mothers accept the healthy exercise which goes with what is usually called "kicking"; but few realize the extent of the learning which goes on at the same time. We have seen that by 3 months most infants have coordinated their limbs to a point where their legs move in a smooth, rhythmical bicycling motion, and the waving of their arms is fluid, without the jerkiness which characterized the early weeks.

Soon after, the infant learns that he can alter this motion; change the rhythm; start and stop his legs at will. He learns, for example, to kick both legs together instead of alternating them. He finds that that motion is the quickest way to get his covers off, or a good way to make his carriage bounce. Certainly he is exercising, but he is also learning that those limbs are part of him; that he can control them.

As he waves his arms around, apparently aimlessly, he is also practicing all the skills which go into reaching out for things and grasping them (see Chapters Seven and Nine). At 3 months most infants have discovered their hands by touch and by eye simultaneously. They watch their hands playing together. But the infant's notions of his own *control* over his hands are probably still very primitive. If he is watched carefully, it can be seen that he greets his own hand with pleasure when it moves into his view; plays with it dedicatedly for a while, but then, when it falls out of view, he accepts that it has gone; he makes no attempt to turn his head and look for it, nor to raise it into view again. He has not yet learned that objects still exist when they are out of sight, nor that his hand is not an object, but part of himself.

Over a few weeks of concentrated hand play, the infant gradually learns that he himself can make his hands come and go. Again if he is carefully watched, this stage can often be spotted. The infant plays with his hands for a while, and then stops, with both hands held in the air where he can see them. He drops both arms to his sides, so that both hands vanish; and then he lifts them again, and looks from one to another. A lucky observer may even see the next stage: this time the baby does not just bring about the miracle of the reappearing hands, he drops the arms to his sides, turns his head to find one of them, and then watches it all the way back to the center again. By about 5 months, it is usually clear that the infant has got his hands thoroughly under control, in the sense that he knows where they are even when he cannot see them, and can bring them back into sight at will. But for some weeks more he will continue to look as if he "checks up" on them, taking the fist he is sucking out of his mouth for visual inspection, or glancing at the hand that is supporting him as he lies on his tummy on the floor.

Once his hands are under this much control the baby uses them to explore other parts of his body. He may pull and twist his ears or his hair, finger his navel, grab his own nose, but it is play with the genitals that is most often noticed by the parents. The penis is an obvious "handle" for a little boy at the grasping stage to get hold of. The vulva makes interesting folds for a little girl to explore. This kind of play is no different at this stage from play with other parts of the body. Yet even at this early age parental attitudes often make it different. The genitals are normally closely covered by diapers and plastic pants, so that play with them is concentrated into moments when the baby is naked. Many parents misinterpret the baby's renewed discovery of his genitals each bathtime, and see him as waiting for a chance to get at himself. Furthermore what the baby does with those organs is often alarming to parents accustomed to adult sexual parts. An infant penis is extraordinarily elastic: the little boy may pull it out, twist it around his fingers, in a way which makes his father shudder. Furthermore, that infant penis becomes spontaneously erect from time to time. Genital play when the penis is erect may look to the parents like true masturbation, and be treated as a moral, or at least a modesty issue. The Newsons [170] reported a widespread incidence of smacking for genital play, even at this age, and many mothers reported that by one year babies were aware of parental disapproval and looked to see if the mother was watching before touching themselves.

At around 5–6 months, babies who are given plenty of physical freedom often transfer their fascination from their hands to their feet. As we have said, the infant often catches a first glimpse of his feet when he begins to lift his head and shoulders off the floor while lying on his back. At other times he catches entrancing sight of them as they wave about on the end of his kicking legs. For about 3 weeks, the infant's free kicking time may seem dedicated to getting hold of those feet. And it is a problem. If he lifts his head and shoulders to get his hands nearer his feet, those feet go down out of reach; if he lifts his legs to bring the feet closer, his shoulders go down. Getting hold of his feet challenges everything he has been learning during this 3-month period: his muscle power, his coordination of one bit of his body with another, and his ability to judge distances and accommodate his vision to things which are moving about. Success often comes at around the half year birthday, with the feet captured, and put in the mouth for thorough examination. A passion for feet is seldom popular with mothers—there are few things more difficult than changing the diaper of a baby who *will* suck his toes.

16

USING HAND AND
EYE TOGETHER

AT 3 MONTHS, babies still behave most of the time as though their looking and their touching systems were entirely separate. The baby will often look at an object within his reach without attempting to reach out for it. And he will often manipulate an object put into his hand without lifting it up so that he can look at it. Yet, as we saw in a previous chapter (see p. 98) the baby is learning about things while he looks at them, even without handling them. And he is rapidly learning how to get hold of them too. By the end of this 3-month period he will be able to reach out swiftly and accurately for anything which is within his reach, and pick it up. Only tiny objects, which require the fine juxtaposition of finger and thumb, will still defeat him for a few further weeks.

We have already seen how extremely selective babies are in their choice of *what* to look at, what to expend their attention on. Some years ago, much research focused on the question of how much infants who could not yet handle objects could actually understand about them just from looking. Common sense and the work of yet earlier decades had led to the supposition that such qualities as shape—especially three-dimensional shape—solidity or size would escape the infant until he could both look at objects and touch and feel them. In the late sixties and early seventies, fresh work began to suggest that infants had an inbuilt understanding of at least some aspects of the nature of objects so that when a child came to handle a particular object for the first time, its properties did not come as a complete surprise to him. In 1972, for example, an elegant study of the infant's understanding of relative size was published. J. S. Bruner and B. Koslowski [41] studied infants aged from 10 weeks to 22 weeks. They were shown two balls within easy reach. The balls were identical, except that one was so small that the infant could have grasped it in one hand, had he been capable of getting hold of it, while the other was much larger, so that the infant would have needed to clasp it in both arms. Even the youngest infants tended to react to the small ball either by clasping one hand tightly with the other, or by holding one hand hovering in mid-air. Their reaction to the large ball was quite different. They tended either to open their arms wide, or to make wide-sweeping swipes toward it. Clearly, even without tactile experience, the babies had some ideas of relative size, by eye alone, and some idea of the grasping methods suitable to objects of different sizes.

There was considerable excitement about this kind of research and many other aspects of the infant's understanding of the nature of objects were subsequently explored. Projects were carried out, for example, to see whether infants "understood" the solidity, or graspability, of objects, by showing them real objects, pictures of objects, and projected shadow-images of objects. But such detailed inquiries concerning isolated aspects of the infant's object-world generally proved unsatisfactory. Bower [31] believed that he had established both that infants "expect" seen objects to be solid and that they are capable of demonstrating this, by swiping at the "objects" and showing distress when their hands pass straight through what is actually a shadow-image, at a much earlier age than had been known before. But his results, and the results of many other studies with a similar orientation, proved impossible to replicate. With hindsight some of the reasons seem obvious.

Since all normal babies *eventually* come to understand the nature and likely behavior of a vast variety of objects within their worlds, any inquiry which is specifically directed at the question of when and how they ac-quire this understanding must concern itself with the *earliest age* at which it can be demonstrated. Demonstrating an understanding requires the baby to *do* something; to react in some clearly observable and measurable way when he is shown the experimental object. We cannot know what a young baby knows unless he shows us that he knows it. These researches therefore involved the continuous invention and refining of methods of studying infants. And however ingenious the chosen method, there was seldom any way in which the researcher could prove that the earliest age at which he had observed the chosen reaction reflected the earliest age at which such a reaction could have taken place, rather than merely the earliest age at which he had been able to measure it. Furthermore, *a reaction* to a given stimulus—an infant's adjustment of his rudimentary grasp to the size of a seen object, for example—need not be at all the same thing as his *recognition* of that stimulus. A baby might be able to differentiate, visually, between a large and a small ball without acting upon the information by doing anything with his hands and arms. Even if both the ability to discriminate between the balls *and* the ability to act upon that discrimination are both present in the individual baby, he may not *wish* to demonstrate the fact. Every parent who has ever tried to persuade a child to repeat an outstanding performance for a new audience will recognize this very real problem. Put a little more scientifically, it may be that the infant's performance is contingent upon any combination of many factors which are outside the scope of the experiment or the control of the experimenter.

To say that this line of inquiry was abandoned would be to put it too exactly, but certainly the theoretical orientation of leading researchers to the whole question of infant coordination of seeing and doing has changed. The accent, now, is not on studying the ages at which specific reactions to specific experimental stimuli occur, but on regarding the very young baby as a highly complex creature in whom the potential for "intelligent" behavior is probably inbuilt and whose development forms a continuous process from birth. This view has in no way reduced the desire to study the processes of this development but it has radically changed what is studied, how it is studied, and the conclusions drawn from those studies.

One interesting new strand constitutes a recognition of the importance of the baby's *physical* behaviors in what are normally thought of as cognitive, or intelligent, performances. Bruner [41] was already moving toward recognition of this factor as long ago as 1972. He believed that the information infants get from looking at things and the information they eventually get from touching things are already genetically mapped upon each other. The infant "knows" what to grasp, and he "knows" how to grasp. His principal task in this area is to learn how to *order* his grasping actions, how to get the sequence right, and how to allow for his own length of reach. Bruner makes the excellent point that it is likely that infants would be genetically programmed to know some of the qualities of objects that they see, and some of the appropriate ways of handling those objects, but it is most *unlikely* that they would be born knowing the length of their own arms. Babies after all come in a large variety of shapes and sizes, and they grow extremely rapidly. Any genetic programming about their own arm reach would therefore be highly inefficient; the infant would have to unlearn the length of his own arms as he grew.

Observation certainly suggests that both order and reach are vital factors during these months. Often infants will reach out toward an object, make careful, painstaking adjustments of the position of their hands in space until they actually touch the object, but be unable to grasp it because they have already closed their hands. They have the order wrong. Similarly infants will often look at an object, bring their hands together directly beneath it, and then grasp one hand with the other at chest level. They have carried out the whole process of grasping, and in the correct order this time, but they have not extended their arms enough to reach the object.

The concentrated hand play which is typical of these months probably serves a valuable purpose in giving the infant information about his own length of arm, his grip, his reach. By 3 1/2–4 months, infants almost always watch their own hand play. The purely tactile manipulation of one hand by the other gives way to very deliberate, visually guided play, with the hands being brought together, taken to the mouth, returned to within eye sight and so on.

Trevarthen has taken the matter further. In a recent series of studies [215] he pleads for what he terms a "psychology of movement." He believes that most developmental psychologists either ignore, or assign a comparatively low place to, the study of motor activity, and that by doing so they may be blinding themselves to a vitally important factor in infant development. He points out the obvious, but often ignored, fact that a baby can only see something if he looks at it and that he can only look at it by moving in such a way that his eyes are lined up with the object. The same is true for almost every imaginable selective act. If the baby is to taste something he must make the movements which take it into his mouth; if he is to feel something he must get it into his hand or get his hand or some other part of his skin surface to it. Trevarthen believes that the space within which acts of the separate body parts can take place may be neurologically mapped within the brain of the newborn. While his actual perception of sights, sounds, and so forth must be prepared by complicated input-processing systems, his *access* to those stimuli depends on how he moves to adjust himself to receive them.

Trevarthen does not believe that movement is the only important factor in infant behavior to which we have unwittingly blinded ourselves. With many other leaders in the field he believes that the whole business of rigorous scientific experiment concerning specific aspects of infant "intelligence" may have come about too early so that we have focused on the particular before we had adequate knowledge of the whole. Just as a computer can only process data which has been fed into it, so a researcher can only produce answers to questions which his experiment was designed to ask. The computer will not tell you that your data is inadequate or misleading. Neither will the experiment tell you that you asked irrelevant questions. If an experimenter sets out to discover, for example, what infants do with their hands and arms when they see this or that, or this rather than that, or this at the same time as or before or after that, everything except the experimental object and the infant's hands and arms is ignored. Such an experiment cannot make allowance for things which the infant may simultaneously be hearing, like traffic outside the laboratory; for the facial expression, physical tension, or indeed the absence of the mother; for the feel of the experimental chair; the infant's mood; his prior experiences; or even what he is doing with his feet. As soon as it is accepted that specifics, such as the relationship between hand and eye, are part of a whole, which is a complete baby, such experiments seem so selective as to approach the absurd.

Rigorously scientific experiments in this area were important in their time because observational studies of young babies had proved so unreliable that developmental psychology as a whole was being brought into disrepute. People had relied on mothers to report their babies' behavior, to keep diaries and lists. The "findings" tended to tell us more about the mothers than about the babies. Others had observed infants themselves, using check-lists to mark off occurrences they were interested in and sometimes using time-sampling techniques to try to account for all the behaviors of a day by recording them for, say, one minute in every half hour. Again, such studies tended to produce results which, while interesting, were not reliable as a different observer often perceived and recorded what was going on in a different way. But the desire to look at babies in their own settings has remained and in the past few years technology has produced new methods. A variety of film and video-techniques, voice-activated recorders, and reflecting devices make it possible to watch the whole child, with or without another person and/or toys, food, or other accessories, and to produce records of what went on which can be analyzed not only by the experimenter but by anyone who wishes to examine, dispute, or re-interpret what are seen as the "results." It is against this technological background that a new wave of naturalistic studies is building. Trevarthen states that

> the art of the new experiments is in letting infants express themselves more naturally and in recording their choice of reaction more directly than before. Unfortunately, when controls and recording devices are set up to obtain quantitative data on a restricted range of questions, the findings may give a distorted view of infant intelligence. Putting an accent on discrete problem-solving and task-perceiving powers of infants, both problem and task being set by the experimenter, . . . have obscured the spontaneous, innate aspects of infant behavior, by which the mind of an infant regulates its own growth in more complex (i.e. naturally-occurring, non-laboratory) circumstances.

Encouraging babies to interact freely with their mothers, albeit observed by sophisticated gadgetry, has already produced some fascinating results. Trevarthen himself has found, for example, that there is a definite stage at which infants seem to have had enough of the kind of play with their mothers which can best be described as communication-for-its-own-sake. Instead of engaging in the kind of intimate, dyadic behavior described earlier they withdraw their gaze from the mother's face, refuse her social advances, and instead gaze fixedly at a toy or other immediately available object. It is as if they had finished talking about talking and now were ready to talk about something else. This impression is strengthened by the fact that infants currently behaving in this way with their mothers (or other principal caretakers) will still indulge in one-to-one talk-about-talk with *other* adults. It seems possible that the business of getting to know the most important person is sufficiently accomplished for the infant to be ready to expand from that relationship, but other people, being less well known, still merit full attention to the exclusion of the object world. Bruner carried out a study with a colleague [191] whose results seem to support those of Trevarthen.

It has been well established by studies of this type that when mothers are playing with their babies, from birth onward, they typically follow the infant's line of regard with their own eyes so that they can monitor what the baby is looking at and respond accordingly. In this study Bruner and Scaife found that there comes a time when the infants use a similar mechanism to attract the mother's attention to an object. If the baby is "thinking about" a toy on the table beside him, he will deliberately detach his gaze from his mother's and direct it instead at the toy. In the many filmed sequences, this behavior led directly to the mother also looking at the toy and usually to her speaking to the infant about it, picking it up, offering it to him or in some other way acknowledging and *joining in* with his interest in it.

While a search for age-dating plays little part in studies of this kind, it is interesting to note that in both these studies the babies were around 16–18 weeks when these interactions took place. This is, of course, just about the time when a baby is likely to become physically competent in handling objects.

But while sophisticated observation of spontaneous behaviors forms one strand of the modern researcher's determination to study the baby-as-a-whole, a great deal of rigorous experimental work is going on too. Instead of designing experiments to ask whether babies of such and such an age can demonstrate that they know this, that, or something else about a given set of stimuli, such workers are basing their studies on much broader developmental concepts.

The scope and complexity of this body of work is beyond the compass of a book of this size but is excellently overviewed by Kagan in the opening chapters of *Infancy: Its Place In Human Development* [120]. Kagan states that "the infant enters the world prepared to attend to changes in physical stimulation in all modalities." While much earlier research was devoted to demonstrating that infants do, indeed, from a very young age, pay renewed attention to a stimulus which changes (whether the stimulus is a toy, a tune, or a taste), Kagan does not believe that it is legitimate to assume that the number of physical differences between one stimulus and another is even a rough index of their psychological differences to the infant. Once an investigator might have shown infants a red ball, a blue ball, and a blue block and analyzed their differences from each other in two dimensions: their form and their color. On this basis he would have assumed that the red and blue balls were more alike than the red ball and the blue block. The first pair differ only on the dimension of color where the second pair differ both in color and in shape. But Kagan points out that the real world seldom offers an infant a stimulus which differs from others in only one dimension. Such an analytic approach makes research work simple but tells us little about real people in the real world. He believes that "one of the most important competences of the central nervous system is the ability to detect the similarity between an event and a mentally stored representation of past experience, and to form a new schema or to alter an old one in a way that reflects the relation between the contemporary perception and the older knowledge." He is interested, then, in the ways in which very young infants build up their first "schemas"—coherent perceptions of objects—in the way and rate at which they become able to remember yesterday's schema when faced with a fresh one today or next week, and in the global features of objects and other experiences which make them noticeable and memorable to infants. "A theory of perception and discrepancy must therefore accommodate dynamic changes in knowledge over time . . . viewing knowledge of events as continually emerging, coherent wholes, rather than an unstable composite of unitary dimensions."

Whatever the infant "knows" about objects, or whatever misapprehensions he may have about their nature and behavior, he will certainly become comparatively adept at handling them during this 3-month period. By the time he is 6 months, all questions about whether he learns to understand what he sees by touching it, or to understand what he touches by seeing it, or about whether he learns both together or merely practices what is genetically inbuilt in him, become academic. By that age interest will focus on what he *does* with what he touches (see Chapter Twenty-two).

As we saw in Chapter Nine, the sequence of the development of reaching out and getting hold of objects is less rigid than are most developmental sequences. In this sense the development of hand-eye coordination is unlike the development of motor abilities. The child must learn to control his head before he can sit up; he must roll from his back to his side before he can roll from his back to his tummy. But he may learn to swipe at objects before he learns visually guided play with his hands, or he may leave out one of the stages of reaching altogether. Furthermore, while all developmental sequences are to some extent open to environmental speeding up, it seems that hand-eye coordination can be speeded up more by appropriate stimulation than motor abilities can be. But this may be because in our society babies are usually given as much motor stimulation as they can use and therefore develop their physical abilities as fast as they can, while they are often not given the optimum amount of visual-manual play, and can therefore develop hand-eye coordination faster if they are offered more.

Returning to the normative studies of Burton, White, Castle, and Held, described on page 104, the stages which most babies will pass through in learning to get hold of objects can be summarized as in Table 5. The "age at first appearance" is the earliest age at which any baby in the sample was seen to accomplish the maneuver. The "age range" encompasses both that first and the latest age at which a baby first performed the maneuver. The age range is as wide as it is because both highly stimulated "experimental babies" and the understimulated "con-

TABLE 5. SUMMARY OF REACHING-OUT BEHAVIOR

Behavior	Average age at first appearance	Age range
Swiping at objects with occasional hit	6 weeks	6 weeks–3 months
Raising one hand toward seen object	8 weeks	8 weeks–3 1/2 months
Raising both hands toward seen object	8 weeks	8 weeks–4 1/2 months
Glancing between raised hand and seen object as if measuring the gap visually	8 weeks	8 weeks–4 1/2 months
Turning body toward seen object presented to one side	2 1/2 months	2 1/2–5 1/2 months
"Piaget-type reach": glancing between raised hand and object, with progressive correction of gap, finally achieving touch	3 1/2 months	3 1/2–5 1/2 months
"Top-level reaching": lifting hand directly to object without intervening visual corrections	4 months	4–6 1/2 months

trol babies" are included. But this does not mean that it can be assumed that ordinary family babies will come midway between the two extremes. As we saw in Chapters Eleven and Twelve both the stimulation offered by homes, and the stimulation taken by infants, vary widely.

Any individual infant may miss out on one of these stages, or pass through it so rapidly that his mother never notices it. Indeed the middle stages of glancing between hand and wanted object, measuring the distance, adjusting the reach, seldom are noticed except by those who observe babies with some care.

For practical purposes, then, all that matters is that at the beginning of this age period the baby will swipe at objects, occasionally hitting them. Somewhere around the middle of the period, he will slowly, painstakingly, succeed in touching things. Toward the end of the period he will reach out efficiently and swiftly for what he wants.

As we have seen, research suggests that the provision of appropriate stimuli can accelerate the infant's acquisition of these skills. While we have no reason to suppose that this acceleration is of long-lasting benefit to the baby, it can be of immediate benefit to the mother, and *therefore* to the baby. Infants in this age group definitely suffer from boredom. The provision of the kind of toys which allow them to practice these vital skills can go a long way toward keeping them entertained at a stage of life when the possibilities of physical play without the mother's help are still limited (see Chapter Eighteen).

Swiping at objects can provide happy entertainment for 10 or even 20 minutes at a time, several times a day, while the infant is at the swiping stage. Unfortunately few homes and even fewer institutions provide suitable objects. A soft, light object, which cannot break however hard it is bashed, needs to be hung within 1 foot (30 cm) of the bridge of the infant's nose. This goes against many people's instincts. They feel that hanging something so close to the baby's face may encourage squinting. Some also feel, perhaps, that "hitting" should not be encouraged. In one day nursery, all the infants of this age group were put in the garden in carriages for the afternoon. We hung woollen balls on long cords from trees above their carriages. Every time a swipe connected, the ball swung, and the tree twigs moved gently. The staff had their most peaceful afternoon in the nursery's history. Occasional exclamatory gurgles were all that could be heard, instead of the usual cacophony of fury from babies put down when they were not ready for sleep.

In the middle stage, when the baby may occasionally succeed in touching an object, if he is given time, his problem is usually adult impatience rather than lack of suitable objects. The mother may offer him a rattle or other toy. He advances his hand, looks at it, looks at the toy, moves the hand fractionally and repeats the process. His longing for the object is clear in his whole demeanor. All too often the mother does not wait for him to achieve success. She either shoves the object into his hand because she wants to do something else, or she gives it to him because she does not like to see the extreme (and, to her, frustrating) effort he is making. Either way she aborts the incident. Very often the baby's successes at first will come when the mother is not actually *offering* him anything and therefore does not notice that he is trying to get something. Perhaps she is sitting with him on her lap, talking to someone else. The baby may have the 2 minutes he needs to succeed in getting hold of the beads around her neck.

If the mother can be patient when she offers something, the right timing for help is when the baby has succeeded in making his hand and the object connect. Often, at this stage, he will have closed his questing hand before it reached its target. Then he does need it put into his hand. Otherwise the success in getting *there* is lost because he still has not got *it*.

Once the infant can reach out and get hold of things, he will reach out and get hold of anything which is within his reach. And his reach is often surprisingly long, with all his new rolling over and craning up abilities. Some of the hazards of this stage are obvious. If the mother has not quite taken in the extent to which his abilities have suddenly developed, it may be her hot cup of coffee he reaches out for, or the iron, or his father's chisel. And, of course, anything he does get hold of will go into his mouth. His mouth, just as much as his hands and eyes, is an organ of exploration. But babies should not eat cigarettes, forks, kittens, buttons, money . . .

On the other hand babies need to be allowed to put more than bottles, pacifiers, and teething rings into their mouths. All too many mothers limit the objects their infants are allowed to handle because they feel it is unhygienic for the baby to mouth everything. Such an attitude leads to extreme tedium for the baby, who wants new and different things to feel and handle. Nor is it a logical attitude. Once the baby is spending some time on the floor, his own hands—which he will suck whatever his mother feels about it—are just as likely to be grubby as the saucepan lids, pieces of paper, and wooden spoons which he so longs to be allowed to play with.

At this early stage, the infant's approach to objects is almost always two-handed. He traps things between his two palms, and scoops them up. It follows that his most active play with objects will take place while he is securely supported in a sitting position so that both his arms are free. A baby chair with its own tray is ideal.

All through this age period the infant can cope with only one object at a time. Even at 6 months, if he takes one small cube, and is then offered another, he will drop the first in order to take the second. The first cube falls because his attention transfers to the second. He cannot yet deliberately let go, or hand back an object. When the mother wants something back she must take it—offering another in its place if she wants to avoid a commotion. At this age, the main interest for the baby is in *getting* objects, and holding them and sucking them. He needs to see and feel and hold as many different things as possible. He is not much concerned, yet, with what he can do with an object once he has got it. Very few 6-month babies are tool-users.

17

LISTENING
AND BABBLING

ALTHOUGH BABIES IN THE EARLY WEEKS of life do make sounds other than crying, it is in this second three months that most will produce positive spates of varied sound. Just as the 4–5 month infant is seldom still when he is awake, so he is seldom silent unless pausing to consider an interesting novelty or leaving sound-space for a partner to reply to him. All the new social, physical, and hand-eye adventures of this age period tend to be accompanied by the infant's sounds, and the sounds themselves become increasingly expressive of a wide range of emotional tones.

Although an enormous amount of research has been done in recent years into the acquisition of *speech* (see Chapters Twenty-three and Thirty), linguists remain remarkably silent on the subject of early sound-making. Most would probably acknowledge that cooing and babbling must *have* an important role in later speech acquisition, but few seem interested in trying to discover what that role is, or in analyzing the components and developments of those sounds. Most of the exciting recent research in this area therefore comes from workers primarily interested not in sound-making, or even in speech for its own sake, but in communication in its wider sense. C. Trevarthen [216], for example, has carried out sophisticated observational studies of infants freely interacting with their mothers. Unconstrained by a strict experimental design forcing the observer's attention to specific points to the exclusion of others, yet with the use of highly sophisticated audio-visual recording and analysis equipment, he has found that infants and their mothers habitually engage in what can only be viewed as "an intricate prototype of human communication." These 3-month "conversations" were by no means entirely verbal on the part of either mother or infant. Both partners used facial expressions, gestures, and movements as well as sounds. But the baby's sounds were definitely part of the interchange.

Trevarthen believes that there was definite communicative intent in both the mothers and babies he studied. But it was not communication *about* anything; the babies did not respond to objects in a similar way, nor even to communication from their mothers which involved objects. It rather seemed that the communication was for its own sake; talk about talk; mutually reinforcing for both partners. Many mothers believe that they talk *to* their infants; many accept that the more they talk, the more their infants will talk. But these studies suggest that what mothers are really doing is talking *with* infants and that at least part of the reason for the greater vocalization of babies who get lots of talk may be simply that they are frequently offered a partner for the communication game.

Mothers and babies communicating in this way fall into a conversational rhythm such that, while either partner may initiate the interaction (perhaps by catching the other's eye and smiling), each then takes turns, so that the vocalization, smiles, expressions, and movements of each mesh into those of the other as if they danced together to the same tune. Babies tend to lead, mothers to follow. The actual voice-tones used by the baby are expressive and varied but high-pitched and lilting when compared to later speech. Mothers use similar tones and rhythms and the fact that their responses "match" to the babies' sounds seems to be an important factor in keeping the interaction going. Trevarthen asked some of his mother-subjects suddenly to "answer" their babies not in their usual imitative way but with a deliberately low-pitched adult sentence. The babies were instantly silenced; many looked puzzled; some cried.

What are the actual sounds that the 3- to 4-month baby is weaving into this kind of communication? The study of infant babble is more difficult than it might first appear. If the babbling sounds of many infants are recorded on tape, the listener tends to analyze the sounds in terms of his own language, or at least in terms of "language" as a whole. The bits of the babble which he tends to note will, inevitably, be those bits which most closely approximate words. If babble is analyzed by methods which avoid this kind of obvious bias—by sound spectrograph, for example, which reproduces the sound waves in a visual graph form—the researcher is still left with information whose significance it is remarkably difficult to assess. He records what the infant utters. He can compare that with the utterances of many other infants. But it is still extremely difficult to find out whether the *baby* could hear the difference between one of his own sounds and the next. And it is even more difficult to guess whether the baby *intended* to make one sound rather than another.

At 3–4 months, most of an infant's babble consists of open vowel sounds. He says "aaaa" and "ooo." Often he is described as "cooing," and indeed he may sound very dove-like. The researcher notes the first occurrence of consonants being added to these vowel sounds. He hears the infant begin to say "Paaa" or "Baa" or "Maa." The addition of consonants makes the cooing sound much more like words, in any language. But does the infant hear the difference between "ooo" and "mooo"? If he does, does he intend to say "moo" rather than "ooo"? Usually it is impossible to know. But we do know that the open-vowel cooing comes before consonants are added, and that the consonants P, B, and M are almost invariably the first ones added to them.

As we saw earlier (see Chapter Ten) the mechanisms necessary for hearing and for producing non-cry sounds are present in the infant from birth. They mature rapidly during the early months, and the infant's ability to control his own sound-making therefore parallels the maturity of his vocal apparatus. Infants seem to be programmed to attend and respond to human speech-like noises just as they are programmed to attend and respond to human face-like sights. It used to be thought that they must also be in some way programmed to practice their own sounds because it was noted that, while being talked to would certainly increase their sound-making, it was not a necessary condition. It was found, for example, that the babies of deaf parents, who were not verbal, still increased their sound-making in this age period just as others did. Unfortunately, so do babies who are themselves totally deaf and therefore unable to receive even their own sounds let alone anyone else's. But does the fact that such babies, cut off from the specific stimulus of hearing speech sounds, nevertheless increase their babbling necessarily imply that they are pre-programmed to increase their sound-making? Not necessarily; it seems possible that if early babbling is as intrinsically communicative as researchers like Trevarthen suggest, it may be stimulated by the other facets of communication which are part and parcel of these early communications. Sounds at this early stage may not be a *specific* reaction to speech sounds but a *global* reaction to social intercourse. Certainly parents need to be alert to this possibility if they have any reason whatsoever to think their child may be deaf. Before about 6 months, babble does not mean that the baby hears. Since early diagnosis of hearing loss is both important and difficult, parents need to assure themselves that as well as "talking" with them, the baby also turns his head to look for someone who speaks from behind him, or reacts to sudden sounds made well outside his eye-line [142]. If there is any cause for anxiety at all, it is best to have the baby's hearing expertly tested as home diagnosis can occasionally be tragically mistaken. One parent, for example, reassured himself about his daughter's hearing by *whispering* from behind her and finding that she turned to him. He thought that he was offering a minimal (i.e. a very quiet) sound-stimulus when in fact a whisper uses high frequencies and is therefore often detectable, as in this case, by an infant with marked hearing loss in other frequency ranges.

Looking around to identify the source of a sound is behavior which must suggest that the infant has coordinated his listening and looking systems and that he has some expectations concerning the likelihood of being able to see the source of a sound. Piaget [178] dated this as a 3-month development, saying that only after this age will most infants make a deliberate visual search for the source of a sound. He explains the tendency of younger infants to look at *something* when they hear a sound in terms of the auditory stimulus being also visually exciting although not yet coordinated with it. But there is much continuing controversy here. Bower [28], for example, believes that basic coordination between sight and sound exists in the infant from birth and is merely refined by learning and experience. McGurk [156], on the other hand, found no evidence of such coordination in 1-month-old subjects and a competence which rapidly increased between the ages of 4 and 7 months.

While all infants increase and diversify their babbling during these months, careful analysis by sound spectrograph has shown marked differences in the number of different sounds made, and the richness of their use. Highly stimulated infants are far more vocal than less stimulated ones. O. C. Irwin [113], for example, found that infants in this age group from higher-social-class families produced more and richer babble than did infants from families of lower social class. J. Kagan [123] confirmed this curious finding, but only for girl babies. Boys babbled the amount they babbled irrespective of the mother's social class, while girls babbled more the higher her social class.

Kagan carefully reviewed the apparent relationship between social class, sex, and early babbling. He concluded that middle-class mothers tended to talk more with their infants than working-class mothers and that (as we saw in Chapter 12) all mothers tended to differentiate in their handling of the two sexes, giving their sons much rough-and-tumble play and their daughters more talking and looking play. A highly talkative mother who concentrates on talking and looking interaction is likely to produce a highly vocal baby, while a less talkative mother who concentrates on rough-and-tumble play is likely to produce a less vocal one. It therefore seemed to Kagan that the sons of working-class mothers could be expected to be the least vocal babies and the daughters of middle-class mothers the most vocal babies (see Chapter 30). We must bear in mind the evidence, albeit preliminary, that there is an inborn, neurophysiological difference between boys and girls which may have a bearing on the kinds of interaction which they typically invite as well as receive (see p. 140).

Nevertheless it is clear that all infants "talk" most when they are communicated with by a familiar adult. As we saw in Chapter 10, the talking-reaction of a 3-month baby is to a talking *person* not just to a sound. Ringing a bell in response to a baby's utterances did not keep him talking, but talking to him did. In the second 3 months he becomes even more selective, he learns to distinguish not just between a human voice and other sounds but between individual human voices. This auditory discrimination closely parallels the developing visual discrimination in which the infant first learns to distinguish between human faces and other objects and only then learns to tell the difference between one face and another.

While the coordination of seeing and hearing has to be perfected during this age period, the infant also has to learn to respond to stimuli applied to only one sense at a time. If he continued to require the total communication complex of sound, smiles, facial expressions, and gestures, which stimulated him to "talk" in his first months, he would never be able to learn to use a telephone!

Kagan and Lewis [122] conducted a series of experiments with infants of 6 months in which they offered a variety of purely auditory stimuli. They played the infants a random intermittent tone, some jazz music, and a prose passage which was read by an unfamiliar male, an unfamiliar female, and the mother. Careful measurements were taken of the infants' heart-rate changes, motor activity, vocalization, crying, and fretting in response to these different sounds.

By this age the babies not only responded differently to each sound episode but responded in a highly appropriate way even without any visual cues. The meaningless tone was largely ignored; the music evoked rhythmic movements in some, while the strange male voice evoked some puzzlement or fretting. The strange female voice and the mother's voice, on the other hand, evoked strong positive responses and most of the babies treated the disembodied voices as if they were indeed callers on the telephone. Every time there was a pause in the reading, the babies answered with a stream of babble.

But while it is clear that infants at the upper end of this age group recognize and respond to the social intent behind talking even when nobody is present, and that they begin to reply to this social intent with a socially intended response, there is no direct imitation of the *content* of adult speech. Babble contains syllables which sound like words, and parents are therefore inclined to pick out these word-like noises and assume that the infant is trying to imitate the actual words he hears around him. This is a clear case of the listener imposing his own knowledge of a language on his interpretation of the child's sounds. The American parent recognizes babble which sounds like an approximation to an English word; the Italian parent recognizes the sounds which are close to an Italian word. Each ignores, as "mere babble," the sounds which approximate words in the other language. In fact babble is universal. Babies do not make every sound known to man in the course of their babbling, because there are still many sounds which they are physiologically incapable of making. But they do make equal numbers of sounds typical of every known language. Nakazima [168], for example, studied groups of Japanese and American babies. The two languages, Japanese and American English, are extremely different from any linguistic point of view. Yet even using spectrographic analysis, Nakazima could find no differences whatsoever in the babble sounds produced by the two groups of children. The sounds made by the two groups remained identical right up to the time when the first words were being produced at around 1 year. There was no Japanese babble, no American babble, just babble.

So it seems that being talked *with* by an adult partner is critical in stimulating a rich flow of communicative babble in the infant and that, by the middle of his first year, he can respond vocally and with discrimination to isolated talk sounds. But it is also clear that what the adult partner offers, at least at this early stage, is not language *teaching* nor even sounds to imitate. Adult partners imitate baby sounds far more than babies imitate adult sounds and attempts to offer adult talk in place of baby-adapted talk lead to the flow drying up. What the adult seems to be offering is partnership itself; pleasurable interaction; a sensitive patterning of stimulus-response flowing backward and forward between the two.

18

BOREDOM AND
THE NEED FOR PLAY

THE PERIOD FROM 3–6 MONTHS is often a comparatively easy one for mothers. The alarms and tribulations of caring for a newborn are over; the baby is socially rewarding, often turning a routine diaper change into a joyous social occasion by his brilliant smiles and persuasive babble, and yet he is still not mobile. The mother can still put him out of danger and expect him to stay put. And she can still expect at least some periods of peace during the day while he sleeps.

Two related specters can ruin this period for both mother and child. The first is the infant's boredom. The second is the mother's fear of spoiling him.

Whatever a baby *can* do, he is going to want to do. His drive to practice new skills is enormously strong, and it has to be. Without that drive he could never overcome the fearsome difficulties of his own immaturity and become competent. So during these months he needs and wants to practice his motor skills: lifting his head, trying to sit up, trying to balance when someone else sits him up, trying to roll over, experimenting with near-crawling positions and so on. He needs and wants new things to look at and new things to reach out for. He needs and wants to handle objects, and mouth them, get to know them. Above all, he needs and wants more and more social contact with adults, especially those who are special to him; he wants to smile and talk and play.

The baby has, then, a full program of activities mapped out for these months. But very few of them are activities which he can start alone, or conduct without help for more than a couple of minutes at a time. His abilities are too new, his incompetence is too great for him to be able to entertain himself.

Placed on a rug on the floor, the infant may occupy himself with kicking, playing with his hands, looking at his toes, and exclaiming over the joys of life for several minutes. If so, the mother is lucky. She can get on with her own affairs. But it is just as likely that as soon as the infant is put on his rug, he will try to roll over, trap the underneath arm so that he can neither complete the maneuver nor go back, and then cry for help. And he is likely to repeat the whole process as soon as he *has* been helped. If trying to roll over is his chosen activity at that moment, he is not going to abandon his efforts just because it irritates his mother to have to keep rescuing him.

Put in a baby chair, with objects he has not seen a thousand times already on the tray before him, he may occupy himself for some time, looking and touching and eventually mouthing them. But he is just as likely to knock off the tray the one that interests him most, and then cry.

Placed in his carriage with objects hung above him, he may hit and swing them delightedly for 20 minutes. Or he may try to get hold of one, discover that he cannot because it swings, and cry.

Almost everything the baby of this age wants most to do requires adult help. He has very little control yet over himself or his world.

Often social play is the only thing the baby wants. He does not want to play with objects, to look at things, to kick and play physically. He wants to interact with his mother. Where giving him a toy will sometimes pacify and please him and sometimes not, giving him mother will always succeed. Where he may or may not enjoy himself on a rug on the floor, he will unfailingly enjoy himself on his mother's lap. Where his own activities may make him smile and talk or may not, pleasure in his mother's activities will always do so. Without fairly constant help and attention and plenty of freely given social play, he gets bored; when he is bored, he gets cross.

It is difficult to imagine what it must feel like to be so totally dependent on someone else for almost every activity; difficult to conceive of having no autonomy, no independence, of being utterly in someone else's hands for day-to-day happiness. Of course there is no real parallel with any adult experience, because an infant's expectations are not the same as an older person's. Nevertheless, an experienced infant's nurse had her view of an infant's life radically altered when she had a stroke, and lay for some weeks more or less helpless in bed. She could not speak and, for a while, she could barely move. When she recovered, she picked out as supremely irritating the very things which adults do to infants without thinking about them. She mentioned her desperate efforts to communicate with people, by facial expression and the few sounds she could make. All too often the people turned away, unaware that she was trying to communicate, or too impatient to work out what she was trying to "say." She mentioned, too, the fury which she felt when people looked after her physical needs as if her body was an object, swiping a wash cloth across her face before she had had time to see that a wash was imminent, or chatting with somebody else while dealing with her incontinence. She likened people's attempts to provide her with entertainment to her own previous behavior with infants, too: "They would switch on the television, and say to themselves, 'There, that should keep her happy,' but it would be a program I had seen before—it was just like handing a baby a rattle every time it grumbled, without stopping to think whether it could possibly have any further interest in that same old toy."

Some mothers find it very rewarding to be so necessary to their infants socially as well as physically. They take pride and pleasure in the baby's pleasure in *them*, and pride and pleasure also in keeping the baby interested and "busy" whenever he is awake. Other mothers react quite differently: they feel that the social demands of these months are not legitimate in the way that the demands of the neonatal weeks are. They can accept ravenous hunger or discomfort as a valid reason for demanding attention, but they cannot accept boredom or loneliness in a similar way. They feel that if he is comfortable in his pram, and has a rattle to play with, the baby *ought* to be content, that he has no right to demand more of them.

In extreme cases a really vicious circle begins. The baby fusses because he is bored, and the mother decides he is getting spoiled. So instead of offering him more company and fun, thus dealing with the boredom, she offers him less because he has "got to learn." Offered less, left to fuss and then to cry alone, the baby eventually goes to sleep. But next day he is even quicker to fuss. His needs are not being met, and he begins to anticipate boredom and loneliness whenever he is put in his crib or carriage or playpen. As he gets more difficult, so the mother's attitude hardens. She will not give in to him. He becomes, in her mind, a demanding monster whom she has to defeat.

Sometimes such a pattern of sadness lasts between mother and child until, with mobility, the baby becomes more able to *take* what he needs; able to crawl after mother; to find things to handle and explore. Then, at last, he may calm down, and the mother may feel she won the battle with her spoiled infant. The tragedy is that it was a totally one-sided battle in the first place.

A baby in this age group does not know how to demand more than he actually needs. His needs and his wants are still the same thing. If he wants company, it is because he needs it. If he needs a new plaything he will also want it. He has not the sophistication to "try it on." You cannot "spoil" a child so young that he has no idea of other people's feelings, no idea of right and wrong, appropriate and inappropriate, no idea of other people's rights. If such a child is given the attention and the help which he shows he can use, he will demand less because he is busy and happy, not more and more. Busy and happy is, of course, the point. If a baby is contentedly watching life from his infant seat, or studying his hands or a mobile while he lies in his crib, then he is making it clear to his parents that he does not need (or want) extra stimulation at the moment. If a rush of affection leads either parent to pick him up all the same, it will do no harm. But if a misplaced guilt leads the parents to feel that the baby should never be left to pursue his own contented small activities, so that they continually intrude upon him when he chooses to be quiet, they unwittingly deprive him of the baby equivalent of "time to stand and stare." Just as the ideal is to follow the baby's own cues as to when he needs attention, without being haunted by the spoiling specter, so his own cues as to when he is happy to be peaceful should be followed without the parents being haunted by a specter of neglect.

Of course the family's practical circumstances make an enormous difference to the ease with which this stage (and all other stages) can be handled. Ideally, the baby needs several complete changes of scene during his waking day, whether these are from house to garden to street, or simply from room to room within the house. And he needs many changes of physical position and type of activity, as well as lots of different objects or "toys." When he tires of lying quietly in his carriage watching the trees, he will welcome a sit in his baby chair with objects to mouth. When he tires of those objects, he will probably be happier with a complete change, to kicking on the floor. When that becomes boring he may be happy sitting in his crib with objects in his lap. And all the while, the changing scene—his mother doing interesting things, friends coming in, other children playing—entertains him as a cinema entertains adults. When everything else is boring, mother, interacting directly and exclusively with him, is riveting. An infant only gets bored on his mother's lap if she ignores him and talks to someone else while he sits there.

Space, money, friends, and not too many other demands make it easy for the mother to give her infant this sort of day. Poor accommodations, other young children, demanding and inconvenient domestic responsibilities make it infinitely more difficult.

Simply in terms of time, the mother who can do a week's shopping in the family car and store it in a large refrigerator, pop the day's washing in an automatic machine and call running a vacuum cleaner over carpeted floors housework has an enormous advantage over the mother who must push the carriage daily to distant shops, line up in a launderette, and wash linoleum. Somehow these simple facts are too often ignored in research into child rearing.

But while practical circumstances are important, feelings are much more so. There are probably as many women making a good life for themselves and their families, despite real deprivation and difficulty, as there are women who can neither be happy themselves nor make anyone else happy, despite every social and economic privilege.

Depression after birth is now widely accepted in our society so that nobody is surprised if a woman weeps ceaselessly in her first couple of post-natal weeks. But from the letters and conversations I have had during the past 2 years, it seems that depression at this later stage in motherhood is probably just as frequent, certainly as painful, and seldom recognized.

Two main themes emerge from these communications. The first concerns a woman's image of herself. If that image can comfortably encompass being somebody's mother—as something added to her sense of self rather than as something taken away—then she has a head-start toward enjoying being her baby's other-half. Many women find that, while their image of themselves as pregnant or at the center of the drama of birth, was acceptable, it does not carry over into the daily (and nightly) routine of baby care. Such women say that they were horrified to find that they felt diminished, in their own eyes, by their semi-confinement to home, their loss of earnings, and the loss of identity and social contact which so often go with giving up a job. Others say, even more bitterly, that they feel that they could have accepted themselves as mothers—as whole, complete human beings playing a new and important role—but they quickly discovered that they were diminished in other people's eyes. It is against this sort of background that decisions about a way of life that will be right for both mother and child are so difficult to make. Some women had been determined to care for their own babies at least throughout the first year, yet found their conviction and confidence sapped within this first quarter. Others had been determined to return to work as soon as possible, yet, faced with separation, found either that suitable day-care arrangements were non-existent or that they were no longer sure that they wanted to leave their babies. Hardly surprisingly, a large number in each of these groups simply found themselves staying at home, not because they wanted to or because they were enjoying life but because they could find no alternative. A smaller, but equally miserable, group found themselves back at work and resenting that way of life too. It does seem that however a woman organizes her life-plus-baby, the most vital point is that the life should feel like a complete whole rather than a set of desperate, lonely, overworked compromises. Being at home with a baby is not a "way of life" unless it *feels* creative and satisfying. Equally, holding down a job and coping with child-care and domestic responsibilities around the edges is not a "way of life" unless all the roles feel knitted together into a single piece.

The second theme is related to the first because it concerns all the people who are, or should be, important to the mother-baby pair. It does seem that, while many women are excellently supported during late pregnancy, birth, and the newborn period, such support tends to drain away as the baby reaches this age. I have been told of partners who, deeply involved with the *new* baby and more intimate with the mother than ever before, at about this time returned to a preoccupation with their outside work and hobbies which they classified as "normal life" but which felt, to their wives, like complete desertion. Relatives also tend to gather, literally or telephonically, to see a new family member in the world. But once he is securely settled, they too tend to return to normal; and that normalcy often excludes the mother and child. Friends are, perhaps, the worst offenders. Often they are attracted by the drama of birth and by the novelty of a new baby so that even those without children of their own or any real interest in maternity will visit and cosset and gossip with the new mother. But people lead busy lives. There comes a time when those friends can no longer face the trek to the mother's home. No doubt they would still welcome her if she could join them for lunch in their usual work-day haunts. But she cannot bring the baby to the pub, or can she?

Many, perhaps most, women need to feel loved, cared for, and valued themselves if they are to love, value, and care for a dependent baby. It is almost as if the mother is giving out so much warmth and nurturance to the child that she needs her supplies regularly filled up if she is not to feel drained and exhausted.

If a mother does become depressed, she will almost inevitably turn in upon herself. If she does so she will become less able to respond to her baby's social advances, slower to spot his cues, and less inclined to offer herself to him. The less the baby gets from her the less she will get back from him and therefore the less pleasurable point there will seem to be in her baby-adapted way of life. In extreme instances, as these months go by, a vicious circle can be set up between mother and child. On the rare occasions when the mother forces herself to make social advances to the baby he actually appears to reject them. He may turn away to a toy or the cat; he may make it clear that he prefers his less available but more responsive father. He may even wound the mother by greeting occasional but cheerful visitors with a kind of joy he seldom offers to her alone.

Partners, relatives, and friends can all help a mother to avoid this sort of situation, especially if they can foresee the possibility of it arising. New people can help too. The woman who is, for the first time in her adult life, going to lead a home-based life with her child, will probably get more support, more genuine sharing, from others who are leading similar lives within carriage or stroller pushing distance than from the old friends who are still commuting. Similarly, the woman who is certain that she wants to work and/or must work outside the home may well find more sympathy for her particular needs from an employer who happens to be willing and able to offer part-time work, flexi-hours, or simply an accepting attitude to workers who are mothers. What will not help is the attitude from all her special adults which seems to say "You've had the baby; you're a mother now; get on with it," and which labels those who cannot do so with the "bored housewife syndrome."

Just as vicious circles can be set up between mother and infant during these months, so can beneficial ones. The more a mother does enjoy interacting with her infant, the more the baby will respond and therefore the more she will feel inclined to give him time and attention. This was made very clear in the pilot study reported by David and Appell [54].

They made detailed observations of the minute-to-minute interaction, at home, of 25 infants, with their mothers in Paris. They found a very wide variation in the amount and the nature of the interaction between different mother-baby pairs. But they also found that almost all that variation was due to differences in the behavior of the *mothers*, not of the babies. Whenever a mother made a social advance to her infant, by smiling at him, talking to him or picking him up, the baby reacted with pleasure and affection, smiling back, stroking her, babbling, and generally rewarding her. No baby was ever seen to ignore a maternal advance unless he was fast asleep. But many mothers, on many occasions, failed to respond to advances made by their infants. Sometimes they simply failed to notice his brightening face as they came within view; sometimes they walked straight past him as he "greeted" her. It was the same mothers who most often failed to respond to their infants socially, who told the interviewers that they were bored with baby care.

Child developmentalists all pay at least lip service to the idea that a child's experiences in his earliest months and years are important to his later development as a person. This proposition is notoriously difficult to prove, scientifically, because such a host of other relationships and experiences interpose themselves between the baby in his mother's care and the child he later becomes. It is impossible to prove that a 5-year-old is as he is because of the way he was handled as a baby. It is even impossible to demonstrate a relationship between specific aspects of infant rearing and later characteristics. It may seem logical that the 7-year-old who sucks his thumb was one who was severely weaned as a baby, but it cannot be proved. Many eminent research workers have tried and failed to show this kind of relationship.

Many people have now reached the conclusion that this whole question of the general atmosphere which prevails between mother and child is probably more important than any specific practice. It looks as though what the mother does, in terms of weaning, or toilet training, or methods of discipline, matters much less than how she does it, in terms of how much she enjoys the child. Of course these nebulous variables of "enjoying a child" or "being comfortable in the role of mother" are very difficult to define and therefore to measure, but some research data, excellently reviewed by Ainsworth [1], suggest that the effort of definition and measurement is worthwhile. The atmospheric variables affect and describe the immediate happiness of mother and baby. But they also appear to have far-reaching effects in terms of the child's later development.

H. R. Schaffer and P. E. Emerson [196, 197] closely studied and assessed the development of babies of 18 months. There was wide variation between one baby and another on all aspects of development and in degree of attachment to the mother. But there was no relationship at all between the current development and attachment of any one baby and anything which his mother had done in earlier months about feeding or weaning or toilet training. On the other hand, they found a very clear relationship between the babies' current development and attachment and the readiness with which the mothers responded, and always had responded, to their crying. There was an equally clear relationship between the current development and how often mothers did start, and always had started, social interchanges with their infants. The highly attentive, responsive, socializing mothers were the ones who had the infants who were well advanced in all fields and strongly attached to them.

The importance to infants' happiness and optimum development of sensitive responses and social initiative from their mothers has even been demonstrated in Israeli kibbutzim, where infants see very little of their parents, being principally cared for by professional nurses. J. L. Gewirtz and H. B. Gewirtz [97] found that in this situation infants did not become particularly attached to the nurses who fed and cared for them all day. They reserved their principal attachment for their parents. The nurses were too busy with groups of infants to be able to give much individual attention to any one child. The parents had only a short daily period with their infants, but devoted it to social interaction with them. The concentrated social attention seemed to mean more to the infants than the continuous physical care.

Mothers can be bored, too; they also need to play. In an ideal world no woman would ever have a baby unless she really knew that she wanted to spend two or three years being somebody else's other-half, and every woman who did have a baby would find all the stages of infant care rewarding. But in the real world some women find themselves condemned to what can feel like a prison sentence. Circumstances and personalities combine in infinitely varying ways to produce this unhappy situation: isolation may be the top floor of a high-rise block with broken elevators, or it may be a feeling of missing out in the adult world. Boredom may be not enough to do or not enough to do that feels like fun. Overwork can be three children under five in inconvenient surroundings or a depressed lack of activity which means that trivial chores pile up relentlessly. The point which is relevant to an infant's development is that happiness and contentment lie between him and his caretaker. If his mother cannot, for whatever reason, enjoy his company then, in the long term, she cannot provide for his happiness either. Conversely if he *is* happy and responsive, he offers her the best possible chance of enjoying mothering him.

To separate a mother and baby who *are* enjoying themselves through each other is tragic, but partial separation between a pair who are not making beneficial circles may be a good thing. From the infant's point of view *somebody responsive and sociable* is a must. If that cannot be the mother, or cannot be the mother on a full-time basis, then it must be somebody else or somebody additional. An *extra* loving adult, whether it happens to be his father, his grandmother, a mother's helper, or a babysitter, will not deprive a baby. What may deprive him is being alone with a mother who is withdrawn from involvement with him, or being in a nursery group where there is no one person who can be consistently involved with him.

SIX MONTHS' SUMMARY

By 6 MONTHS the infant is not only increasingly complex and individual, he is also so emotionally bound up with people, especially the mother, that his actual behavior is intimately tied up with hers. His crying may be almost non-existent or it may be frequent—depending on his rapport with the mother. His motor play will be optimal only if she gives him opportunities and help. His dexterity in getting and handling objects will partly depend on what she offers him, while his "talking" will be more frequent and more varied the more she talks with him.

But by no means is all the variation between the stages reached by 6-month babies under the mother's control. Even at this age those differences between the premature or slow-starting babies, and others, may remain. If a baby gets off to a slow start, he still has to go through all the stages of all aspects of development. Although, once his newborn troubles are over, he may go through some of them faster than most, he is still likely to show a lag at least in some areas. Once again, then, these pointers to the behaviors which are likely at 6 months are only useful in the light of detailed knowledge of which earlier stages the baby has already passed through.

Behavior	Likely stage reached at 6 months	Comments
Feeding	3 meals and a fourth bottle or breast-feeding per 24 hours.	The most usual pattern is for the fourth milk feeding to be a late-night one. The fifth milk feeding early in the morning may not have been given up until 4–5 months. Some mothers may prefer to continue this feeding and drop the late-night one. Either way the remaining meals will approximate ordinary family mealtimes.
Food	Puréed solids at all 3 meals. Some finger foods such as zwiebacks, apple quarters, or cut-up vegetables.	Balance of quantity between milk and solids still very variable, depending on when solids were introduced, and the infant's preferences. Milk intake should not drop below about 1 pint (570 ml) per day.
Feeding method	Most infants will be taking some milk from a cup. The infants who were breast-fed will mostly be weaned from the breast by now: some to a bottle, some directly to a cup. Solid food given in high chair or baby chair rather than on mother's lap.	Infants who are not offered breast or bottle will tend to take less milk. Infants will wish to wield spoon, albeit inaccurately. Will like to pick up and self-feed pieces of food.
Food preferences	Often marked. May prefer liquid or crisp textures, reject thick purées.	Infant will not starve himself. Brief sucking at beginning of meal may lead to acceptance of solids which would otherwise be rejected.

Behavior	Likely stage reached at 6 months	Comments
Weight	Gains very roughly 5 oz. (145 g) per week from 3–6 months, i.e., baby born weighing 7 lb. (3.2 kg) will now weigh roughly 15 1/2 lb. (7 kg).	Consistent gain far more important than high gain. May gain extremely rapidly following illness. High gains are no virtue under other circumstances.
Sleep	Roughly a 12-hour night, barely interrupted by a late feeding, and either two or three separate naps of varying length.	Sleep needs are as variable now as earlier, but likely to be consistent with earlier ages, sleepy babies continuing to need more than wakeful ones.
Crying	Discomfort usually causes whining before actual crying begins. Full-throated *sudden* crying only usual following fright or pain. Night crying may be due to nightmares. Daytime crying often due to boredom or loneliness. Unless really upset by long neglect or frank illness, always stops crying when picked up by mother.	Amount of crying largely depends on sensitivity of baby (to noise, etc.) and on sensitivity of mother to his cues. Crying is no longer a normal part of the infant's day as it still was at 3 months. He now has other signaling mechanisms at his disposal if his caretakers are alert to them.
Teething	Lower central incisor is cut, on average, at 6 months.	Normal children can be born with a tooth, or cut no teeth in the first year. Teething is not an indication of overall development. Teething may cause a sore gum, dribbling, occasional fretfulness. It does not cause changes in stools, fevers, rashes or other signs of illness. Cutting of teeth is not an indication for weaning from breast or bottle.

Behavior	Likely stage reached at 6 months	Comments
Motor activities	Rolls from stomach on to back. 1–4 weeks later rolls from back on to stomach. On back, raises head from flat surface. Strains forward if propped sitting.	Ages are variable, the order is not.
	Uses all four limbs in rhythmic smooth kicking. Lying on stomach alternates head-up position, with chest lifted by forearms or hands, with bottom-up position, with legs bent under him. May momentarily manage to keep both head and bottom up, thus being in crawling position. True crawling is unusual at this age,	Takes obvious pleasure in gross physical exercise.
	but some progress on floor may be made by slithering and/or rolling.	Safety precautions are needed, as progress across the floor is unpredictable.
Sitting	Lying on back, pulls himself to sitting using adult's hands as handles only. Can sit with minimal support to lower back. May sit alone, leaning forward to use own hands for support.	Likes to sit, where he can see the world, most of the time he is awake. Needs pillows around him, as still topples unexpectedly.
Standing	Tries to pull himself to standing when on adult's lap. Held standing, takes full weight; typically "bounces" as alternately straightens and relaxes knees.	May virtually refuse to *sit* on lap. Many infants regard laps as trampolines at this age.

Behavior	Likely stage reached at 6 months	Comments
Grasping and manual play	Concentrated play with own hands is dying down; may be partly replaced by discovery of own feet, which are handled and put in mouth. Reaches swiftly and accurately for objects, usually using two-handed approach. Objects usually picked up using palmar grasp; cannot yet take small objects between finger and thumb.	Objects are always explored by mouth as well as by hand.
	Drops first object if given another. Cannot voluntarily let go of objects.	Little use yet made of objects apart from exploration.
Social responses	Very marked. Infant prefers people to any other objects and his mother to any other person. Smiles often, laughs, responds to talk with talk. Often tries to instigate social interaction by smiling or talking or waving toward mother. May object when left, especially by mother. Anticipates normal happenings, "greeting" mother when she comes in, expressing excitement at meal or outing preparations.	Heavily reliant on mother for play and entertainment as well as for physical care.
Hearing and speech	Turns his head and body toward source of sound. Clear pattern of answering with sound when someone talks to him. Babble now	Even deaf babies babble. Infant's *reaction* to sound is only indication of normal hearing.

Behavior	Likely Stage Reached at 6 Months	Comments
Hearing and speech (*cont'd*)	contains distinct consonants, and may begin to be intonated. Talks most either when being talked to, or when happily alone, often when he wakes in the morning.	Infants who are talked to a great deal will be more vocal than others. Girls may be more vocal than boys.

PART IV

FROM SIX TO TWELVE MONTHS

Broadening His World

19

THE INFANT
WITHIN THE FAMILY

DURING THE SECOND HALF OF THE FIRST YEAR, the relationship which
mother and child have made tends to be put to the test. The infant does
not develop as rapidly during this period as he did in the first half year,
but the developments that take place have a dramatic impact on his
mother and the rest of his family. If the mother's relationship with the
infant is basically positive, each of them enjoying the other's company,
the drama is exciting even if exhausting. But if her relationship with the
infant is already to some extent unsatisfactory—perhaps due to her fear
of his becoming over-demanding and spoiled—it can seem horrific.

During these months, the infant becomes mobile. His achievement
of mobility is the logical extension of the motor abilities he acquired
earlier. But the handling of a mobile infant in Western society is *not* a
logical extension of the patterns of care the mother arrived at earlier.
Non-mobile infants in our society can be, and are, put down out of harm's
way and left for varying periods while their mothers do other things than
care for them. We expect to have both our hands free and our backs
unburdened. And we expect to be able to move freely around our houses.
But as the infant learns to roll, to slither, to crawl, to pull himself to
standing, and to climb, these expectations have to be revised. Ordinary
domestic settings become death traps for the infant, for he acquires his
mobility in fits and unpredictable starts, without a vestige of extra good
sense to go with it. His mother has to have sense and foresight for both
of them, with new abilities and therefore new dangers arising literally
from one day to the next.

Previously the infant may have fitted quite smoothly into the domestic setting established before his birth. Room had to be found for his
various "holding devices"—his carriage, crib, chair, and so on—but oth-

erwise things could be as before. In these months the parents have to spend both ingenuity and perhaps money on safety precautions. Perhaps one of the most useful purchases is the "gerry carrier." This is a device which enables the baby to be carried on the mother's back in a frame. The baby is close to the mother, can peer interestedly over her shoulder, while she has both hands free for the performing of routine household tasks. While these are not yet common in many parts of Europe, they are increasingly widely used in the United States. The design of the carrier has now been improved, so that the baby can safely be installed in the carrier on the floor and the mother can then lift the baby onto her back. Although a baby is obviously safe as well as interested and entertained while thus carried, babies become heavy. Furthermore there are tasks which it would not be safe for the mother to carry out with the baby so placed. Such possibilities as spattering hot fat from a stove do not have to be emphasized. So other safety devices are needed too. Unless there can be a special play area set apart for the baby when he starts to crawl and explore, the whole family's convenience must suffer in order that he can have a safe place to play. It may be necessary to install dummy electric plugs, stairs may have to be protected with stair gates. The trouble with such safety devices is that they tend to cause inconvenience to all other members of the household who must step over and reach around them as they go about their daily lives. Furthermore, the actual organization of living rooms must change too. Ornaments, phonograph records, books, must be banished on high or be chewed or broken. Coffee tables can no longer be used for hot cups of coffee; tablecloths can only safely cover empty tables.

The infant spent earlier weeks painstakingly learning to pick things up. Now he can, and he will. Anything he can reach he will take, and anything he takes, he will chew. Two cigarettes might kill him. A cup of coffee will scald his soft skin where it would barely redden his mother's. Even where real dangers are anticipated and avoided, there are continual minor annoyances. Wastepaper baskets are up-ended, cushions are pulled off chairs, stray letters are chewed to illegible pulp, and the sleeping cat's tail pulled.

Earlier on the infant often got bored, but could be harmlessly entertained if his mother would give her time and thought to occupations for him. Increasingly in these months he thinks of his own. And somehow they are seldom the ones his mother considers suitable. He wants to play with the trash in the trash basket, and finds his mother's scoldings and bodily removals funny. Again and again he crawls toward that basket looking at his mother from time to time over his shoulder. In the end either the trash or his mother's temper must go.

He becomes increasingly able to anticipate and to remember. His brightening and his rapid crawl toward the door when he hears his father's key in the lock may entrance both his parents. But the clamor he sets up for ice cream whenever he is taken to the shops is another matter.

His mother used to buy him an ice cream as an occasional treat, and enjoy his pleasure in it. She may not at all enjoy his demanding it as a right.

Along with all this, the infant's vocal range is rapidly increasing and being put to good use. He no longer divides his sounds between crying, grumbling, and pleasant cooing. He learns to shout for attention, to scream his anger or frustration, to clamor at his mother to stop talking on the telephone, or to his father, or to his sister, and talk to *him.*

So the infant increases his impact on his immediate surroundings, and demands increasing, continuous, watchful care from his mother. At the same time he is likely to demand increasing social interaction with her, and to push their whole relationship on to a more and more emotional plane.

By 6 months, the infant who has been making it clear for weeks that he knows his mother from other people, begins to single her out for more and more special attention. Yarrow [227] has shown that where at 4–5 months an infant may treat his mother and a strange woman to equal shares of smiles and talk, by 6 months he will probably ignore the stranger altogether, or give her a somber stare. All his smiles are now reserved for the known and loved person. Ainsworth [2] found that at around 6 months there were a whole range of behaviors, both gross and subtle, which infants began to reserve exclusively for their mothers. Infants who were in a room with several familiar adults and the mother would always strive to follow if the mother left, but would never try to follow anyone else. If the infant was worried, he would bury his face in his mother's skirt —but not in anyone else's. Playing with the mother, the infant would pat her face, play with her hair, and explore her body; such intimacies were granted to no one else. Even certain facial expressions and sounds seemed to be reserved for the mothering person alone.

Most mothers regard such special behaviors as positive signs of the infant's affection for them. They are gratifying, flattering to the mother. But other emotional changes which are less easy to tolerate tend to arise soon after them. The negative side of the infant's passionate attachment to his mother often begins to show itself in the two separate but related phenomena usually known as "separation anxiety" and "stranger anxiety." The baby not only shows his mother special signs of favor, he also objects increasingly strongly whenever she leaves him, and he often objects also to contact with anyone whom he does not know and love.

Separation anxiety and stranger anxiety have been, and remain, the subject of much argument and research. It was in 1965 that Spitz published a review of the evidence and the theory which he had derived from it [207]. Spitz maintained that these two anxieties were really separate aspects of a single development in the infant: his new ability to differentiate his mother or mother-figure from other people. He argued that as soon as a child "knew" his mother he would become strongly attached to her and that as soon as he was thus attached he would naturally object to being left by her. Fearful reactions to strangers were ascribed to the infants equating the presence of an unknown person with the absence of the loved one.

With the hindsight of much more recent work, the details of Spitz's theory fail to form a convincing whole. Stranger anxiety seldom even starts to manifest itself before 8 months, while separation anxiety, with a more variable starting time, usually peaks later still. In order to argue that both arose from the baby's new discrimination of his mother from all others, Spitz had therefore to maintain that this discrimination was only normally possible for a baby in the last third of his first year. This is, of course, in direct contradiction to the large body of work already mentioned, which clearly shows that babies are capable of telling their mothers from other people months earlier than this. Spitz was seemingly reluctant to accept that separation anxiety could occur earlier than stranger anxiety and could be due to a different set of phenomena in the infant. He maintained that stranger anxiety *must* be induced by fear of separation from the mother because most infants had no other reason to be afraid of strangers, never having experienced hurt at the hands of an unknown person. This runs counter to the large body of research which shows, both for human infants and for the young of other animals, that strangeness is in itself a cause for fear. If it were not, we should all be able to cuddle newborn lambs and calves. Spitz ignored this data and he denied that infants' fear of strangers is easily elicited when they are actually sitting in their mothers' arms and therefore most unlikely to anticipate separation from them. This last point has been amply demonstrated by workers such as Morgan and Ricciuti [160] and Decarie [56]. Contact with the mother often delays or damps down an adverse response to a stranger, but it certainly does not prevent such a reaction in most infants at some ages.

But if Spitz's unifying theory of "8-months anxiety" has not stood the test of time, it was nevertheless vitally important in stimulating other research into these problems. Almost every important work on the subject uses some part of Spitz's thinking even while it contradicts the rest. Which part is accepted and which is rejected depends on the theoretical position adopted.

Bowlby sees both separation anxiety and stranger anxiety as emotional phenomena which are qualitatively different yet linked by being rooted in the infant's attachment to his mother. For him, it is not necessary to suggest that the baby's ability to recognize his mother occurs at the same time that he first exhibits distress at her leaving him, because he sees the relationship between mother and baby as one which grows and deepens. Bowlby first published this point of view in detail in the first volume of his trilogy, *Attachment and Loss*, in 1971. The final volume, *Loss*, published in 1980, surveys work on the subject both past and ongoing [33]. Kagan and his colleagues do not see these anxieties as being based on the development of an emotional relationship but on the development of the infant's cognitive abilities, especially those associated with memory. Very briefly, the theory is that when the child becomes able to generate a "picture in his mind" of a recently past event such as mother being in the room, he will, when faced with a new event such as mother's absence from the room, compare the two. If he is unable to resolve the discrepancy between the two, he will be liable to distress.

Although a great deal of fascinating work has led Kagan to this view [120] he is clearly aware that it cannot account for every aspect of separation anxiety and stranger anxiety. He himself points out that a baby of 10 or 12 months will often start to cry as his mother moves toward the door. Such a child does not yet have two discrepant events to compare, so it cannot be the discrepancy itself which upsets him. Kagan's answer is to postulate that with the ability to remember immediate past events and compare them with present ones goes the ability to predict future events. That leaves the child crying because he anticipates discrepancy—change—*and is uncertain how to deal with it.* The question of the child's ability to cope, to take personal action to deal with events is a very interesting one to which we shall return. In the meanwhile, while Kagan and his colleagues strive to keep these anxieties within the sphere of the infant's intrinsic cognitive development rather than his emotional relationships and feelings, they do have to acknowledge that mothers are special. Infants seldom react with distress when a familiar piece of furniture is removed from the room or when a strange one is introduced. Discrepancy between the recently remembered past and the observed present is therefore not *in itself* distressing. Their answer lies in introducing the concept of "salience" (importance to the child) and the idea that very familiar and salient events are better "articulated" (held in the memory) than less familiar and less salient events. The removal of the sofa and its replacement would not cause distress because sofas are probably neither salient nor well articulated. Mother is both. It seems but a short step from Kagan's salience and articulation to Bowlby's attachment and love.

It seems likely that future work will show that both these theoretical standpoints have validity and that their usefulness will increase as the proponents of one view become able to accept and integrate the other. In the meantime those who are concerned for the well-being of individual children may find some crumbs of practical application from the research cake to add to their own common sense in observing and reacting to their children's apparent needs. It can be useful to parents to have some idea of the age at which their child is likely to begin to suffer from anxiety when his mother or other caretaker leaves the room, and, if he does so suffer, for how long he is likely to do so.

Many babies of 6 to 7 months clearly note the comings and goings of their mothers and, if secretly watched, seem to indicate displeasure each time she vanishes. The baby's face may sober, his waving arms stop, the toy he was mouthing drops and he may gaze fixedly at the door through which she passed. But actual protest is unusual at this early age.

Obvious distress, with crying, seldom begins before 9 months and both the likelihood of its occurring and its intensity if it does occur, rises for several months after that so that the peak is around the first birthday. There is some evidence to suggest that the babies who start to be distressed by separation at the earliest age are those who are furthest advanced in their social and cognitive development. Some authorities suggest that this is because such children are developmentally more mature than others. Other authorities suggest that their overall advancement *and* their early protests at separation are both rooted in a close and stimulating relationship with the mother or her substitute throughout the early months. Once a baby does display this distressed behavior, his anxiety over being left is likely to last well into the second year, but the frequency and intensity of his distress will vary with circumstance.

It is the variability of individual circumstances which make it so difficult to study or comment on this kind of anxiety in real life. The reactions of an individual baby on a particular day depend on a vast complex of variables, including those which are themselves difficult to assess, such as his mood or his fatigue. But they also depend on practical variables so peculiar to one baby in one setting that it is almost impossible to make generalizations. The research worker can only record the behavior of the baby, and use that behavior to "place" him on some scale of separation anxiety. He can arrange that the separation experience should be the same for all the research subjects, but he cannot arrange that all the infants should be in a similar mood, nor that the controlled experience should be just as novel for all. Some everyday situations make these difficulties clear.

At 6–8 months, when separation anxiety may be expected to be building up, an infant may be an efficient crawler, or still totally immobile. If he is mobile, he will be accustomed to dealing with his mother going out of sight by attempting to crawl after her. If, at home, he is accustomed to being able to follow her about, he may be confident and secure, and therefore not very anxious. At the same time, a physical barrier, such as being in a playpen, or behind a closed door, may shock him, frustrate him, more than the same barrier would shock an immobile child who has not yet known the joy of being able to follow.

Similarly some fortunate infants are accustomed to a daily life situation where they are seldom left by the mother when they are awake. Domestic arrangements may be such that kitchen, play-space, garden, telephone, and front door all adjoin, so that the mother seldom needs to go further out of sight than around the corner. Such an infant may not manifest much separation anxiety. The mother may believe that he is not anxious in this way. But if she had to move to a house where the infant spent most of his time in a room quite separate from her work-space, she might discover that he instantly became very anxious indeed.

Again, some infants have been accustomed since birth to accepting a variety of substitutes as well as the mother. In an experimental situation, the mother's prearranged departure from the room may seem to him similar to her daily departure for work. His reaction may be to look around for her substitute, rather than to yearn after her.

Clearly then, the experimenter, however carefully he sets up a controlled situation of temporary separation from the mother, and however carefully he records the infant's reactions to it, cannot fully understand his results. The baby's reactions are dependent not only on his mood, but also on minutiae of his normal daily life which even the most skillful retrospective interviewing cannot hope to elicit.

In the interests of a happy life for all, it is usually worth avoiding anxious protests over separation whenever possible. If a baby, despite being in the "sensitive" age group, has never protested at his mother's leaving the room, it is worth trying to maintain that comfortable state of affairs. If, on the other hand, a baby has made it abundantly clear that his anxiety threshold is low in this respect and the intensity of his distress high, it is equally worthwhile to avoid evoking, or at least to minimize, it. Attempts to deal with separation anxiety by firmness—by detaching the baby's clinging arms and putting him in a playpen, for example—almost always backfire. It does not take long for a baby who is anxious when mother leaves the room to learn to associate the sound of the front doorbell ringing not only with her imminent departure but also with that play prison. He may soon panic whenever his mother tries to put him in the pen, even if, on this occasion, her only motive is to keep him safe while older children rush in. Attempts to counteract separation anxiety by actual punishment may relieve the mother's feelings for the moment but will almost always add to her burdens in the longer term. The mother who reaches a point where she can no longer stand the baby crying every time she leaves the room to put away the ironing, to go to the lavatory, to check the oven, or whatever, may finally become so impatient that she dumps him in his crib and shuts the door on him "just until I've finished what I have to do." Once again the baby may quickly come to associate being put in his crib with lonely separation from an angry mother, rather than with peaceful sleep. Sleeping problems are infinitely more difficult to cope with than daytime separation anxiety so the mother will pay an extremely high price for her morning's peace.

Most infants only react extremely to vanishing mothers when they actually see them depart. The infant may be entirely content to wake alone in his crib, and talk and play until his mother comes to him. Equally if he was absorbed in play when she left the room, he may be unalarmed when he realizes he is alone, and only begin to search and worry for her after several minutes. Often sound is a reassurance. The infant can hear his mother moving around in the next room, or hear her speaking on the telephone. He knows where she is, knows that she has not vanished out of his familiar world, and therefore he does not demand her until he needs her for something. On the other hand, the mother of a highly anxious child who makes a practice of slipping away while he is busy may make matters worse. Often one can see this happening when the child is left to sleep in his crib or in his carriage. The mother settles him, spends some moments fiddling, just within his view, perhaps with the toys that hang on his carriage. Then, at a moment when the child is looking at the trees overhead, or getting his fist to his mouth, she slips away. A yell of betrayed fury follows. And if the pattern is repeated often enough, the infant may come to anticipate this kind of surreptitious departure, so that he begins to fuss at the mere sight of carriage or crib, knowing that they spell desertion. On the whole, with most infants, anxiety is less if the infant is told, by word, intonation, and gesture, when the mother is going to leave him. She may adopt a ritual of departure, such that she puts the baby down, tucks him in, adjusts the carriage hood, hands him his teddy bear, says, "See you soon," and leaves. There may still be tears, but they are tears at being left, not tears at being betrayed.

Separation when the infant is awake and up is usually best handled by avoidance whenever that is possible, and by calling the infant's attention to it when it is inevitable. The anxious infant who never knows whether he is going to look up and find his mother gone, can become the infant who keeps so constant an eye on his mother that he cannot play. If she must leave the room, and cannot take the baby with her, the mother can say she is going, and use whatever phrase the infant is accustomed to—"Won't be a minute" or "Back soon"—and then continue to talk to the infant as she carries the laundry downstairs, or whatever. Again the infant may cry, but his confidence is rebuilt a little each time his mother reappears as promised.

Separations lasting hours or days rather than minutes raise different problems. The infant at the height of his attachment to his mother, and anxiety over separation from her, will not easily tolerate such separations. His understanding of time and of space is negligible. He cannot hold in his mind a picture of his mother, nor of where she is. He cannot grasp the landmarks so useful with older children, such as, "Mummy will come by lunchtime." If she is gone, out of his sight, for longer than his short memory-span then, as far as we know, she is gone entirely from the infant's point of view. She is not where she usually is. She does not do for him what she usually does. And he has no way of understanding that the change is temporary. Some people scoffingly refuse to accept this. They may say, "You surely cannot believe that the baby whose mother goes out for the afternoon believes that she will never come back?" Of course the infant does not *think* this. He does not have the concepts with which to put such an idea together. But equally he does not have the concepts with which to put together the idea that she is sure to come back soon, that she loves him and would not desert him. All he can *know* is that she is gone. And it seems likely that since he is not yet an autonomous person, who can function without the adult care he is used to getting from his mother, he is left with an empty aching void, and a confused sense of loss of his own identity. His other half, his support, his control, his interpreter of the world is missing.

Infants should not be expected to span hours or days without a completing adult half. On the other hand they cannot, at least in our culture, have their mothers constantly with them. Mothers increasingly want and are expected to fill other roles as well as the mothering one. Ideally most people would like to see this dilemma solved by an equal participation in baby care from both parents. The child then has two attachment figures and a better chance that one of them will be available to him most of the time. In practical terms the ideal is not realizable for more than a tiny minority. However much couples believe in equal partic- ipation, however much fathers want to share equally in the baby's care, the majority of them cannot do so. Society is in the middle of a double bind over this. The mass media extol father's role yet employers still expect him to be present at his post throughout working hours. Books about child care stress the father's vital importance to his child, yet he cannot be physically present during his baby's waking hours except on holidays and on weekends. The participation of fathers has changed child care; it has changed the whole atmosphere of family life. But it has not yet come anywhere near to solving the problems of the baby's depen- dency. Sadly, for many men, the simple fact that they are *not* around the baby nearly as much as their wives often means that they are not entirely acceptable to their offspring as mother-substitutes. What the baby misses when his accustomed mothering figure goes away is her very familiarity; her predictability; the expressions of her face, intonations, games, partic- ular jokes, and so on. A father who has made a special effort to be present at home, because his wife will not be, often cannot provide this familiar- ity. It comes from hours and hours of routine daily interaction; the inten- tion to be fully participant is not enough.

A few couples manage to mix their work lives and their family lives together so that bringing up the children is just one important part of a totally joint lifestyle. Some may be couples who run a joint venture and live on the job—storekeepers, small farmers, or market gardeners, for example. Some may be students, living a jigsaw puzzle of study, part-time work and child care. Increasing numbers, during this economic recession, may have to rely on casual work and survive periods when neither is employed. If their morale is not too low, their babies may benefit from having one or both parents around even when those parents would much prefer to be out and earning. But most of the couples who can arrange to share their baby's care between them will be at the other end of the spectrum of advantage: professional people who freelance or are free to bring their work home or to choose the hours they spend at their jobs. Most parents have to rely on conventional jobs requiring attendance during office hours and often requiring additional hours spent commut- ing. They have to accept that they live in a society which still expects either that the mother will shoulder the major part of day-to-day child care while the father works, or that the child will be "taken care of" in some other setting while both parents work. Ours is still a society in which most people would be amazed if a father stayed home from the office because his child was sick and one in which colleagues and bosses do not expect to have to think about workers' children.

So if two parents are still prevented from sharing the care of one dependent baby between them, what is the answer to the dilemma of the mother with a child in this age group and outside commitments? I do not believe that there is one answer—only a range of compromises, some less desirable than others. I think each family has to work out a profit-and-loss account for itself over this issue and that doing so has become very little easier since this book was first written.

A great many women have to work. They do not do it for something called "personal fulfillment" but for something called money. If the family budget cannot balance without both parents' earnings or if the mother is solely responsible for the child, the economic argument has to take priority and the best possible arrangements made for the baby's care. But even this is not a clear-cut situation. At what level of income does earning take priority over child care? Some single mothers say "thank god for food stamps; they're the only thing that make it possible for me to keep the baby with me and survive." Some say "the food stamps help but there's no way you can keep two people on that." Some say "Food stamps? I haven't fallen that low yet I'm glad to say." If people are to experience their lives as decent, they have to be able to live somewhere near the standards they expect. Nobody has the right to sit in judgment on someone because the life they feel to be poverty would be affluence to someone else. Nevertheless while the woman who feels she has to work because she feels she must have the money must certainly be helped to do so, the woman who would rather be at home with her baby should be helped to do that, too. More money spent enabling mothers *not* to work if they prefer to be at home with very young children would undoubtedly be money well spent.

But what of all the others? The many women who—while they could certainly use the money—mainly want to work for other reasons? The rapidly expanding day-care movement is beginning to provide answers for those whose children are approaching pre-school age. Day care within the community, staffed by people who are part of children's lives outside as well as inside the center, can be excellent for these children and can help their parents toward a warm, close network of local friends, too. But for babies and young toddlers, group day care is almost always second best. Babies need an individual relationship with an adult who is completely sensitized to them, subconsciously in tune with them, familiar with all their cues. They need it on a one-to-one basis and they need it pretty well all the time. It is within and through this relationship that the baby learns all the most important lessons of his life, from language to loving.

While he is having this intensely personal relationship with somebody, the baby can also get a great deal out of additional relationships. It is good for him to learn that other people are different; that they do things in different ways, say different things, sing different songs. It is good for him, too, to learn to trust additional people and to rely on them. But floating populations of other people are only useful to him as extra to his basic person or people. They will not do instead, either emotionally or developmentally. Furthermore the child in this age group does not want, or benefit from being part of, a peer group. Human beings are not born in litters, and they are not ready to get anything out of group care, group play, before they are around two. Children who are just toddling can teach each other nothing. They cannot listen to each other; they are not ready to learn to respect each other and they have not the ability to put themselves in each other's shoes. A child of three can learn that it hurts when his hair is pulled and that he hurts others by pulling their hair. A baby of 15 months only knows that he himself is hurt: the effect of his own retaliation is totally lost on him. He is not ready for this kind of social learning. Various studies of young children in day care have shown that it has no ill effects on either infants or their relationship with their mothers. But while it is natural that mothers who need or want to make these arrangements for their babies should seize on such work with delight, it is important to look critically beneath the hopeful headlines. A lot of the research data applies to children older than the ones we are discussing here. The headline "Day care makes sociable kids!" appears over a photograph of 2- and 3-year-olds playing together. They are sociable *now* but how many of them were in the pictured facility before their first birthdays? "At last, the answer for working mothers!" announces another banner headline over a description of a new facility. But how many of those working mothers are really free to throw themselves wholeheartedly into a career job? Careful inquiry usually reveals that most of the women with the younger children leave them during hours which permit only a part-time job located nearby. The most careful large-scale study of the effects of day care on *babies* was published in 1978 [120] and showed no ill effects, indeed no significant differences at all, between the babies reared at home and those who spent their parents' full-time working hours in the center. But even this study must be read with care. It shows what can be done but it is very far from describing what is usual. A special day-care facility was set up for the study and staffed by professionals delighted to be included in it. Every imaginable facility for the excellent care, education, and happiness of babies and toddlers was built in and it suffered none of the staff changes or financial stringencies which bedevil most day-care centers. Each baby had his "special" caretaker who, working always in close cooperation and daily contact with his mother, served him as a substitute. If all babies whose mothers want to work outside their homes could be cared for to this standard there might be no problem; but while a community center might aspire to do this, there is no hope of such facilities becoming generally available. How could it be economic to provide one highly trained and experienced woman for every child whose mother (perhaps far less highly trained or paid) wanted to work?

Most of the children *of this age* who are in full-time group care do no more than survive the experience without visible damage. The fact that a child survives does not mean that the group care is good for him. It does not mean that he positively benefits from being in the group. So while parents may decide that they have the right to opt for day care for their baby so that they can both follow the jobs or careers they want, they need to realize that they are making the decision for themselves, not for the baby. If the day-care arrangement they find works out, if the baby settles and does not seem upset, if his basic relationship with the parents seems still secure, then they have got away with it. The profit and loss account is positive for the parents and neutral for the baby and that is a reasonable deal. But that profit and loss account is never going to show a *positive* for the baby in this age group, however much the parents may wish to convince themselves that it is good for him too; better than being smothered at home; more stimulating, more fun. They need to wait a year or two before all that will become true.

If mothers have a sufficiently high opinion of their own role, they can usually see that if they want to leave their less than 2-year-old regularly, what he really needs is a substitute mother. If he is not to go on having his mother or father to relate to most of the day, every day, then he needs somebody else. A few people still have grandparents both willing and available. A few more pay au pair girls or mothers' helpers. But perhaps the most usual satisfactory arrangement is the simple swap, the family next door or down the road who will love your baby if you will love theirs.

When the first edition of this book was published, I said that I felt the pressure on mothers to leave very young children in order to work was going too far. At that time, in the upsurge of the women's movement, there was a strong feeling that any woman who elected to stay home with a baby *ought to* feel bored or unfulfilled and was in some way letting down her sex. In the late seventies that kind of pressure eased a little. Most women's groups now recognize that real liberation must include the freedom to have and care for babies as well as freedom from having that role imposed. But where a mother must work or wants to work while her children are very young, the American solution still seems to be group care, whereas in most of Western Europe other solutions are preferred. In Sweden, for example, ideals of equal parenting are given legal backing in six months' statutory-paid paternity leave and then in job protection for fathers who want to remain at home full- or part-time. In Czechoslovakia many infants' groups have been disbanded in favor of a supervised system of "day-fostering" under which approved women care for three or four infants in their own homes. In Britain there are far more infants who are cared for by Day-Minders than in day centers and, while this partly reflects a shortage of centers, it also reflects the choice of many mothers who feel that an individual mother-substitute matters more to their baby than purpose-built facilities. We need to remain open-minded, to be willing to consider and to try a variety of options. Ultimately, though, the solution to meeting the rights and needs of both babies and women will probably come through enabling them to remain together during the first two years of known dependency and then providing liberal re-training and part-time programs so that mothers can easily return to work. With excellent contraception and liberal abortion laws, couples who do not want children need not have them. For those that do, a 2-year commitment for each child is not very long.

Even where a baby is being cared for within his family there is a great deal to be said for arranging that he have the opportunity to become attached to some other available person. There is a considerable amount of research which shows that children in this age group who protest bitterly if their mothers leave them either alone or with a stranger, remain calm, or protest only minimally, if they are left with a known (and presumably liked) person [133]. Data also show that such separations cause least distress if they take place in completely familiar surroundings [188]. There are certainly clues here for mothers planning separations, whether they are for regular work outside the home, for occasional time away from the baby or for longer trips caused by illness or family emergencies. Perhaps the most important clue is that the baby should, if possible, be left with someone to whom he is attached. That means that a mother planning a return to her profession needs to take the time to allow her baby to make friends with his future mother-figure *before* he is expected to accept mothering from her. It also means that every family, however determined the mother is to take full-time charge of her children, needs to ensure that there are other adults to whom they are attached. Emergencies strike, by definition, without warning. A child who is well-attached to two parents may seem well-provided-for. But should one parent be desperately ill in the hospital, the other will certainly want to be away from the baby, visiting and coping. There needs to be at least one other available adult to whom the baby is attached so that if disaster should strike he is left on a life-raft rather than struggling in a sea of complete despair [185].

The other important clue concerns familiarity of place. The ideal seems to be that the anxious baby should, whenever possible, be left in his familiar home surroundings. It is probably because au pairs care for children in their own homes that those children survive the constant changes of caretaker as well as they do. Most child-minders prefer children to come to them, but if all the adults concerned can be patient, the baby can become familiar with his minder's home before his mother ever leaves him there. Temporary and/or traumatic separations can almost always take place in the home if parents realize that this is preferable. Going to stay with Granny while mother has the new baby will probably cause far more upset than having Granny stay at home. Similarly, it is usually a mistake to take a baby to the airport to see a parent off or even to take him in the car to the railway station or to hospital reception. Everybody will stay calmer if good-byes are said in the living room.

Clearly stranger anxiety, even if it is not the *same* as separation anxiety, is closely related to it. In ordinary daily life, association with strangers is often part of a separation experience. If a child is left with a strange babysitter, and objects, it is impossible to know whether he is objecting to his mother's absence or the stranger's presence. Mothers' reports about their children's anxiety with strangers are often similarly confused. The baby may object to the clinic nurse undressing him. The mother thinks it is because she is strange, but it may be because he dislikes being held still for undressing, or even because he anticipates an injection such as he had at his last visit.

Morgan and Ricciuti [160] carried out a complex series of experiments with 80 children between 4 and 13 months. These studies have produced some hard facts out of the confusion.

They found that, overall, fear of strangers was less frequent (when the factor of separation from the mother had been excluded) than is usually thought. Furthermore anxiety became more frequent with increasing age, being almost absent in the 6-month babies, and reaching a peak at 1 year. It would certainly, from this sample, have been inappropriate to label it "8-months' anxiety."

At 6 months there was only one mildly negative reaction to the stranger. All the other babies of this age not only accepted the strangers, but became increasingly sociable as they approached and talked to them. And they were happy to respond to the strangers' advances whether they were seated on their mothers' laps, or in a baby chair some feet away from her.

Slightly increasing numbers of 8-, 10-, and 12-month babies evinced some degree of distress at the presence of a stranger. This distress was increased both in the number of babies it affected, and in intensity, both by distance from the mother, and by closeness to the stranger. By 12 months, babies could only tolerate the stranger if there was distance between them, and physical contact between baby and mother. Even so, more than half the 12-month babies were clearly uneasy. Any attempt by the stranger actually to touch the older babies evoked anxiety. On the other hand, smiling and nodding to the baby from a distance, playing a sort of "peek-a-boo," evoked a pleased response from almost all of them.

Recent studies [189] have confirmed the finding that babies, even at the 1-year peak of stranger anxiety, react better to strangers who offer them interaction than to those who sit impassively. Many authorities believe that this is because an impassive adult offers the baby no action-cues: provides no answer to the question "what should I do, faced with this strange person?" Not knowing what to do, the baby feels helpless and is therefore more likely to feel fearful. Offered friendly smiles and talk, some familiar kinds of re-action are suggested to the child, who will often respond happily. Perhaps the traditional way for visitors to avoid making babies shy—ignoring them—is not, after all, the effective way.

Taking this study, together with the existing literature, it does seem that we may over-estimate the tendency of infants to fear strangers in *themselves*, and underestimate the importance of what those strangers do. Some adults are shyer than others. But even the least shy would be disconcerted if a total stranger strode up in the street and hugged them. Similarly infants are often labeled as "shy of strangers" because they object when their mothers hand them over to admiring friends to be dandled, or weep piteously when a passing stranger tickles them in their carriages. Mothers who try to force their infants to accept physical advances from people they do not know probably increase their tendency to shy away. Just as detaching the arms of a clinging child only makes him more inclined to cling, so forcibly handing him to someone he does not want to go to can only increase his determination to keep away. If the child is allowed to go voluntarily from his mother's side to examine a strange visitor, not fearing physical capture onto her lap, if he is allowed to play peek-a-boo with strangers in shops, safely perched on his mother's shoulder, and not anticipating being handed over by her, he is far more likely to feel secure about exploring people. It even seems likely that he will eventually go more willingly to playgroup or nursery school or the houses of his friends.

Some mothers do not see the emotional demands which infants make during these months as "demands" at all. They are so attuned to the infant, so well rewarded for their sensitive mothering by his flattering attachment, that they meet the needs without thinking about them. Such mothers tend to talk constantly to their babies, to interact with them a great deal, to be always on the alert, noticing the infants' smiling gestures as they pass, and pausing to share what their babies are showing them even as they go about their own affairs. Many such women would feel it downright rude to walk down the street with the baby sitting facing them in a stroller and *not* chat. They would find it impossible to sit and read a book while the baby watched them. But other mothers feel more detached from the infant. They do not see him as a person, a companion —albeit a young one. And therefore they have to make a deliberate effort to meet the high emotional needs of this age period. In extreme cases the mother may consciously resent the infant's dependence and his refusal to accept other people. If a mother once begins to feel sucked dry by the demands of the infant, his behavior can fuel her resentment almost hour by hour. She goes to answer the door and he cries; she returns and calms him and tries to do the ironing while listening to the radio—he shouts for attention. A friend comes for coffee and the baby refuses to get off her lap or to keep quiet while she chats. When the friend leaves the mother goes to the bathroom. The baby screams and, if he is mobile, probably thunders piteously on the door. The mother becomes more and more convinced that she is being destroyed as a person in her own right. She is increasingly impatient of the infant's emotional demands; and the more she rejects them, the stronger they become.

We do not know why some mothers find it easy and some find it difficult. The reasons must be as diverse as the experiences and personalities of all mothers and all babies put together, so there will never be generalized answers. One factor can be the reaction of the father to the baby's extreme dependence on mother. Fathers who have been highly involved with the care of the baby from birth are usually so attuned to him emotionally that they can accept his emotional demands and respond to them. If this is so the father is likely to come in for his own share of clinging. He too may be flattered by tears when he departs. But it can work the other way. Participant fathers can be jealous in a situation where, having shared the baby's care, they do not share fully in his attachment. And fathers who have had less to do with the child's care may be in even worse shape. The more the baby demands from the mother, the more the husband may feel shut out: shut out from the relationship between baby and mother, and also from his own relationship with his wife. Obviously situations of this kind place the mother under extreme stress. She is, quite literally, in a love tug-of-war. All too often she finds herself unable to give either father or baby what he needs. Her husband's jealousy makes it impossible for her to tune in fully to her baby. Her baby's needs make it impossible for her to tune in to the husband. The baby has ceased to be a shared responsibility and pleasure and become a barrier. Research in progress on both sides of the Atlantic suggests that far from strengthening a marriage, a baby usually strains it to its limits.

Whatever the reasons for the mother's ease or difficulty in coping with this stage in the baby's development, the pattern does seem to repeat itself over the generations. Mothers who have been closely and sensitively mothered themselves find it easier to give this sensitive mothering to their infants, who will, in their turn, find parenthood rewarding. The converse—insensitive mothering following insensitive mothering— emerged clearly in a study of battered babies [105]. Parents who physically damaged their children, through "punishment" or "rough" handling, and who were unable to control their tempers (much though they usually wished to be "good parents") seemed to lack in their own lives what E. Erikson [75] called "basic trust." They had no sense of their own worth, and could not make their children feel valued. They did not believe that other people could understand them or meet their needs, and they could not understand nor meet the needs of their children. Perhaps "basic trust" is the prime benefit of the baby who, hour after hour, day after day, finds himself adequately cared for, adequately understood, sensitively responded to and enjoyed by the mother, and anyone else who is regularly involved in his daily life.

Happily not many parents batter their babies, producing physical injury which requires medical attention. The actual numbers cannot be assessed since doctors vary in their alertness to the possibility of battering when they see an injured child, parents vary in their readiness to seek medical aid, and hospitals vary in their readiness to report or record such incidents.

But a surprisingly large number of mothers not only physically punish children of this age group, but are prepared to say so to an interviewer. In the Newsons' British study [170], for example, 62 percent of mothers reported that they had smacked their babies before they were 1 year old. Of course the smacks ranged from a reminding pat on the hand, through a stinging slap on the legs, to a few real blows. But the *concept* of physical punishment for babies was clearly present. And it is a peculiar one.

A baby of this age who is punished cannot, realistically, be being punished for anything other than being a baby, or having a momentarily neglectful or forgetful mother. His behavior is under *her* control; his "goodness" is *her* business: it is an essential part of her mothering job to keep him safe and acceptable within his home setting. When he breaks an ornament he does so because his vital curiosity tells him to examine it, his neurophysiological control is too immature for him to examine it gently and his memory span is too short for him to remember that his mother told him not to. His mother forgot to put it out of his reach. Punishment seems irrelevant. Many mothers would accept this, but still say, "He ought to know better than to tip his dinner out of the dish all over my nice clean floor!" But why should he? A few minutes before, the mother herself was helping him tip bricks out on the floor. Is he supposed to share his mother's ideas about play materials versus eating materials? And as to that clean floor, the mother spent half the morning swooshing bubbly water over it; is the baby supposed to *understand* that soapy water cleans things and gravy dirties them?

Often the stresses which lead a mother actually to punish her baby arise out of his effect on other family members. Sometimes fathers are appalled by the asocial behavior of infants whom they see very little, and do not understand. Grandmothers may imply that babies in their day were not allowed to behave like this or like that. The mere presence of an irritated father or disapproving grandmother can make the mother far less tolerant than she would be if she were alone with the baby. Feeling that his behavior is reflecting badly on her, she may be more than usually inclined to slap him and dump him weeping in his crib. Again, older children may complain bitterly (and with reason) when handfuls of their hair are pulled out. The mother has learned to avoid this hazard for herself, but she may feel that justice demands that the older child should see the younger punished. All mothers have to work out the delicate tightrope of their family relationships for themselves. But punishments, at this age, are almost always pointless. The baby will mind the smack, but he will not understand the reasoning behind it. And because he does not understand it, the punishments are liable to escalate. If he is smacked for playing with an electric plug, he will forget in a few minutes. When he returns to the plug his mother is liable to smack him harder. The third time he does it she may lose her temper. It is far easier to avoid starting to punish than it is to stop in the face of what appears to be defiance.

And some punishments are dangerous. A smack that was intended to be gentle can catch a child off balance so that he bangs his head. Shaking him can produce a whiplash effect. His head is still heavy relative to his neck, and actual brain hemorrhages have been reported as a result of the brain banging inside the skull [45]. The mother may also pay dearly for less violent punishments. Being isolated from the mother as a punishment can suddenly increase a child's separation anxiety to fever pitch, so that for weeks he can barely be persuaded to let go of her skirt; being put to bed as a punishment can start sleeping problems.

Somehow the mother has to find ways of staying on the infant's side; of refusing to allow herself to feel against him; of nipping her own resentment in the bud and finding other ways of venting her stresses. Unfortunately our society's ideal is of the mother who mothers sensitively and likes it. To admit that you cannot or do not enjoy this stage of mothering is to admit to a kind of failure. Yet the various units which have been set up to *prevent* baby-battering, and the research groups which have studied mother-child relationships within this age group have all found that mothers were relieved simply to be allowed to admit to being irritated, without feeling censured. It is not easy being the other half of a developing person who is not yet a social being. If welfare authorities, husbands, and friends knew this, and could admire mothers for managing it, rather than taking it for granted as "natural," that in itself would make the job seem a little easier. After all, any difficult job seems more bearable if one is encouraged to be proud of oneself for doing it well.

20

MORE PHYSICAL
FUNDAMENTALS

FEEDING, SLEEP, AND TOILETING are the three main areas within which the physiological needs of infants are met. As such they are obviously important. A child who is not reasonably cared for in physical terms cannot develop fully in other areas. Yet in Western societies the importance of these physical-care issues tends to be over-stressed, especially once the newborn period, during which they are vital, is over. Eavesdropping on mothers chatting together at a welfare clinic, a baby's meals, his sleeping habits, his "progress" in toilet training are continual subjects for riveting discussion. But a mother's attempt to discuss her baby's motor progress, his language development, or his social understanding tends to receive only cursory attention. Hospitals, even those which pride themselves on their forward-looking arrangements for play and emotional care for sick children, put these a long way down the list of budget priorities. Excellent physical care always comes first. Even day nurseries—with some honorable exceptions—tend to show off their tiny toilets, their airy cribs, and their attractive menus. The visitor must ask if he wants to know how the children's other needs are catered for.

There is no doubt that any infant who can be persuaded to follow his mother's wishes in these areas makes her daily life comparatively easy. If he will eat what she puts before him, sleep when she puts him to bed, and accept her toileting program, her child care will be smooth. This is probably why success in any of these areas is such a subject for congratulation between mothers. A baby who will do these things is a "good" baby. His mother is, by definition, a "good" mother: she has not spoiled him or let him get away with anything. If such a good baby is also happy, active, alert, and intelligent, well and good. But if he is not, he is still a good baby. On the other hand if he is alert, active, and happy, but a fussy feeder who sleeps little and soils much, he is definitely *not* good. He will be fortunate if he is allowed to remain happy.

A concern with issues which make the job of rearing an infant easier is obviously fair enough. But it is important that all those who are even marginally concerned with infant care should realize to whom these things are important. They matter to the mother, her convenience and her pride, far more than they matter to the baby. Just *because* eating and sleeping and eliminating are basic physiological functions, the infant, given normal care, will look after them for himself. If he is offered a reasonable diet, he will eat enough to keep himself well; he does not care whether his dinner constitutes a "balanced meal"—it is his mother who cares. As long as he is not subject to acute physical or emotional stress, he will sleep as much as he needs to. He does not care if it is 5 A.M. when he finishes his night, but his mother does. Nothing but full-fledged disease will make him harm himself from constipation; he will pass a bowel movement when he needs to and only his mother cares whether it goes in a pot or his clothes. Very few normal children from ordinary families in Western societies reach school age starving, exhausted from lack of sleep or incontinent. But many well-nourished, rested, continent children reach school emotionally impoverished, verbally incompetent, physically ill-coordinated, and pitifully ignorant of the world and how it works.

Perhaps we should readjust our thinking a little, so that we sort out which issues are important to maternal convenience, and which are truly important for the child. The baby who makes good use of his time awake is just as "good" for himself as the baby who goes to sleep on schedule is "good" for his mother. From this standpoint mothers are at least as much to be congratulated on finding a new entrancing game for their infants as for finding a new baby cereal they will eat.

FEEDING

Traditionally, weaning is one of the major maternal preoccupations of this half year. It was during these months that infants had to be persuaded gradually to relinquish the breast or their bottles in favor of increasing quantities of solid food, with milk from a cup. But from the kind of information discussed in Chapter Thirteen, and from observation of mother-baby pairs, it is clear that this pattern has changed. Infants are now normally given a wide range of solid foods from a very few weeks of age, so that their diet even at 3 months approximates the diet of a 9-month baby a generation ago. Very few are breast-fed at all, and only an infinitesimal number are still breast-fed by 6 months. And the bottles are often not withdrawn. They simply stop being receptacles for "feedings" and become receptacles for comfort drinks. Even where a mother does determinedly wean her infant from the bottle, she is more likely than ever before to provide him with alternatives. Pacifiers, for example, are widely used in the United Kingdom by all social classes, while learning to drink from a cup is eased by the use of cups with spouts from which the infant half sucks, half drinks. Present-day grandmothers can probably still remember exactly when they weaned today's mothers. But those mothers find it very difficult to say when they wean *their* babies; it depends what you mean by weaning.

The tendency to allow the infant bottles of milk at bedtime, or even bottles of milk *ad lib.*, while building up his diet toward a full mixed one, leads to some nutritional difficulties. As we saw in Chapter Thirteen, no assessment can be made of any infant's food requirements until his milk intake is known. Once that milk has become a comfort and a beverage, rather than a food, even the mother may not know how much the baby actually drinks. If he drinks a good deal of milk, as we shall see, it is neither sensible nor desirable to expect him much to increase his intake of "real" food, for he will only get fat. On the other hand if the bottle has been taken from him, or if it has been filled with juice rather than milk, so that his milk intake has dropped drastically, he will genuinely need far more solid food than before.

The food requirements of the infant (whether he is a hungry or less hungry child) do not rise in direct proportion to his age. In the early months he grew faster than he does in this second half year. His requirements were therefore proportionately higher then than now. This is reflected in the official recommendations for the food energy to be provided for groups of infants in this half year as compared with the first. It is thought that groups of infants between 3–6 months of age should have made available to them 52 kilocalories per pound of their bodyweight (115 kcal per kg). Between 6–12 months that recommended figure drops to 49 kcal per pound (107 kcal per kg).

As we have continually stressed, the needs of any individual infant may be very different from any group average, but, nevertheless, individual needs will, to some extent, be related to individual weight. While a small baby *might* need more food than a larger baby of the same age, the larger baby is *likely* to need more food especially if he is genuinely large —long as well as heavy—rather than obese and possibly rather inactive.

An average birthweight baby who has consistently gained weight at the expected rate will probably consume around 800 kcal each day, rising to around 1000 as he nears his first birthday. Obviously no parent is going to be foolish enough to try and count the baby's calorie intake, but it is worth noticing that he needs only a quarter more food at a year old than at 5 months. Many feeding difficulties start because unreasonably large helpings are served to babies when they start to join the family meals.

Apart from very gradually increasing calories, the infant needs no more of any particular nutrient than he did at 0–5 months of age. The protein, vitamins, and minerals which he should have available to him all remain the same. He could, therefore, be fed just as he was in the earlier period except for the question of milk. Most babies, by 6 months, will no

TABLE 6. DIFFERENCES BETWEEN THE OVERALL NUTRIENTS RECOMMENDED FOR GROUPS OF BABIES
AND THE INTAKES OF INDIVIDUALS FROM VARIOUS QUANTITIES OF UNMODIFIED COW'S MILK

	Total Calories kcal	Protein g	Minerals		Vitamins					
			Calcium mg	Iron mg	A µg	D µg	Thiamine mg	Riboflavin mg	Acid mg	C mg
Recommended group provision	895	22	600	6	450	10	0.3	0.4	5	20
Infant taking 32 oz. (915 ml)	320	0	0	6	100	10	0	0	0	20
Infant taking 20 oz. (1 pt) (about 600 ml)	535	4	0	6	230	10	0.1	0	0	20
Infant taking 10 oz. (1/2 pt) (about 300 ml)	710	13	260	6	340	10	0.2	0	2	20

Note. Cow's milk usually contains a trace of vitamin D, but this is too small and too variable to be a reliable contribution to the diet. The vitamin C content may be high in summer, but how much reaches the infant's digestion depends on season, cow's diet, heat treatment of milk and exposure to sunlight. For practical purposes it is best to treat cow's milk as containing no vitamin C.

longer be given an infant milk formula, but will be drinking liquid cow's milk like the rest of the family. As we saw on page 228, liquid cow's milk does not provide the vitamins and minerals the infant needs, without supplementation. Furthermore, the infant's milk consumption may drop due to weaning, or at least to a change in his mother's attitude to his bottle-feedings. Table 6 tries to highlight the importance of milk in the baby's diet and the impossibility of sensibly planning his solid meals without taking his milk consumption into account. It sets out the recommended intakes of various nutrients for *groups* of babies and contrasts these with the nutrients which an individual child will get from various quantities of unsweetened liquid cow's milk. Assuming that the baby continues to drink roughly 32 oz. of milk, but that it is now the ordinary milk bought for the family, he will need more calories, almost all his iron, and vitamins A and C. The vitamins are available and recommended by all pediatricians and health centers for babies of this age, but it is difficult to know how many families actually buy and regularly use them. In the United Kingdom they have been available for years at a specially subsidized price, and it is known that only a small percentage of families avail themselves of this health measure. The supplementation is vitally important.

The use of vitamin C-containing fruit juices for babies is widespread and if these are used then a deficiency is extremely unlikely whatever else the baby does or does not eat or drink. A single jar, for example, of any of Gerber's strained juices will yield at least 40 mg of vitamin C, and this is well above the baby's daily requirement.

Vitamin D is a much more difficult problem. "Enough" is vital to a growing child. Without it his body cannot efficiently use the calcium and phosphorus which enable him to build strong bones and teeth. The result can be hypocalcemia which, left untreated, may progress to frank rickets and permanent deformities. "Too much," on the other hand, can be dangerous. Hypercalcemia can lead to the formation of extra bony deposits, osteomalacia.

The margin between "too little" and "too much" vitamin D and its associated use of calcium by the body is confused by the fact that human beings manufacture vitamin D for themselves when bare skin is exposed to sunlight. If there is plenty of sunshine and the infant spends time in it, even if only his arms and face are exposed, he may need no dietary vitamin D at all. If there is no sunshine or if the infant is seldom out of doors, his need for vitamin D may be urgent. In recent years health authorities have veered back and forth between this Scylla and Charybdis. Some cases of hypercalcemia were reported and the levels of vitamin D in fortified infant foods were reduced as a result. But cases of frank rickets, and of hypocalcemia likely to lead to rickets if left untreated, have also been reported. In 1972, for example, a study of 569 children in the British Midlands revealed 17 with frank rickets with major deformities of the bones while 40 percent of the children studied showed at least some degree of hypocalcemia [107]. In 1980 Brooke [39] and his colleagues reported on a study of 67 Asian women and their newborn babies. This study showed that a low consumption of vitamin D during pregnancy was related to low vitamin D concentrations in the baby at birth, together with sub-optimal formation of the bones of the skull and, in 5 of the infants, to symptoms, from birth, that meant rickets would inevitably have developed if treatment had not been instigated.

Dark skins are adapted to protect people who live in sunny climates. People with dark skins who live in comparatively sunless climates are therefore particularly at risk of rickets. The skin pigment protects them, in this particular too well, from the little available sunshine. But people do not only vary in the amount of sunshine which is available to them or the amount of that sunshine which their skins can absorb, they also vary in the extent to which they expose themselves to sunshine. Racial and geographical differences are therefore complicated by cultural ones. Dark children living in close-packed city streets in New York have more than enough sunshine available to them in summer and very little in winter. If they habitually play outdoors in the summer months, they may build sufficient stores of vitamin D to carry them through the cold and cloudy winter, but if their parents shun the street or stoop as a play-place and have no yards or parks to offer, they may lack sunshine all the year round. Ethnic minorities, especially those who have recently arrived in the host-country and have not yet adapted to its lifestyle, may be at greater risk of vitamin D deficiency than their skin color alone would suggest. In Britain, for example, many Asian mothers spend most of their time indoors and keep young children with them. In the United States the same is true of Vietnamese families. Both groups are at greater risk of deficiency than are their much darker-skinned neighbors of West Indian origin but British or American lifestyle.

With so many climatic and social variables to consider, as well as the wide variation in individual susceptibility to under- or overdosage, it is extremely difficult to give generally applicable advice on vitamin D intakes. This has recently been recognized in Britain, where official reports published in 1980 and 1981 [59] place a heavy responsibility on baby clinic staff to adapt overall recommendations to individual circumstances. The milk sold in Britain for family consumption is not fortified with vitamin D, so the need for supplementation usually begins as soon as a baby stops taking infant-formula. But it is left to the health professionals to decide whether, in a particular family, a baby should have supplementary vitamin D even while he is drinking fortified formula (because his other circumstances make it likely that he is vulnerable to deficiency) or whether a toddler will be better off without extra vitamin D because he eats fortified baby cereals and spends most of his days outside in sunshine with few clothes.

In the United States the position is different because all milk is fortified with vitamin D. Until recently this valuable health measure made rickets virtually unknown even among the dark-skinned urban poor. Now, however, doctors are alert to the possibility of vitamin D deficiency among the increasing numbers of children who are forbidden milk—or allowed only minute quantities—because of allergy. Children who are fed on formula based on soy rather than cow's milk and are then weaned onto a diet which excludes dairy produce will require careful supplementation to ensure that their weanling—and later—diet provides the vitamin D (and calcium) which was included in that infant-formula but may now be lacking. A major group of nutrients, such as dairy produce, should never be excluded from a child's diet without continuing medical advice.

Lack of vitamin A is almost unknown either in the United States or in Britain. Pharmacists tend to express more concern about overdosage than underdosage. Nevertheless people do require some vitamin A and most babies will be the better for a carefully controlled supplement unless they eat a great deal of cheese-fortified margarine, liver, or are regularly given fortified "infant dinners."

Iron needs are difficult to assess as iron is stored in the liver and is used and re-used by the body; it is lost only very gradually in excretion. A child who has adequate iron stores may need very little dietary iron to keep them topped up. On the other hand a child whose stores are already depleted—perhaps due to his mother's inadequate diet during pregnancy and/or breast-feeding, or perhaps due to physical injury leading to blood loss—may become anemic if he does not get enough. Providing iron is not simple either because the body will only absorb and use certain kinds. Unless a doctor diagnoses iron-deficiency anemia in a baby and prescribes for him iron-fortified baby cereals, the occasional egg yolk and, if he will eat it, some liver from time to time, will keep the baby adequately supplied. Mothers of liver-hating infants who detest eggs may find it useful to know that chocolate is also a comparatively good iron source. Drinking chocolate contains around 3 mg in every two teaspoons, while cocoa powder contains even more. Chocolate to eat (provided that it is real chocolate rather than "chocolate flavored candy") has around 1 mg in every bar.

Dropping the milk intake to a mere 1 pint (about 600 ml) per day makes a difference to the infant's remaining dietary needs mainly in terms of simple calories. He must now get more than half his total calories from solid food, instead of only a quarter. But in other respects that pint of milk still protects him from deficiencies. His protein intake falls just under the recommended intake, although it is still above the minimum. But in practice such a small protein lack could not fail to be filled by his solid food, whatever items of diet were chosen to fill his calorie gap. His intake of calcium is still adequate and consumption of the B vitamins is almost so. The trace of thiamine which is missing on paper will again certainly be made good by the traces present in almost all ordinary foods. His need for vitamin A supplementation has gone up, and his position with respect to vitamins D and C remains the same. The infant can still therefore be fed so as to satisfy his calorie and iron needs, just so long as he receives regular vitamin supplementation.

Mothers who buy infants of this age expensive protein foods—choosing "high-protein" cereals, and trying to persuade the baby to eat meat and fish—do him no physical harm, but he does not need this added protein. And if they are on a tight budget, they may be giving him protein foods he will simply waste, biochemically, rather than giving them to older children whose bodies actually need them.

Dropping the milk intake to 1/2 pint (about 300 ml) per day does radically alter the nutritional picture. The infant now lacks some of what he might need of almost everything. Above all, his protein and calcium intakes are now below safe levels, and these vital nutrients are not easily available as supplements. If such a child will not take more milk, then he must be treated as completely "weaned." His milk must be regarded only as a valuable extra, and he must be fed a complete diet, just as an older child is fed. Chapter Twenty-five, on feeding in the second year, may be useful.

In practice a milk intake as low as 1/2 pint is unusual at this age unless milk is being deliberately excluded from the diet. Mothers often report that the child takes this quantity when they mean that he drinks that much in liquid form. A considerable amount of milk goes into ordinary cooking. A further bout of kitchen experimentation showed the quantities of milk needed to prepare some very ordinary foods often fed to infants in this age group.

Using proprietary baby cereals, the amount of milk absorbed proved variable, but none took less than 2 oz. (60 ml) of milk, and most took 3–4 oz. (90–115 ml) to produce a serving of four slightly heaped tablespoons.

Scrambling an egg yolk, to the soft consistency preferred by most infants, used 1 oz. (30 ml) of milk.

Mashing a half potato to a soft texture used 1/2 oz. (15 ml) of milk, while a serving of potato soup, or other creamed vegetable soups, took 2 oz. (60 ml).

Cornstarch pudding or tapioca pudding gets most of its food value from the milk with which it is made, while some infants will like Jello for dessert made up with milk instead of water.

Of course the actual amount of milk *consumed* by the infant, in the form of foods of this kind, will depend on his appetite. Many infants will not eat portions of this size; or a good deal may go on his chin, or the floor. But over a whole day, most mothers who cook for their infants will find that they have *served* him a good deal of "concealed" milk.

Clearly baby cereals are again an excellent help in feeding the infant who drinks little milk. They take half a feeding bottle to mix one portion; when mixed they provide around 120 calories, 5–6 grams of protein, 150–200 mg of calcium, about 3 mg of iron and all the missing B vitamins.

As we saw in Chapter Thirteen, almost all mothers studied in recent years have stated that they use ready-prepared infant foods, in cans and jars, almost to the exclusion of home-cooked foods. Where milk is still meeting most of the infant's vital nutritional needs, the exact composition of these canned foods need not concern the mother very much. They will certainly contain adequate calories and she knows that his vitamins must be supplemented anyway. But where an infant is taking little milk, some thought does need to be given to what he is getting in his canned dinners. They are often criticized for being too starchy and too sweet. The latter charge is a valid one. The infant who is accustomed to strained or junior fruits will probably refuse freshly stewed apples, even with a reasonable addition of sugar. His canned varieties are more like jam than fresh fruit.

But the charge that the canned dinners contain too much carbohydrate is rather different. Often it is an economic rather than a nutritional charge. When you buy a jar of "Junior Beef Dinner," you buy 7 grams of protein, equivalent to a flat tablespoon of lean minced stewing beef, and yielding 69 calories. The remaining 54 calories in the jar are made up of a little fat and a lot of starch. This does mean that you are buying rather little actual meat for your money. Clearly the exact composition of the meals should be stated on the jar, so that mothers could see exactly what they were buying. If an infant is gaining weight too fast, so that the mother wants to keep his carbohydrate consumption down while still ensuring his other nutrients, she must clearly cook for him herself, rather than buying composite meals which allow of no adjustment. But then if she were dieting herself she would not expect to do it on bought steak and kidney pie. But in other circumstances, the balance is not an unreasonable one in nutritional terms. A return to the kitchen produced the following comparisons between a widely available canned infant dinner, an equally available infant supper, and their home-cooked equivalents (see Table 7).

Both the home-cooked lunch and the home-cooked supper would be regarded as "ideal" by most people. Yet the lunch yielded only a little more protein than the canned variety, and it had a few more calories too. Similarly the home-cooked supper yielded one third more protein than the can, but one third more calories as well.

These findings hardly support the charge that the canned foods are "all starch" and "much too fattening" and that they have "no goodness in them." A baby would have been more inclined to get fat on these home-cooked dishes than on their canned equivalents, and while he would have got a little more protein as well, it would almost certainly have been protein he did not need. After all the baby on 1/2 pint (300 ml) of milk per day is only taking 11 grams of protein less than the "safe level" for his group. One such jar of dinner together with one serving of baby cereal amply fills that theoretical need. After that it is most unlikely that he requires or benefits from more protein; he only needs more fuel-food, more calories to satisfy his appetite. Mothers who want to use convenience foods but are worried about what is in them are better catered for

TABLE 7. COMPARISON BETWEEN TWO PROPRIETARY CANNED INFANT MEALS AND
THEIR HOME-COOKED EQUIVALENTS

Canned meal	Home-cooked meal

"Beef Dinner"	1 oz. (30 g) cooked, lean minced stewing beef
	  69 kcal, 7 g protein
	half a medium-sized potato, mashed
	(1 tablespoon)
	  45 kcal, 0.8 g protein
	One small carrot, boiled and mashed
	(1 dessertspoon)
	  23 kcal, 0.7 g protein
	One tablespoon stock, to mix
	Negligible food value

Total 3 tablespoons of food
  123 kcal
  7 g protein
	Total 3 tablespoons of food
	  137 kcal
	  8.5 g protein

While the home-cooked meal does yield a little more protein (1 1/2 g) it also yields more calories (14). In real terms the differences between the two meals are nutritionally insignificant. A somewhat fattier meat or smaller carrot would be enough to cancel the difference out.

Canned meal	Home-cooked meal
"Cheese and Egg Supper"	1/2 egg 1/4 oz. (7 g) American cheese 2 oz. (60 ml) milk Baked together to make a custard

Total 3 tablespoons of food
  75 kcal
  4 g protein
	Total 3 tablespoons of food
	  110 kcal
	  6.5 g protein

Here the difference between the protein content of the two meals (2.5 g) is almost exactly matched by the difference in calorie value (35 kcal). Each meal yields about 2 g of protein for every 35 kcal. The infant who eats the home-cooked meal is therefore simply getting more to eat than is the infant who eats the canned meal. Spoonful for spoonful the home-cooked meal is more concentrated, but the constituent balance is almost identical; only the bulk is different.

than they used to be. Among the ranges of more expensive babyfoods are now many single-item jars—containing only a meat or a single fruit or vegetable—as well as jars which are guaranteed not to contain substances which are banned from the diets of babies with common food-allergies. In the United States the labeling of babyfoods is both comprehensive and reliable. Mothers who will take the time to read those content-lists and can spend the money to buy from the quality ranges will probably be able to find what they need.

Some infants prefer home-cooked foods, and some mothers enjoy preparing them. If this is so there are all kinds of benefits, both nutritional and social. Nutritionally they are better than "complete dinners" in that they are flexible. More potato can be given if the child is extra-hungry; less sugar can be added if he is having diarrhea; carbohydrates in general can be cut down if he is gaining weight too fast, or the concentrated calories of some extra fats can be added if he is gaining weight slowly and cannot eat much bulk.

Socially, home-cooked meals may be better in that they enable the baby to share (with suitable mincing and manipulating) what the rest of the family is eating. And they enable him, too, to get used to a variety of flavors and of textures at an early age.

While it is not fair to say that canned infant foods all taste the same, they do tend to be extremely bland if they are for the main course, or very sweet if they are sweet at all. Perhaps more important, their texture is consistent from meal to meal. Baby cereal mixed runny or stiff is still perfectly smooth. Canned dinners progress from strained, through junior to toddler, but the minced texture of the junior foods is consistent, and the chopped-up quality of the toddler foods is consistent. And there are no contrasts: no crisp toppings of browned cheese on a canned cheese entrée. An infant who expects all his food to have this sameness may find it very difficult to adapt to that "good mixed diet" toward the end of his first year.

But if the mother does not want to take the time to prepare baby-foods, and if the infant accepts canned varieties, there is nothing nutritionally wrong with them. And there is no doubt that they do save an enormous amount of time. All the mother needs to do is to make sure that she has some idea what she is feeding to the baby. If she intends to use jars extensively, it might well be worth her writing to the manufacturers of her chosen brands, asking for their analysis sheets of different varieties. The idea is not that she should make any attempt to balance the contents of a jar against her baby's nutritional needs, but simply that she should avoid being fooled by the descriptive names given to these foods. These names give no clue to the overall food value—in terms of calories —or to the protein richness of the particular meal. Similarly named "main courses" may literally contain half as many calories or half as much protein as each other. Often the puddings contain more calories than the main courses, while the "breakfast" and "supper" jars vary even more unexpectedly. The unwary mother tends to assume that an "egg-and-bacon breakfast" will be roughly equivalent to a "scrambled egg breakfast." But she would be wrong. If enough people asked to see the manufacturers' analyses, they might begin to realize that mothers will buy a dinner in a jar, but not if it is a pig in a poke.

Whether or not a mother uses prepared babyfoods, at around 6 months the infant must be given the opportunity to learn to chew food. Often it is assumed that he will not chew until he has teeth to do it with.

Often also it is unthinkingly assumed that once he has his four front teeth he is ready to chew. In fact the critical period for learning to chew seems to pre-date the appearance of any teeth at all, and chewing is certainly not assisted by those first teeth, which are for biting, not for grinding.

In the early months the infant sucks his food; then he learns to let semi-solids slide down his throat. But he still has to learn to use his jaws to convert genuinely solid foods into swallowable textures and he is certainly ready to start by 6 months. Obvious foods for practice chewing are peeled quarters of raw apple, strips of raw carrot, pieces of toast, zwiebacks or the occasional cookie. At the same time, even if the infant's main food is still proprietary babyfood, some vegetables should be given him diced up rather than mashed, so that he can practice picking them up with his fingers, putting them in his mouth, and chewing them. The new experiences of taste and texture tend to be far more acceptable to the baby if he has them under the control of his own fingers than if they are dumped in his mouth from his mother's spoon.

Around 6 months is also the time when many babies begin to imitate people around them—and often especially their mothers. So again this is the time when the infant should be given every opportunity to start to feed himself with a spoon, preferably while his mother is eating her food too. Some infants, who *have* been given the chance, can feed themselves completely by 9 months.

As the infant takes over responsibility for feeding himself, both with his fingers and with a spoon, his own appetite, his eager eating, becomes again the reliable guide to the quantities he needs, which it was in the earliest weeks of life when he was given only milk. Once the infant is competent at feeding himself when he is hungry, or when he particularly likes the offered food, or when he is racing his older sister, he should be regarded as competent on *all* occasions. There is no curious quirk of infant development which makes a child able to feed himself his favorite dessert, and unable to feed himself shepherd's pie. Mothers recognize this if it is put to them, but they still tend to say, "I just help him a bit at the end, you know, when he is getting bored," or "When he's tired, I feed him." Feeding him when he can feed himself is asking for later trouble. An infant who is too bored to bother to eat is not hungry enough to need to eat. And if he is too tired to feed himself he is overtired and should sleep first.

Finger foods rapidly progress from being entertainment, practice, and education for the baby and become *food*. The slice of toast which at 6 months he mouthed and sucked may be eaten to the last crumb at 9 months—all 72 calories and 2 grams of protein of it, not to mention that butter. . . . It is at this point that "snacks" may begin to amount to a significant proportion of the infant's daily food—and a misleading proportion to the researcher, because mothers often do not count them,

TABLE 8. IMPORTANT CONSTITUENTS OF SOME "SNACK" FOODS

	Portion	Calories	Protein g	Other significant constituents
Milk chocolate	Children's bar or half a 2 oz. bar or 16 M&M's	164	2.5	70 mg calcium; 0.5 mg iron
Vanilla ice cream	smallest cone	55	1.2	40 mg calcium
Plain sweet cookies	2 cookies	141	1.6	Some calcium, iron, B vitamins
Chocolate cookies	2 cookies	142	2.0	Some calcium, iron, B vitamins
Currant buns	1 bun	190	4.4	0.5 mg iron, some D and B vitamins
Plain cake (pound type)	Small slice	122	1.7	Some iron and B vitamins
Banana	Half small banana	22	0.5	
Raisins	Heaped tablespoon	71	0.5	0.5 mg iron
Potato chips	Individual packet of approx. 23 g or just under 1 oz.	145	1.8	Trace elements varying according to brand and added flavorings

when they are asked what the baby has eaten in the past 24 hours. Recent surveys, large and small, all suggest that snacks are now the rule not the exception. Infants commonly have cookies or zwiebacks on waking in the morning. A mid-morning snack of cookies and a drink is universal, and most also have a mid-afternoon snack, perhaps of cake or more cookies. In addition, a high proportion of infants get some sweets every day— often on a daily trip to the store—and ice cream or ice pops on most days. Table 8 gives the more important constituents of such foods. They are often thought of as "impoverished," but this generalization is meaningless. If snack foods are intended to give the infant calories and pleasure, there is nothing the matter with them nutritionally. But, of course, they cannot give pleasure without giving calories. So if they make the infant unenthusiastic about his real meals, they can *lead* to an impoverished diet overall. Similarly if they do *not* make him unenthusiastic about his real meals, they may make him fat.

SLEEP

Sleep tends to be a major preoccupation among mothers of babies in this age period. As we have seen, caring for the infant becomes increasingly demanding, both physically and emotionally, in the second half year. As the baby gets older, and especially as he begins to be mobile, the mother can accomplish less and less while he is awake. His naptimes and the evening when he is asleep may be the only times when she can accomplish jobs which with his "help" are potentially dangerous. They may also be the only times when she can do anything at maximum speed and with maximum efficiency. The vast majority of babies are therefore given ample opportunity to sleep. Great trouble may be taken to ensure that they are warm, comfortable and undisturbed. One can assume that between 6 and 9 months the hours of sleep the infant takes are the hours he needs. He still cannot keep himself awake voluntarily.

Unfortunately the hours of sleep he needs and takes are often not the hours his mother would like him to take. And many mothers are misled in their expectations by the pattern of sleep suggested as necessary by many widely used handbooks of infant care. An average figure, taken from several handbooks published for mothers by babyfood manufacturers, for example, would be 16 to 17 hours for infants between 6 and 9 months. Even Dr. Spock [209], while accepting individual variation in sleep needs, suggests 14–16 hours' sleep at 1 year, and suggests that mothers should do all they can to encourage infants to sleep this much.

What evidence we have suggests that many babies sleep very much less than this. The Newsons [169] found a range, at 1 year, from 9 to 18 hours per day. The average in their survey was 13 1/2 hours. N. Kleitman and T. G. Engelmann [129] similarly found infants averaging 13 1/2 hours at 6 months, and maintaining this figure, with a drop to around 13 hours at the age of 2.

Most babies from 6 months will normally sleep through the night—at least in terms of the hours of sleep, even if there are brief awakenings. Such a night probably amounts to roughly 12 hours of sleep. Any remaining sleep is in the form of daytime naps. The majority of babies from 6–9 months still need two such naps. But they vary in length from 20 minutes of actual *sleep* to 3 hours.

Provided that the infant does not come to associate his crib or carriage with loneliness, or with crossness from his mother, he may well be happy to spend an hour twice a day in it, even if he does not actually sleep for all of this time. Many babies seem to enjoy a period alone, with plenty of interesting things to look at or play with. Often a carriage in the garden, where there are trees moving, clouds, shadows, the occasional bird, is popular. Failing that, toys in his crib, mobiles and pictures to look at, may keep him equally happy. If this pattern can be kept to, it serves the double purpose of giving the mother a little peace and privacy, while leaving the baby free to sleep as and when he needs to.

Occasionally, mothers who are rightly anxious not to make the infant feel that they wish to be rid of him are quick to abandon one of the daytime rest periods as soon as it becomes clear that the child barely sleeps during it. A protesting cry as she leaves, and the infant's struggles to sit himself up, may be enough to make her abandon that nap altogether. In fact, a brief protest on being left is so frequent as to be normal at this age. The infant would prefer his mother to stay. And he states this fact. If he settles down happily within a couple of minutes, all is well. Far more important is to go to him swiftly when he wakes up from a nap, or finally decides that he has had enough rest time. If he is left crying at this point, he is very likely to be put off the whole business of being left alone. He must know that when he needs his mother, she will come.

As we have seen in earlier chapters, and as the range of hours of sleep around the research averages shows, infants vary in their sleep requirements. A baby who goes to sleep peacefully, and within a few minutes of being put to bed at night, or at some point during an hour's daytime rest, can be assumed to have had all the sleep he needs if he wakes after an 8-hour night or a 10-minute nap. In these circumstances the mother has the problem, not the baby. He is awaking because he has finished sleeping. He cannot go to sleep again at will because he is not tired. His mother cannot put him back to sleep again. The "problem" has to be lived with. If the parents try to force the child to sleep more, a wakeful infant is liable to turn into an infant who *does* have sleep problems. A baby who sleeps from 8 P.M. to 5 A.M. every night, and for two periods of 15 minutes during the day is exhausting. Every possible way of helping him remain content, alone, until a later hour in the morning and, perhaps, from a somewhat earlier hour in the evening, should be tried. A sleeping bag— with sleeves, so that there is no way the infant can get down inside it and smother himself—will keep him reasonably warm while he plays in his crib. Carefully chosen toys will go some way toward keeping him occupied. Sharing a room with an early-waking toddler may keep both children occupied first thing in the morning. At the same time the house needs to be organized so that it is as easy as possible for the mother to accomplish what she needs to do during the day, while in the constant company of the wakeful infant. Once the mother can accept that the baby is not going to sleep in the daytime, once she stops feeling that he ought to sleep, and wasting time and emotional energy on settling him and resettling him for naps he does not need, she and the infant can often arrive at a *modus vivendi*. If there simply is no room for the infant to play safely on the kitchen floor, the mother may find herself doing the vegetables in the playroom. If the infant will not stay in his playpen, and she must use a sewing machine, she and the machine can go inside the pen, leaving the infant to roam, safely protected from the needle, outside. Even the typical mode of interaction between infant and mother may be affected by his wakefulness. A baby who sleeps for 2 hours in the morning, waking for one hour before his lunch, may be able to claim his mother's undivided attention for that hour, especially if she knows he will sleep again in the afternoon. So she may play with him, her other commitments already met. But the baby who is awake all morning has to allow her to do other things than play, part of the time. The pair may adopt ways of playing which do not involve the mother abandoning everything else. The mother can talk while she works, smile and make faces, show the infant what she is doing. He, in his turn, because he is so constantly with her, will probably come to accept a situation where he has part of her attention all of the time, where other infants get all of the mother's attention part of the time.

The infant who wakes continually during the night is a different matter. If he wakes before he has had sufficient sleep for the moment, then something is waking him. Babies become increasingly easy to wake from about 6 months onward. The infant who can be shown, sleeping, to admiring visitors at 4 months, will almost certainly wake if people go into his room when he is 8 months. So the reason for the night waking may be a practical one. Often the baby who is still sleeping in his parents' room is disturbed by their coming to bed, their talk and moving around, or even their coughing and snoring. Sometimes infants who have always shared a sibling's room become disturbed by his sleeping noises. Obviously it is worth trying to see whether the infant sleeps better alone. Where there is no separate room for him, his crib can sometimes be carried into the living room once the parents are ready to go to bed.

But a great deal of night waking at 6–9 months cannot be so simply explained. Moore and Ucko [159], in one of the few actual studies of this problem, found that it tended to be the infants who received least attention during the day, and whose mothers were afraid to pick them up when they cried for fear of spoiling them, who woke in the night. Spock, on the other hand, in the new edition of *Baby and Child Care* [208], takes the opposite view. He believes that it is "spoiled" babies who wake in the night and that the more they are "spoiled" by being attended to when they wake, the more frequently they will do it. Most researchers are agreed that some form of "nightmare" is common after 6 months. I put the word in quotes because we cannot, in a pre-verbal child, know what form the night fright takes. All we know is that the child wakes, usually with a sudden scream. No ordinary cause can be found. He appears afraid, is almost immediately reassured when his mother comes to him, and usually goes rapidly back to sleep.

Even if the actual number of minutes the mother or father must spend awake with the child is small, disturbances of sleep, night after night, for weeks or months, are exhausting. Unfortunately, where simple practical measures to ensure that the infant is not disturbed from outside fail, very little can be done to help the parents. The child cannot wake himself up on purpose. There is therefore no possible logic in regarding night waking as a "bad habit" which can be broken by leaving the child to cry. In the vast majority of cases nothing but the reassurance of seeing the parent will settle the baby. And the parents will only lose more sleep by lying listening to him crying before they go to him. On the other hand it is important also that the *parents* should not get into bad habits. When the child normally wakes several times in each night, it is easy to get out of bed, almost asleep, and go into his room at the very first murmur. He may not be really awake. Left for a few seconds he might have settled again. Visited, he will certainly surface.

After about 9 months, a change seems to take place in that infants become able to inhibit sleep at will. This can, and all too often does, raise all kinds of new problems. The mother can no longer decide that if the baby needs to sleep he will sleep, and conversely that if he does not sleep he does not need to. On the contrary, some infants fight their drowsiness until they are so tense and exhausted that they cannot relax into sleep. Over-excitement, fear of the dark, a quarrel with mother at bedtime, can all make the infant determined not to go to sleep.

Problems over going to sleep, as opposed to length of sleep, or waking during sleep, often start with an obvious upset. Yarrow [228] reviews the evidence for disturbances following brief periods of hospitalization. Sleep disturbances following the return home were very common, especially between 9 months and 1 year. Less traumatic events can start trouble also. A holiday away from home can break the infant's sleep pattern, so that he cannot be returned to his old behavior when he gets home. A new room may lead to sleep refusal. Even a shift around of the furniture may cause trouble.

But most often, the tired infant who will not allow himself to go to sleep is reacting primarily to separation from his mother. To allow himself to pass into sleep is to relinquish her altogether. Rather than do this, many babies will cry and scream until she returns, be delighted to see her, accept any entertainment she offers, and then start again as soon as she goes. Others will lie quietly as long as she is in the room, but snap fully awake as soon as she creeps out, settling again when she resignedly sits down once more. A few infants, especially those who have been actually smacked for crying after they were settled for the night, will sit silent in their cribs, listening for the sounds of the rest of the family moving around in other rooms.

Luckily, this is the age period during which infants find within themselves resources to help them relinquish the mother at night. These are ritual behaviors which give the infant security and comfort that are within his *own* control, which allow him to comfort *himself* after his mother has left him. Thumb sucking and pacifier sucking may have been in the child's repertoire since the first weeks of life, but for many children they take on a new significance during these months. At the same time the child may adopt what Winnicott called a "transitional object"—meaning an object which stood in for the mother in her absence—and use this object, often in combination with sucking, to comfort himself. This adoption of a soft, cuddly object, often a piece of blanket, or a soft toy, or old diaper, has been studied by various researchers [210]. But we still do not know what proportion of infants do in fact form such attachments. Those who do, form them in about equal numbers before and after the first birthday, and once the attachment is formed it is invariably extremely strong, so that the child's "relationship" with the object needs to be taken almost as seriously as his relationship with other people. Whether such a relationship is actually good for a child, we do not know. But it certainly does not seem to be harmful. Like many things the answer will probably turn out to be a matter of degree. To be able to use such an object to comfort yourself when your mother leaves you for the night is useful. It must also tend to increase the infant's feeling that the world as a whole is a comforting place; that all comfort need not stem from the mother herself. On the other hand a continual need for the object during the day might tend to suggest that the child was being asked to depend too much on himself for comfort, and was perhaps not getting what he needed from people. Furthermore in an extreme case daytime finger sucking, combined with twisting a blanket around the head, would be likely to limit the infant's exploratory and play behavior.

Much the same can be said about other comfort habits. Many babies relax themselves for sleep by ritualistic rocking, or by twisting their hair or banging their heads against the crib bars. All these habits can be useful self-relaxers, but all can go too far. The infant who chooses to rock by himself in a corner in the daytime is not being offered, or is not accepting, enough stimulation and interest from his environment. The infant who bangs his head hard enough to hurt needs bumpers around his crib. If he then makes it clear that the ritual is no use to him if it does not hurt, one needs to know why he must hurt himself.

Some ritualistic comfort can be quite deliberately provided by the mother for infants who find it difficult to settle at night. A regular and pleasant bedtime routine is often the start of it. The regularity makes sure that the infant knows when bedtime is coming up; the pleasantness makes sure that he reaches his crib as relaxed, as happy, feeling as securely loved as possible. Many mothers find that the deliberate ritualization of their good-nights, their curtain-drawing, the amount they leave the door open and so on helps their baby to release them gradually, rather than feeling that the mother has walked out on him, leaving him emotionally in mid-air. The danger is that once a little ritual has begun, the infant builds and builds on it, until it is effectively putting the parting off for an hour or more.

TOILET "TRAINING"

Toilet training is a human universal. All infants have to learn not to soil in or near the living space. But the extreme interest, the concern, the anxiety which the whole topic arouses is by no means universal in time or in place. In the London of 300 years ago, chamber pots were in use;

people did not void on the floor of their houses. But neither did they have our horror of the sight of feces. Those same chamber pots were happily emptied out of the windows into the open sewers in the streets below. And many a busy man gave audience while enthroned for defecation. In the rural village cultures of today children are taught to go to a special place outside the compound. But while they are learning, most of their "accidents" take place outside where they are already rolling in the dirt. And there are few clothes to worry about. Even in the rural parts of Western societies there tends to be a greater tolerance for the actual dirt of excretion. If children are usually muddy, if there are animals always around, if half the farmyard is trampled into the kitchen at every meal-time, there is likely to be far less fuss about a wet or soiled pair of pants.

In sophisticated societies, with their rest rooms, their swept streets, their diapers and plastic pants, the whole business of excretion has been as much concealed as a constant human function can be. The child who, because of his youth, will not conform, is under heavy pressure.

Any attempt to persuade a baby to void into a potty rather than a diaper is usually referred to as toilet "training." But often this is a misnomer. Toilet training can only correctly refer to the process by which a child is taught to respond to his own need to void, by telling or signaling to his mother, or going himself to the potty or lavatory. This teaching cannot even begin until the infant is old enough, mature enough, to *recognize* his own need to void. Only very rarely can the infant identify the signals from his full bladder or rectum before he is 1 year old. So the attempts in this half year are not *training* at all.

If it is not training, why does it "work" some of the time and for some of the parents who attempt it? In early infancy sphincter control is a reflex matter and, during the period *before it can come under the child's conscious control,* the reflex can sometimes be conditioned. In parts of the world where diapers are not available but living-spaces must nevertheless be kept clean, very young babies often become conditioned to passing a bowel movement when they are "held out" in a particular way. In the West it is not enough that the infant pass a movement when he is taken off his mother's back, unwrapped and held out in the open air: he must pass his movement on a pot. When this happens it is because that sphincter has become conditioned to the stimulus of the potty-rim against his buttocks.

During the years when "potting" small babies was common practice, an extensive literature on the method of conditioning and another literature on the results accumulated. Both sets of literature were excellently reviewed in T. Berry Brazelton's classic paper "A Child-Oriented Approach to Toilet-Training" [37]. Brazelton showed that the conditioning was necessarily negative rather than positive as there was no intrinsic reward for the infant in passing a movement or urine in a potty rather than a diaper. He also showed that the incidence of difficulties later in infancy was extremely high. Although most modern parents accept Brazelton's own approach to toilet training and would agree that true "training" is neither possible nor desirable in early infancy, some still put the potty in the right place at the right time to catch movements and urine.

Many infants have, from the beginning, a fairly regular voiding pattern, being especially likely to pass a movement immediately after feeding. Furthermore their urine-retention time is very short, so that if they wake dry from a nap, or return dry from an outing, it is a reasonable guess that they will urinate shortly afterward. Some mothers take advantage of these patterns, and pride themselves on having a few daytime diapers to wash.

Being "caught" in this way is most unlikely to bother a 6-month baby. He will let go and void when he needs to, wherever he finds himself. If the mother puts him on the pot simply to save herself washing, or to protect chafed skin from wet diapers, there is probably no harm in it. But unfortunately few mothers are so cool about this emotional subject. They tend to feel very strongly about "success," being filled with pride and pleasure when the potty is used, disappointed when it is left empty, and irritated when the infant immediately soils or wets his diaper. Reactions of this kind are likely to communicate themselves to the infant and may store up trouble for the true training period which still lies ahead. Furthermore, the more successfully mothers "catch" their infants, the more likely they are to decide that they have "trained" them. The mother puts the baby on the potty after breakfast each morning and he produces a movement; she catches urine at mid-morning, at lunchtime, and after his afternoon nap. At suppertime he produces another movement. For weeks on end only naptime and nighttime diapers may be used. By the time he is 9–10 months, she is quite convinced that the whole toilet-training business is vastly overplayed, and that she has succeeded from the beginning. Other mothers congratulate her and ask the secret. She is almost certainly in for a nasty shock. Far from being trained, her 9-month baby simply had not begun to care where he put his body products. At around a year he begins to become aware of them; aware of the feelings they give him; aware that they come out of his body and belong to him. At the same time he is increasingly involved in crawling and toddling, so that sitting on a potty (or indeed sitting still anywhere) becomes a very undesirable activity. The smooth successful "catching" pattern becomes totally disrupted, and the mother finds that, just like other mothers, she now has to toilet train her baby. And, as we shall see, the early catching success does not mean that true training will be easier or quicker than it would have been if the infant had been left in his diapers until he was ready to learn.

Because of the secrecy and emotionality which we attach to elimination, finding out what mothers actually do about training their infants is beset with difficulties. If mothers are asked what is happening at one given point in time, they tend to over-estimate the infant's "prowess"; if they are asked later on to remember his toilet training, they tend to look back through rose-tinted spectacles. Survey results have, therefore, to be taken with a large grain of salt. But those which report a *late* start to training, or *late* success, are likely to be more accurate than others. A mother is unlikely to say that her infant was still in diapers at three and one-half when he was not. But she is very likely to say that he was out of them at two when he was not.

The accuracy with which researchers can report on toilet training is affected also by the changing fashions in infant handling. Overall changes tend to take place consistently throughout a society, so that, for example, the attitudes epitomized by Truby King [146] have given way to those epitomized by Spock [208] or Leach [139].

But within that overall change, taking several generations, change also takes place more quickly in some sub-groups or socioeconomic classes than in others. Average figures, given by a survey, may therefore reflect a wide range of practices all current at the same time in different groups. And, since the production of survey results takes a long time, they may fail to reflect the current practice of those who have moved on to new ideas since the survey was made. The studies quoted below show very large numbers of mothers starting to "train" their babies during this half year. Yet if it were possible to carry out a swift survey now, there is little doubt that it would show far more mothers leaving out the catching stage altogether, and delaying training well into the second year.

A study in California [104], reported in 1966, showed that a few mothers still started training in the early months while just over 50 percent delayed until 18 months. Similarly in Great Britain C. M. Drillien's [66] study of 518 Scottish babies showed 90 percent of all mothers starting training during the first year. The Newsons [170] found 83 percent of their sample had begun before the first birthday, while 20 percent had sat their babies on potties in the first few weeks of life. Now, in both countries, the vast majority of parents reckon to delay training until it can be true training; until the child himself is able to take responsibility for recognizing his need for the potty and for using it. Yet there are always some who seem to have missed out on a change of this kind. There still are babies who are "held out" (over a potty) after feedings in the first 6 months. There still are toddlers who are routinely placed on the potty whether they willingly consent or not.

Clearly we cannot generalize about how many mothers will train their infants at different ages. It will depend on who they are, where they live, what their friends do, what their mothers and their doctors and their neighbors advise.

But whatever they do, and whenever they do it, the training is aimed at producing a child who will reliably and independently use a potty or lavatory instead of a diaper or pants. Unfortunately there is no controlled study which directly compares the age at which this happy state is reached in children who were placed on the potty early or late. But deductions can be drawn from various studies: all suggest that the age at which the mother starts to place her infant on the pot, or truly to train him, has no bearing whatsoever on the age at which he will be "trained." C. M. Drillien, for example, found no relationship running in either direction. Her early-potting mothers had 2-year-olds who were neither wetter nor dryer, cleaner nor dirtier than the late-training mothers. The Newsons followed up their study of 1-year-olds with a study of the same children when they were four [169]. Again they could find no relationship between early or late toileting, and reliability or unreliability at 4 years. Finally, in a rare experimental manipulation of ordinary daily life, T. B. Brazelton [37] actually encouraged the mothers of 1170 infants seen in private practice *not* to start any form of potting before their children were 2 years old. All were reliable, at least by day, within 4 months of the start of training.

The only suggestion that the commencement of toilet training can be left over-late comes from a paper [117] reporting a longitudinal study of infants who became bed-wetters in later childhood.

Children whose training commenced when they were between 15–19 months were somewhat less likely to be enuretic between 6 and 8 years than were children whose training was delayed until they were around 2 years. While this might suggest an optimum time for beginning toilet training (although there is no suggestion of "the earlier the better"), the children in this study were being reared in an Israeli kibbutz with training carried out as a group procedure by nurses, rather than individually by parents. We do not know the significance of this type-of-rearing variable. Since the 5 percent of earlier-trained children and the 15 percent of later-trained ones who were enuretic at 6–8 years are described as inse-cure and over-active, it is possible that the timing of the start of training had little to do with the eventual result. In an earlier study by Dimson [62] 165 families were studied who, between them, had 225 enuretic children and 174 who became reliably dry by the pre-school period. These children could not be distinguished in terms of the age at which their mothers started to pot or to train them.

It does seem, therefore, that early potting is most unlikely to lead to early successful training. The majority of infants will be more or less reliable in the daytime by the middle of their third year, whether they are first put on a potty at 6 days, 6 months, or 16 months. Simply in practical terms, early potting seems a lot of effort for not much reward. With a little frivolous arithmetic, one can work out that the mother who starts to place her baby on the potty at 6 months, and does so six times a day until he is two will have potted him 3276 times. Each time she will have had to undress and redress him. And, since she will often have been unsuccess-ful, she will have used a good many diapers as well. On the other hand the mother who leaves out the catching stage, and starts training her baby at 18 months, will have used more diapers, but she will only have placed her infant on the potty about 1000 times for the same effect. Since changing a diaper is rather quicker than placing an infant on the potty, the training mother has probably saved herself a good deal of time over the catching one!

But of course practical considerations are not the only ones. Once infants do become aware of their excreta as coming from themselves, they become extremely interested in them, concerned about them, and intrigued by the sensations which voiding produces. If they detect over-concern in the mother, or feel that they are being pressured by her in this extremely personal area, they are likely to react both with a marked negative response to being put on the potty, and with greater or lesser emotional disturbance (see Chapter Twenty-seven).

Once again the available research data are unsatisfactory. Many attempts have been made to relate anxiety in children to too early or too severe toilet training, or to relate a general miserliness and emotional withholding in adulthood with problems over constipation during the toilet-training period. Generally speaking such attempts have failed, because, as we have said before, the *atmosphere* in which the mother trains her child is likely to be far more important to him and his emotional well-being than what she actually does, or the age at which she does it.

Most researchers show that a marked resistance to potting or to later training arises in at least 30 percent of infants, whether the mother starts early or late. The Newsons [169], in a coda to their 4-year-olds' survey, had the impression—although they attempted no statistics as they did not believe the mothers' reports were necessarily accurate—that resistance arose less often with infants whose training had been delayed well into the second year. But they point out that the mothers who were prepared to delay training their infants for that long were also likely to be mothers who would be sensitive to the infants' feelings about the matter, and would withdraw pressure at the first signs of unhappiness.

If potting is begun in this half year, it is important to realize how likely it is that voiding will become an angry issue between mother and child, and how impossible it is for the mother to win any pitched battle she may enter.

The infant in this age group is not capable of becoming clean or dry out of virtue. He does not recognize the signs of impending voiding. He does not know he is about to pass a movement or to pass urine. He therefore has to accept his mother's whisking him off to the potty, apparently at her whim.

The infant cannot, of course, begin to understand what the mother is up to, or why. Later, when he knows he is about to void, he will realize that this is why he is put on the potty. Later still he will understand that his mother actually prefers him to perform on the potty; later again he will understand why. But at this stage the whole matter is totally incomprehensible.

If, by happy chance, potting can be incomprehensible but fun, the infant may accept it as just another part of his life. But it is difficult to make it fun. Most infants dislike sitting on a potty anyway, as they feel insecure without the solid floor or a supporting chair. Most of them hate being unexpectedly interrupted in the middle of play, most wake from naps in a bad temper and resent anything the mother does at that moment except cuddle them, and a great many dislike being dressed and undressed. If any or all of these factors do irritate the baby, they are the more likely to make him angry because they recur so frequently. If a mother is going to place her baby on the potty at all, she is likely to do so at least six times a day, and she may well do it much more often.

If the infant does object to being put on the potty, and his mother tries to insist, she will very quickly find that she has joined in a battle which there is no way for her to win. Just as it is physically impossible to make a child eat if he refuses, so there is no way to make him void in a potty if he refuses. If the mother is prepared physically to force him to stay on the potty she still cannot make him use it. Within a few days of being made conscious of the matter as an issue between them, the infant will have learned simply to withhold his movement until he is allowed up —and then to pass it on the floor or in his clean diaper. If this apparently willful bad behavior makes the mother cross, it only strengthens the balky infant's determination not to give in. The battle can reach such proportions that it dominates the whole relationship. And all before the infant was physiologically mature enough for training. It seems a high price to pay for a lighter laundry load or disposable-diaper bill in the earlier months.

21

BECOMING A BIPED

THE ACHIEVEMENT OF MOBILITY, first as a quadruped, then as a biped, occupies a very great deal of the infant's time and energy during this half year. The process of getting moving comprises three distinct, although overlapping, phases. Firstly the infant must learn to sit alone, balancing himself, without aid from chair-back or cushions. Having achieved this, he will develop some form of progression across the floor, which for brevity we will call crawling. Once this is established, the infant will begin to pull himself to standing posture, with furniture, crib bars or human hands for support. Once he can stand on his two feet, he is on the way to walking.

A. Gesell [93] points out that sitting up alone is not only the obvious mid-point between lying down and standing up, it is also the developmental mid-point in terms of neuromuscular control. Control starts from the top and moves downward. The new infant must learn to control his head as it wavers on his weak neck. Once his neck can cope with his head, he becomes able to control and hold up his shoulders and upper back, so that held in sitting posture the rounded sag in his spine is only at waist and hip level. A little later still, he can keep his whole back straight. Only his hips and legs still remain to be disciplined.

Most infants are at just about this stage at 6 months. Many of them are ready to sit in that they have their heads and backs in control, but few of them can yet balance in the sitting posture. Placed carefully on the floor, they can be balanced for a few seconds, but then the outstretched hands of parent or researcher prove their worth.

R. Griffiths [99] tested 571 normal infants between birth and 2 years, in order to construct a scale of normal development; 150 of those babies were between 4 and 9 months at the time of testing. She found that during the sixth month almost all could sit up with minimal support from a cushion in the small of the back, and protection from sideways falls. At 7–8 months most of the infants could sit on the floor, but could not be left sitting because they still tended to overbalance unexpectedly. In her sample, it was during the ninth month that most babies became able to sit on the floor and play. This age-dating has been confirmed, for an American sample, by the Gesell Institute's results, published in 1980 [7].

Some infants, during the 7–8 month period, solve the problem of balance when sitting by hunching forward and resting their hands on the floor. This gives a stable, but not a useful position. With his hands taken up with balancing himself and his head bent forward, the infant has neither a good view of the world, nor freedom to play. So even if the infant can remain in this posture indefinitely, he does not really count as "able to sit alone."

Other babies learn to balance themselves without using their hands, but can maintain the balance only until a "wobble" sets in. As soon as they move their heads, or stretch out for a toy, or lean forward, the balance goes and they topple. The sitting, in such a case, is true sitting, but it is still not very useful sitting.

With constant practice the infant, before he is 10 months old, reaches a point where he can retain his balance while using his head and his hands freely; he can even lean right forward, retrieve a toy and regain the sitting position. At this point he can truly be said to be sitting independently.

Constant practice means constant falls. Clearly as many of these falls as possible should be from the floor to the floor, rather than from a high chair to the floor. Chairs which have provided a safe support for younger babies—who maintain a comparatively constant pressure on the seat and the chair-back—may become very dangerous during this phase. The infant sits unsupported for a few seconds, with his back and his arms clear of the chair. Then he relaxes, and hits the chair-back or arm with a thump which makes it rock, or even tip. The floor is the safest place for sitting practice. But even the floor can prove discouragingly hard if the infant's head hits it several times in a day. A simple answer, throughout this period, is to surround the child either with cushions, or with rolled quilts. At 6–7 months the cushions provide that minimal support to the small of the back which will allow him to sit for a few seconds; when he rolls onto his back or forward into crawling position, they also make a soft landing. A little later they may encourage him to try sitting without supporting himself on his hands, and catch him when his own triumph at finding himself sitting leads him to wave his arms and overbalance. Later still, they are there to prevent damage when he leans forward too far for his new-found equilibrium or, worse still, tips straight over backward because something makes him jump. Of course no baby should ever be left alone in the room if he is thus cushioned. If he fell face down into a cushion, he would probably push up with his arms and clear his nose and mouth. But he could fall awkwardly, perhaps with his arms trapped beneath him. He could smother. But provided he is properly supervised (and no baby of this age group should ever be left free alone in a room), cushioning his falls *is* worthwhile. His fontanelles are still partially open; his skull does not provide the protection of an older child's skull; he *could* hurt himself. Furthermore, motor development is partly dependent on confidence; and recurrent bumps can put the timid off for a long time.

Getting into sitting position unassisted is more variable in its timing than the ability actually to sit. By 6 months, most infants will raise their heads and shoulders from the mattress or floor, when lying flat on their backs. Often the infant will do this when he wants his mother to give him her hands so that he can pull himself up to sitting. Since by this time most babies can roll all the way over from their backs to their stomachs and back again, many roll over, find themselves up against the bars of their cribs or the side of the carriage, raise their heads and shoulders, and discover that they can use the bars or sides to struggle to a holding-on sitting position alone. Many a mother has been amazed to spot her not-yet-sitting infant peering toward the house over the edge of his carriage in the garden. Obviously restraining straps should *always* be used, as once the baby can move around this much he could either fall out of the carriage or tip it over. Once this trick is discovered, the infant usually goes on with it, but this still does not mean that he can get himself into sitting position without anything to pull up by. Few babies can do this before they are playing freely in the sitting position at around 9 months. Then the constant practice of going from sitting to crawling position, and of leaning over and righting himself while sitting, gradually teaches him. The most usual method, at this age, is to roll onto the stomach, pull the knees right up, and then move the hands closer and closer to the body, with a final heave that tips the child back onto his bottom.

The development of some form of crawling often parallels the development of independent sitting quite closely in individual infants. At 6 months the infant can almost sit alone; he has just the remaining problem of balance. At 6 months he can almost crawl. If a toy is put on the floor, just out of his reach, as he lies on his stomach, he pulls up with his knees, pushes with his hands and often gets his stomach right off the floor so that he is in true crawling posture. He just has the remaining problem of actually moving forward.

During the seventh and eighth months, most babies clearly *want* to crawl; watching them, one can see that they are thinking forward, see the effort that is being made. But few will actually progress. Often, in the eighth month, the infant is reluctant to lie flat on his stomach at all; he gets into hands-and-knees position as soon as he turns himself over, or collapses from sitting. Often too, he will rock himself on hands and knees. And he may learn to turn around on hands and knees, swiveling to follow his mother as she moves around the room. Some infants develop idiosyncratic modes of getting around by a combination of rocking, swiveling, rolling over, and squirming on their stomachs. It is not at all unusual to find a baby who cannot yet crawl, in quite a different part of the room from the safe corner where he was left moments before.

During the ninth month, at about the same time that he becomes able to sit safely, and play, with his head and hands free and mobile, the infant will begin actually to progress across the room. To the extreme frustration of many infants, first progress is often backward. The infant pushes harder with his hands and forearms than he does with his feet and knees, so, with gaze fixed on a longed-for toy just in front of him, he shunts backward away from it. Fortunately this is a short-lived phase. Once he can crawl backward the baby will soon get his direction right.

So, by the end of the ninth month, the infant is likely to be able to sit on the floor and play, and crawl across the floor to get things or to follow people.

While sitting up and crawling tend to progress together, walking is definitely a later accomplishment. Many 6-month babies very much enjoy the standing position, held under the arms, on an adult's lap. As we have seen in an earlier chapter, many use the lap as a sort of trampoline, pushing down with their feet, momentarily straightening their knees, and then sagging again, in a rhythmic "jumping" movement. During the seventh month, they begin to use alternate feet, instead of both feet together. The infant now seems to "dance" rather than to jump. Often one foot is placed on top of the other, and then the underneath foot pulled out and put back on top. But at this stage the infant does not bear his full weight, nor does he make any obvious attempt at progress. There is none of the longing to move forward when he is held standing, which is so obvious at the same age when he is in crawling posture.

It is usually at around 9 months that this dancing movement begins to give way to a definite placing of one foot in front of the other. The infant may enjoy being held up while he wobbles his way a few "steps." But few babies will support their full weight at this stage; most will be around 10 months before they can be stood squarely on their own feet.

Contrary to Gesell's belief that neuromuscular control moves downward, the infant usually learns to keep his knees stiff, to support his weight, before he learns similarly to control his hips. Characteristically he still sags forward slightly at the hip joints although his legs are straight.

This stage in the development of standing is similar to that point in sitting, at 6 months, where the infant could sit, but not balance. Now he can stand, square on the floor, taking all his weight, but he cannot balance.

Once he can take his full weight the baby will quickly learn to pull himself up to standing. R. Griffiths [99] found that the average age for this was 11 months. Many babies pull themselves up earlier; the norm was 40 weeks in the Gesell Institute survey [7]; probably it is partly a question of opportunity. Many infants, for example, first pull themselves to standing in their cribs—but will not do so if they wear sleeping bags. Others start with the bars of a playpen, but if no playpen is used they must find some other, perhaps less obvious aid. Often the mother herself is the first object used. She may be sitting on the floor with the baby, who crawls to her, and works his way up her clothing until he stands triumphant and wobbly, holding on to her shoulder if she is lucky, her hair if she is not.

Just as newly crawling babies are often distressed by their inability to crawl forward, so newly standing ones are often flummoxed by their inability to sit down again. Sometimes there is a period of several weeks during which the infant pulls himself to standing as soon as he is let loose on the floor, and then cries piteously for help because he cannot let go and sit down again. As soon as he is rescued, he repeats the performance. As with crawling backward this phase does not usually last for long. The infant either learns to let go and sit down with a plop, or he learns to lower himself, more gently, by sliding down his support and not letting go with his hands until he is nearly there. In the meantime there is nothing to be gained by trying to force the issue—by leaving the baby to cry until he finds his own way down. He will, eventually, but he will get down by falling down, and falls at this stage are bad for his confidence. If this phase is tiresome, the solution may be to take the baby out more, in carriage or stroller. He is not yet at the stage where it occurs to him to want to walk when out on an expedition. He will sit, happily, and rest both his muscles and his own and his mother's nerves.

Within 2 to 3 weeks of learning to pull himself up to standing posture, and usually, therefore, during the twelfth month, the infant learns to "cruise" around his support. At the start he is likely to pull himself up so that he is facing the sofa-back or other support and holding on to it with both hands. Maintaining the two-handed grip, he inches his hands along, and follows them with a sideways step with the leading foot. Left straddle-legged, he usually then sits down; indeed it may be this crabwise cruising which first teaches him how to sit down from standing. As greater confidence develops, he begins to move, still sideways, but hand over hand along the support, moving one foot and then bringing the other up to it. With more confidence still, the infant stands further back from the support, so that he holds on more or less at arm's length. By this stage he is using the support purely for balance, and is trusting his full weight to his feet, even during the difficult moments when one foot is in the air in mid-step.

It is only at this stage—usually between 12 and 13 months—that most babies appreciate walking while holding an adult's two hands. At earlier stages they tend to be alarmed by the empty space all around them, and to prefer to move around solid furniture.

At the first birthday, most babies will be moving around on their own two feet in *some* fashion. A few will be actually walking, at least a few steps from one support to another. Rather more will be walking around furniture, letting go with one hand to reach with the other hand for the next support. These may also stand without support for a few moments. Most will still be cruising only where they can hold on with both hands. And a good many will still only be pulling themselves up.

Learning to walk takes most babies about 9 months, from the time they first pull themselves to standing, to the time when they can be said to toddle freely around. It also takes them a great deal of physical effort, and a good deal of what, in an older person, would be called courage. Which adult would spend his time hauling himself to his feet, wobbling, falling down, getting up again, taking a step and falling again, day after day after day? Most people would send for a wheelchair after a couple of weeks. In geological time, as Anthony Smith [206] colorfully points out, being a biped is a very recent development. Our ancestors were quadrupeds, with horizontal spines. Our assumption of the upright posture freed our hands for tool use, and contributed to our superiority over other animals. But we achieved it by adapting a quadruped's skeleton, not by an entirely new engineering design. Every new human being repeats, in miniature, the difficulties of turning that skeletal structure upright. And to some extent every human being suffers from the inappropriate design of his spine for bipedal life, for the rest of his years.

In the first year, babies are physically much better adapted to quadrupedal than bipedal life. Compared with adults, or older children, their shoulders are hunched, their necks short, their rib cages rounded, and their bone mass very high in relation to their muscle mass. During the second and third years, all this is modified. Muscle has been shown, by X-ray, to increase its width at twice the rate that bone width increases during the same period. The rib cage becomes progressively flatter, and the neck longer. At the same time the infant's legs straighten and lengthen relative to his body and arms, and his feet develop arches.

When a baby first stands, he looks so peculiar that his mother is often concerned. His arms appear very long in relation to his legs. But time will adjust this relationship, and in the meantime it serves the child well by keeping his center of gravity low, for balance, while leaving his reach comparatively long. Furthermore this appearance is increased by the child's tendency to straddle his legs and flex his hips, also in an attempt to aid balance. Straight legs, at this age, are the exception rather than the rule. Most infants appear either bowlegged (though some are so encumbered with diapers this is hardly surprising) or knock-kneed. All are flat-footed, and start to walk with the whole sole of the foot put directly to the floor. The arched foot with its heel-toe walk comes later. All these characteristics contribute to the gait we know as "toddling." Another 2 years or so will change the toddler into the straight-limbed, slimmed down, beautifully proportioned, freely moving creature we call a child.

While the sequence of developments, and the ages at which they occur, are as this chapter has described for most children in Western societies, neither ages nor sequence are invariable.

A few infants leave out the crawling stage altogether. Usually such infants learn to sit steadily at a comparatively early age. They learn to pull themselves to standing, from the sitting position, and from then on seem to concentrate their attention on cruising around the furniture. Cruising satisfies their desire for mobility, and they do not bother to crawl. Usually such an infant *can* in fact crawl. If, while he is sitting down, an attractive object, such as a small bright vehicle, is pushed across the floor in front of him he will not haul himself up to go after it, he will follow it at ground level. Infants who leave out crawling are therefore choosing not to crawl, rather than unable to do so.

Some infants go through the crawling phase, but in idiosyncratic ways. A few roll over and over to get quickly across the room, and then squirm the last foot or two to their objectives. Others, especially those who are somewhat late in learning to sit up, lie on their backs, raise their buttocks off the ground supported by heels and shoulders, and progress by "humping." Some seem late in learning to pull their knees up under them, and get around by squirming forward on their hands and elbows, dragging their legs behind them, or pushing with their toes with legs extended. Some never use hands and knees for crawling, but rather move on hands and feet, "walking like a bear." This last form of progression is also sometimes adopted by conventionally crawling babies as a last stage before walking. Finally, babies who learn to sit steadily at an early age sometimes adopt the "bottom shuffle," getting about on one buttock and one hand. This last method does sometimes seem to delay walking. A real expert at the bottom shuffle gets little advantage from learning to walk. A crawling baby cannot look around very well, and has both his hands occupied. But a bottom-shuffling baby has the same visual field (somewhat lower down) as a walking one, and has one hand free. Furthermore he is firmly balanced.

In extremely rare cases, an infant may thumb his nose at the accepted sequence of motor development not by simply leaving one stage out, but by reversing the sequence and learning to crawl, or even to walk, before he learns to sit alone. R. S. Illingworth [109] reports one such case, where a bright, well-advanced girl reached the age of 19 months, cruising well around furniture, walking with one hand held, but quite unable to sit up. In the absence of any other reason, it was thought that she must have congenital shortening either of the gluteus maximus muscle, or of the hamstrings. There are also cases in the literature of institutionalized infants who crawled before they could sit up. These may be due to neglect. If an infant is put on the floor he can teach himself to crawl. But without adult help he cannot get himself up to try sitting; if he is left lying in a crib whenever he is not on the floor he may not even know what sitting up feels like.

Some infants follow the usual sequence of motor development, but show a marked acceleration, sitting alone as early as 4–5 months, and walking independently before 9 months. Sometimes such acceleration is part of an overall advanced state of development. But often—to the bitter disappointment of parents who have been proud of their child's early achievements—it proves to bear no relation to overall development. R. S. Illingworth [109] quotes the example of a boy whom he saw walking alone at 8 months, and who on formal IQ testing at the age of 5 had an IQ of 88—well below the average.

Hot controversy has raged, in recent years, around the question of the motor precocity of African as compared with European babies. M. Geber and R. F. A. Dean [90] studied 113 Ugandan newborns who behaved like European babies of 3–4 weeks. They studied a further 183 children between 1 month and 6 years, and found that sitting alone was usual at 5 months, while the infants tended to pull themselves to standing at 7 months and walk alone at 9 months.

These findings, and many similar ones, were hotly disputed by H. Knobloch [130]. But his sample were American Negroes, where Geber's were Bantu East Africans. His lived in urban America, hers in Uganda.

Ainsworth [2] also found motor precocity in the Ugandan infants she studied. She attributed it, at least in part, to the very close physical relationship between infant and mother. She saw it, therefore, as culturally and socially caused, rather than as a racial phenomenon.

Ironically, E. Pavenstedt [175] has shown that *adverse* social circumstances can produce motor acceleration also. In her study of grossly deprived and neglected infants, she found motor development far in advance of development in any other field. She attributed this, at least in part, to the absence of safety precautions taken for these infants, or holding devices provided for them.

But while there is some evidence accumulating to suggest that social and environmental factors may influence the age at which walking begins, most European longitudinal studies, looking repeatedly at the same infants over time, have shown no social-class or sex differences relating to motor development. The only consistently recurring variable in such studies has been familial: both early and late walking tend to run in families.

While the possibly accelerating effects of extra motor stimulation, of neglect leading to extra motor practice or of genetic variables remain open questions, some researchers consider that specific teaching might lead to earlier independent walking. In the newborn period, infants exhibit a reflex reaction to feeling the soles of their feet touching a hard surface. Held in this position they place one foot after another, as if they were "walking." N. Zelazo, P. Zelazo, and S. Kolb [229] found that infants whose newborn walking reflex was regularly and deliberately exercised, and who were held in walking position for regular practice even after the reflex died away, learned to walk independently some weeks earlier than a control group of infants. It is not yet clear, however, whether it was the specificity of the walking practice, or the more general motor stimulation given to the experimental infants, which led to the earlier walking. Nor is it clear whether the newborn walking reflex was actually maintained, prevented from dying out as it does in most infants, or whether the reflex died out to be replaced by newly learned walking techniques.

There is ample scope for further research into the development of walking. In the meantime, for practical purposes, it is safe to assume that given every opportunity for physical freedom, physical play, and physical assistance from his parents, an infant will walk as soon as he is ready. Over-encouragement to an infant who is not steady on his feet—not ready, in his own view, to walk alone—can be actually dangerous. The skull fontanelles are seldom completely closed even by 1 year. The infant's skull provides far less protection than it will do later. It is not a good idea to encourage falls, and the best way to discourage them is to let the infant decide when and how he will walk.

22

BECOMING
A TOOL-USER

AT 6 MONTHS, the infant has become adept at getting hold of objects. If a toy which he wants is offered to him, he will reach out and take it. If it is placed on a table within his reach, he will stretch out and pick it up. He no longer needs the continual visual monitoring, the glancing backward and forward between his own hand and the object to which he is reaching, which was typical of his behavior a few weeks earlier. His reaching is now what L. Burton, P. Castle, B. White, and R. Held [44, 223] describe as "top-level." The child sees the object he wants, and without needing to look at his hand—which may be in his lap—stretches directly for it. The extent to which the 6-month infant can do without visual monitoring when reaching out and grasping is illustrated by an unusual experiment conducted by T. Bower [29]. He found that if infants were shown a brightly colored and lit object, within easy reach of their hands, they could reach out and grasp it when all light had been extinguished. The reaching and grasping were therefore accomplished completely "blind."

Bower also describes an interesting change in the relationship between reaching out to an object and actually grasping it. In younger infants, as they become proficient at reaching for objects, the reaching and the grasping become a single movement. The infant reaches, and, as his hand comes to the object, his fist closes. If he has mis-reached, so that the fist closes on nothing, he withdraws the hand and repeats the whole reach-grasp sequence. Furthermore, babies under about 6 months very seldom reach to an object *without* grasping. Hence the pulled noses and hair of normal motherhood.

Bower believes that at around 6 months reaching and grasping become differentiated behavior which the infant is progressively able to use together or separately. He has, of course, been able to grasp without reaching since the earliest days of life. But he now becomes able to reach without grasping. Bower sees this as developmentally significant in that once an infant can reach and then grasp, as two separate-but-related actions, he can also presumably learn to grasp and then reach. And that is a prerequisite of tool-use.

This separation of the two actions of reaching and grasping has not yet been satisfactorily proved, experimentally. Bower himself maintains that in younger infants there is no measurable pause between the end of reach and the beginning of grasp; while in infants over 6 months there is such a pause, when the arm has finished its movement and the hand has not yet begun the grasp. But this pause is measured in milli-seconds. The experiments may prove difficult to duplicate.

In the meantime Bower believes that traditional learning theory can provide an adequate explanation for differentiation between reach and grasp. Younger infants reach out and grasp everything they see that is within reach and which they want. But many such "objects" are not in fact graspable. At one time or another every infant can be seen vainly trying to capture a dancing sunbeam, clutching at a soap bubble, or trying to pick up a bright picture from the page of a book. The child's world is full of such visual illusions: things which look solid and graspable, and are not. Bower believes that the older infant has learned this and has learned that to ascertain whether or not an object can be grasped, it is safer to rely on tactile than on visual information. If an object feels graspable, then it is. Our environment does not provide tactile illusions in the way it provides visual ones. Things that feel solid, are solid, even though certain materials may provide surprises by being unexpectedly light, or heavy, for their size.

The older infant therefore looks, reaches, and touches, before he grasps.

Whether or not Bower's theoretical formulation and preliminary experiments in this area prove correct, they certainly make sense in terms of the changes in manual behavior which take place during the months immediately after the infant has learned an accurate top-level reach. Increasingly, at 7, 8, and 9 months, the infant touches things without trying to grasp them. He pats and strokes the table in front of him; his mother may get her hair stroked without it being pulled; the infant can touch a pet rabbit without squashing its ear in his fist. Increasingly, too, he differentiates the use of his individual fingers and thumbs from the use of his whole hand. At 9 months he can reach out and poke an object with his index finger, instead of pushing it with his hand. A little later, when asked to point something out, he will point with that index finger instead of indicating the object with a wave of the whole hand. And in picking things up, he will pre-adjust his hand to the seen size of the object not simply by shaping the hand as he did earlier, but by approaching very small objects only with the thumb and index finger. Before his first birthday he will oppose finger and thumb so accurately that he can pick up a single currant.

Many mammals will use their forelimbs to get hold of objects. The 6-month infant's ability to reach out and take things is still very primitive. It is only the very beginning of the manual dexterity which will eventually distinguish him from all other animals.

At 6 months, the most characteristic "use" which an infant makes of an object is still to put it in his mouth. He may, however, transfer it from one hand to the other. And as he holds it, his fingers will curl around it in a grip which is far more secure than the palmar grasp of the 4–5 month infant.

At this stage, if a second object is handed to the infant while he is holding the first, he will drop the first to receive the second, even if he could comfortably hold one in each of his hands. It is as if his attention span is not great enough to take in two things. The first object is not thrown away, or openly and deliberately rejected, in favor of the second. It simply drops from his hand because his attention is on taking the second.

But the infant's reaction to objects matures quickly. By the end of the sixth month, while he may still mouth the object briefly, he is also likely to do something with it, to make some use of it or some attempt at exploring its possibilities. If the object is a simple cube, such as is used in developmental testing, he may bang it on the table. If it should be a bell, or rattle, which sounds as he picks it up, he may deliberately shake it to make it sound again. Once the infant tends to do something with objects, he is also likely to be able to hold two at the same time. But he is still unlikely to use both together to make a more interesting toy than each separately. He may, for example, wave two rattles, one in each hand. But he will seldom bang the two together so that they combine their sounds to make more.

Few infants over 6 months can get more than passing entertainment out of watching and playing with their own hands. The baby may still suck his fingers or his thumb as a comfort habit when he is tired, worried, or sleepy. And he may still glance at them as they pass across his field of vision. But he knows all he needs to know about his hands as objects. They have become all too familiar. Infants who are reared in boring, understimulating conditions—perhaps particularly in institutions—tend to continue with hand play for longer than other babies, and to develop other forms of self-stimulating or masturbatory play. Such a baby may learn the pleasures of rhythmical rocking or head banging, or he may discover that he can comfort and amuse himself by combining thumb sucking with rhythmical pressing of his thighs together, or rubbing of his genitals against the crib bars. All these comfort habits are normal, in the sense that many babies use some of them from time to time. But extensive use of any of them during waking hours does suggest that the baby is having to provide most of his own stimulation and play. If nothing else is provided for him, he will play with himself. But offered people and objects he will play mostly with them.

Some families do not understand the exploratory nature of early manual play. The infant is offered toys, but only a stereotyped small collection. He may have a string of beads or plastic balls strung across his carriage, two small toys fastened to the bars of his crib, and two rattles and one teething ring which are offered to him when he is awake in his baby chair or playpen. To limit a baby's playthings in this way is like leaving a hospital patient to lie in bed all day with one book which he has already read. For a 6-month baby, the possibilities of such simple toys are extremely limited. Once they have been thoroughly explored, they are no longer entertaining. Failing anything else, he may pick up the rattle and wave it once or twice, just as that hospital patient might idly leaf through his book once more. But then he drops it, and cries.

Providing a baby with appropriate "toys" (not, as we shall see, necessarily objects purchased from a toy shop or even purchased especially for the infant) is worthwhile from everyone's point of view. The baby will discover and learn at his own optimal rate if he is offered materials which fit with his developmental syllabus; the rest of the family will find him more enjoyable if he is seldom bored. Money which is to be spent on his pleasure will give better value if it is knowledgeably spent while the parent who understands what is likely to interest the baby at any given moment can usually find an answer to moments of crisis such as impending fury at being kept still in a crowded train.

The basic and simple message from a mass of far from simple research [118] is that babies in this age period tend to pay most attention to stimuli which are just slightly different from any with which they are entirely familiar. There is evidence to show that this is true of stimuli of every kind. Kinney and Kagan [126], for example, used both music and speech in an auditory stimulation experiment. 7 1/2 month-old-infants heard a french horn play a six-note melody and, once familiar with this "tune," they heard it played on different notes; on different notes and in a different rhythm, and, finally, different notes in a different rhythm played by a different instrument—a guitar. In the speech experiment they similarly heard a rhythmic series of nonsense syllables and, once they were accustomed to that, a progressively changing series ending with different syllables in a different rhythm. In both experiments it was the first and second step changes which evoked the greatest search for the source of the sound and the greatest changes in heart rate. A similar pattern of response, throughout this half year, has been demonstrated when infants have been allowed to get used to looking at particular patterns or objects and have then seen stimuli which varied slightly, moderately, or extremely from that standard. The greatest attention is paid to the moderately different stimulus and infants will make more effort to acquire such a stimulus, too. If the infant's own kicking releases a mobile which is slightly different from one at which he has gazed for hours, he will kick longer and harder than he will kick for that too-familiar or for a completely strange mobile [79].

The theoretical explanation for these findings is that the child in the second half of his first year has developed "schemas" for a number of people, sights, sounds, objects, and feelings. That he has reached the developmental stage where he can call these schema into his mind in response to a new event and try, so to speak, to compare or mesh together the remembered with the new. If there is almost no difference between them, his attention will not be held for long. But if there is a very great difference between them, he will not see any relationship and will not therefore pay attention after his first reaction to the novelty. Reaction to extreme novelty may indeed be negative. Long before any of this scientific work was available, the author purchased for her own baby a small gray rubber elephant with a loud and easily induced squeak. The baby was fascinated; she had had other small rubber animals. But the first accidentally caused squeak produced virtual hysteria. Elephant had to have the squeaker hole taped up until, weeks later, the child had had sufficient experience of making things make noises that she was able to enjoy making the elephant make a noise too.

Infants with older brothers and sisters are usually exposed to just the "right" mixture of familiar and slightly different objects to play with. Bored with his own bricks, the infant may be handed a giant Lego brick belonging to his brother. It is still a brick, but it has interesting nobbles on it, and being plastic rather than wood it makes a different sound when banged on the table. Bored with his woolly ball, the infant tries a rubber one; his tedious old rattles give place to his sister's maracas or a can of model animals which he can shake. Above all, such an infant is able to demonstrate his pleasure in slightly new and different objects; his mother can *see* that he likes the contents of the 3-year-old's toy box better than his own baby toys. But the first baby may not be so lucky. His baby toys may be the only real *toys* in the house. And it may not occur to his mother to share hers with him.

The desire for constant but slight novelty in the objects he plays with does mean that bought toys are often inappropriate for infants of this age group. Families can neither afford, nor store, a continual succession of rattles and balls and bricks and cuddly toys. There are some toys which can be bought now, and used, in many different ways, over a long period. But basic day-to-day entertainment can almost always be better provided from within the existing household. Wooden spoons, small saucepans, boxes with lids, scrumply paper, pieces of material, ribbon and string, will all be pleasurably explored. And when the infant tires of one saucepan, another may please him. It is familiar, but its weight, its size, its color are different. In our consumer society with its ludicrously elaborate packaging, the family's weekly shopping can provide scores of objects which will interest the infant. The stoutest can be stored to make an "odds-and-ends box" for the infant to turn out and repack when he is a few months older. Obviously such *ad hoc* play materials have to be closely supervised. A rattle from a reputable shop may bore the baby but it will not cut his mouth; a pudding container will if he bites it.

The infant's progress as a tool-user does seem to be closely related to the opportunities he is given. Between 6 and 8 months he learns about objects by handling them, and the more different objects he handles, the more he will learn. By around 8 months, he also begins to learn by watching demonstrations. The difference can be most clearly seen in the infant's reaction to pencils and paper, and to toys which can be pulled along on strings. At 7 months, the infant will pick up a crayon; but however much his mother attracts his attention, and scribbles with it, he is unlikely to copy her. He will, if he is permitted, chew the crayon and crumple the paper. But around 8 months, if someone *does* demonstrate the action and result of scribbling, he will definitely watch, and may attempt to copy, although he is unlikely to manage to mark the paper for another couple of months. Similarly, at around 7 months, the infant may manage to pick up a piece of string, attached to a little wheeled toy on the other side of the table. By pulling at the string, he may even draw the toy toward him, but he is unlikely to show much sign of understanding what he has done. Six weeks later, a demonstration will be watched closely and eventually copied. There is seldom any doubt when an infant has understood and deliberately repeated such an achievement. The arrival of the toy is usually greeted with enormous pleasure, grins, and lengthy excited babbling.

By 9 months the infant's reaction to two simultaneous objects has changed completely. He no longer disregards the first in favor of the second nor uses them both but separately. Typically he now brings the two together, side by side, as if comparing them. And he begins to use the two objects together: banging them against each other, putting them down on the table top, picking them up again. But his skill with objects is still inhibited by the difficulty he experiences with letting *go* of what he has picked up. Releasing an object is exactly opposite, in its neurophysiological demands, to grasping. And it involves controlling the fingers separately from the whole hand. Normally it begins to develop at around 9 months, or simultaneously with the beginning of a finger-thumb pincer approach to very small objects, and the ability to use the index finger alone for pointing or poking.

At 9 months most infants can only let go of an object by putting object and hand on to a flat, hard surface. It is in this way that the infant frees his hand from one cube in order to pick up another. The idea of release usually comes before the ability. The infant may respond to the mother's request to "give it to me" by holding the object out to her. But he cannot actually let go of it. Indeed his fingers may remain quite tightly curled around it, so that she has to uncurl them to retrieve the toy. A little later, if she holds her hand flat under his, he may be able to release the toy onto her palm, as he does on to the table top. But he will still be unable to drop it into a container, or onto the floor.

Deliberate releasing of objects usually starts late in the tenth month. It may usher in a phase which the mother does not entirely enjoy. As with other abilities, once the infant can, he will. And that means weeks of toys dropped over the edge of the carriage, food dropped over the feeding tray, wash cloths dropped out of the bath. Many mothers resort to tying objects on to every piece of equipment the infant uses. This may be why, typically, it is in the tenth month that infants get the idea of swinging things on the end of strings, and much enjoy "fishing" over the edge of crib or carriage.

During the eleventh month, all these dawning abilities, together with the child's mobility, are put together in his play. He learns to throw objects away from him, neither dropping them, nor pushing them, but genuinely (if wildly) throwing them. He will throw a soft ball, crawl after it, and do it again. Equally he will behave like a small retriever dog if an adult will throw for him. He learns to push away a wheeled toy as well as pulling it back by its string. His new ability to release objects from the hand makes filling-and-emptying games a top favorite. The various forms of sorting box sold commercially are usually too sophisticated for the child at this stage. But a box and some bricks will be combined and recombined endlessly. The infant may, if he is given a demonstration, even attempt to put one brick on another to make a tower, by the time he is a year old. But here the difficulty he still has in accurate releasing usually foils his attempts. He poises the second brick accurately over the first, but cannot let it go in exactly the right place.

The last three months of the first year should be a time when the infant is encouraged to use these play abilities in daily life, too. Where at 6 months he probably grabbed the spoon with which his mother was feeding him, just because he was an object-grabber, at 9 months he is perfectly aware of its use. His attempts at self-feeding will probably still be extremely messy. But there is some evidence that infants who are prevented from feeding themselves during this vital phase may still be having food ladled into their mouths at 18 months or even 2 years. Feeding by the mother at that age can all too easily become forced-feeding (see Chapter Twenty-five). Messy or not, he should be allowed to do all the self-feeding he can manage, now.

In the bath he can and should have the wash cloth to swish over himself, even if he would still suck the soap if allowed that. In dressing, he knows quite well that shoes go on feet, and will have a go at putting them there. If he is not hurried, he will hold out his arms for a coat or his legs for his trousers. Given the chance, he will imitate many of his mother's domestic activities, presaging the passion for housework which is so typical of the second year.

By his first birthday, the baby can get hold of objects, get rid of them again; retrieve them by a variety of means, including the conceptually difficult one of pulling a string. And he begins to know what to do with them, what they are *for*. He has come a very long way in six months.

23

BECOMING A TALKER

As we saw in Chapter Seventeen, the study of very early language development is an extremely difficult field, and one in which there remains a scarcity of good research. The study of language in this second half year is little better. There are disputes among researchers about what infants utter, about what their utterances "mean," about why they make the sounds they do make and indeed about why they make the effortful transition from sound-making to speech at all. Given that infants do eventually begin to speak, there is further argument about whether understanding of a word must come before that word is spoken, or whether the word can be spoken before it is understood. And all this disputation takes place across many disciplines: as well as linguistic specialists, there are neurologists, physiologists, brain biochemists, psychologists, social psychologists, and philosophers researching in this area.

If few pieces of our knowledge about language development are agreed upon, most researchers would be unanimous on one point: the importance of language. In many ways language is the most vital function which an infant develops. It is the basic tool of being a human being. If rising on to his hind legs and becoming a tool-using biped gave developing man an advantage over other animals, developing speech gave him an even greater one. By using language we can convey information about things which are not physically present, and about ideas which do not physically exist. We can say anything which we can do; say what we cannot do; say what no man has ever done. We can discuss possibilities, projects, ideas which are truly original, outside the experience of man. The knowledge of one generation can be passed on to the next without the new generation having to undergo the experiences or do the finding out for itself. The saving of time and effort and the creative possibilities which all this opens up are immeasurable. They add up to what we call "culture."

A book of this length cannot hope to review research in this field. The difficulty is not only the sheer volume and complexity of exciting work in progress, but also the passionately held, yet contradictory, theories and views to which that work is giving rise. Hazel Francis has made a brave attempt to decide upon and allocate appropriate space and weight to different research groups; her book *Language in Childhood* [85] is recommended. Any reader who is interested in the academic battles which are raging and in their implications for an understanding of language development should turn also to Adrian Desmond's *The Ape's Reflection*, which was published in 1979 [60].

For many generations it was assumed that human language was unique not only in its expression in speech but also in the kind of abstract, conceptual thinking which that speech both demonstrated and facilitated. The Victorians, badly shaken by Darwin's revolutionary statements about evolution, with their then-blasphemous implications of our animality, clung to language and thought (and their associates morals and ethics) as a last bastion of the uniqueness of Man who alone was made in God's image. Later generations, less offended by Darwinism, nevertheless accepted the entrenched ideas of Man's qualitative superiority over other animals. They could observe that no other animal speaks as people speak and it was easy to accept that no other animal could think conceptually either. If the behavior of one species is entrenched as the standard by which the behavior of other species are studied and measured, superiority is easy to maintain at the expense of understanding. Even today, when concern for other species shows itself in burgeoning conservation and protection movements, there is a strong element of patronage still remaining.

But how different are human beings from other animals and does our language and thinking really set us apart? During the seventies it was shown that we share almost 99 percent of our genes with chimpanzees, while pygmy chimpanzees are genetically even closer to us [26]. Chimpanzee organs have already been used for transplantation into human patients and it is clear that a man-chimp is genetically feasible. Many scientists have remarked that the genetic similarity between men and apes is so great that the very marked differences in their appearance are surprising. We are much more like apes than we appear to be.

Findings like these gave new impetus—and for some people, new direction—to attempts to teach human language to apes. In the thirties and forties various baby chimpanzees, such as Gua and Vicki, had been raised in human families, treated as far as possible like human babies. The express purpose of these studies had been to compare the development of ape and human young *and to pinpoint the stages at which the apes got left behind.* Little attention was focused on ape development in itself. Even less was focused on those areas where the development—or the speed of the development—of the apes left the humans far behind. Such apes had learned to understand one hundred or so human words but attempts to teach them to *speak* had failed. The actual production of speech sounds depends on appropriate neuromuscular organization which chimpanzees do not have. Attention was therefore turned to finding other means whereby apes might be able to communicate with people. In the sixties Washoe learned to communicate extensively using American Sign Language [89]. The Premacks [182] then devised a plastic-shape "language" for Sarah. Now some dozens of apes, gorillas as well as chimpanzees, are being schooled to communicate in variations of these "languages" as well as through a variety of ingenious computer-linked keyboards. With these aids some apes can be taught by some people to wield human "words." But controversy about what these findings mean remains widespread. Do they mean that apes do in fact have "language ability," previously considered uniquely human, once they are provided with a means of expressing it? Or is their "language" not really language at all but perhaps something closer to coding? Why can apes wield our language when, as far as observers can yet tell, they use no form of symbolic communication among themselves in the wild? The search for answers to this kind of question is still bedeviled by Victorian attitudes. Those who wish to deflate the human race's view of itself as evolutionarily superior tend to glorify the language of apes pointing out that they must go on record as the very first species to learn the language of another species—us. Those who accept our evolutionary superiority, on the other hand, tend actually to define language as human so that any communication by a member of another species is automatically classified as non-language. At a recent and unforgettable conference, members of the first group demonstrated ape "language" which was at least as sophisticated as that of a verbally well-advanced human toddler, only to have psycho-linguists from the other group declare that the speech of human toddlers is not truly language at all!

Aloof from the battlefield it seems possible to see humans and apes as genetically close yet clearly different. It would seem that at some far distant time their evolutionary paths diverged and led to two separate species. If they are on two different paths then their relative development and performance can be interesting without being value-laden. Most of the misleading thinking about ape "language" seems to arise from a determination to see apes—and their communications—as poor versions of people and their language.

Some members of the ape-species have been shown to be able to use symbols creatively and purposefully. Human beings do this too. But this does not mean that when apes wield symbols taught to them by humans, their creativity and their purpose is used to produce *human* communication. The direct relevance of all this mind-boggling work to our thinking about language development in infants is that the point of words is their meaning; that their meaning is intrinsic to the individual's own psycho-social framework, and, for words to be communicative, that psycho-social framework has to be shared by speaker and listener. When a human attempts to communicate with an ape, these conditions cannot be met. When an adult human attempts to communicate with a very young one, they may, or may not, be met, depending on the stage of understanding and of socialization the child has reached. Many symbolizing apes are taught, for example, the "word" cry. They use this word in situations where they might be expected to be unhappy, as when a beloved teacher leaves or a favorite food is removed. But apes cannot cry; only humans cry. What can that word-idea "cry" therefore *mean* to an ape? *Does* it mean "I-am-unhappy-and-if-I-were-human-I-would-cry"? Or do we only assume, out of our humanness, that this is the message? Symbols for "sorry," "good," and "please" are also commonly taught to apes. Each of these value-laden words is completely linked to human social systems and conventions. The symbols, as taught, clearly mean something to the apes but it seems most unlikely that they mean what their teachers assume them to mean. Studies of apes in the wild suggest that apologies are conveyed for offenses very different from those human beings are taught to regret. Washoe was taught to sign "sorry" when she hurt anybody yet she customarily made this sign whenever anyone was hurt even if there was no way in which she could have been responsible. Furthermore, many of the apes are reported as being fascinated by blood; keen to squeeze people's minor wounds to produce some and in no way "sorry" if the victim then squeaks with pain.

This work throws into sharp relief the importance of shared experience in a world with a shared conceptual and social framework. Human infants learn language which both reflects the objective and social structure of their world and imposes structure on aspects of it which are novel to them. When a chimp signs "dirty," he uses the symbol he has been taught for feces, but we can easily see that he is unlikely to share our view of a muddy floor as also "dirty." Young children are often in a similar predicament when they meet new words or new uses for words. They will only learn to use language richly and freely as and when they can come to share with us the concepts which lie behind them.

Since human beings appear to be the only animals which develop symbolic language spontaneously, neurophysiologists tend to feel that this uniqueness of function is likely to be reflected in a uniqueness of structure within the human brain.

It has been known for years that adult human brains show a difference between the right and the left hemispheres, with a lengthening and thickening of one small piece of the cerebral cortex on one side only. This area is more usually in the left hemisphere and there is convincing evidence that speech processing is carried out there [92]. But such a development within the brain's structure could come about due to its use in language—with the structure being dictated by the function rather than the reverse. Later research shows that it is not so. The asymmetry can be

demonstrated as early as 30 weeks of fetal life [88], and the extra development is more pronounced in newborn girls than in newborn boys, which
is interesting since girls tend to acquire speech more easily and rapidly
than boys. For a while it looked as if an actual brain structure that accounted for language function might have been discovered. But still later
data deny that the brain structure is unique to the human race. Similar
differences between the two hemispheres of ape brains have been found,
and, now that scientists know what to look for, the same phenomenon—
in more primitive form—is being demonstrated in monkey brains too.
Nevertheless this is the area of the brain in which speech-processing takes
place in humans so if we cannot claim a unique anatomical structure, we
have to return to the idea that humans make unique use of that structure
in their language.

Detailed study of functioning human brains was, for many years,
limited by ethical considerations; only during necessary operations or
treatments could it be permissible to open the skull to stimulate various
areas. But, since the early seventies, EEG monitoring has become so
sophisticated that it can "provide the first direct physiological evidence
for localization of language production functions in the intact, normal
human brain" [149]. Using this non-invasive, painless tool, research continues apace. It is important—and surprising—that our mapping of the
brain is still primitive. We have a great deal still to discover.

Work with children who have suffered various kinds of brain damage
makes it seem unlikely that one particular area in the brain will be shown
to be *exclusively* capable of making speech development possible. Bassler
[16], for example, has shown that infants who lose one complete hemisphere of the brain often do better, in terms of speech development and
other abilities, than infants who suffer less severe but more generalized
brain damage. He believes that the brain has functional plasticity such
that if one major part is completely removed, other parts can take over
its function. If, on the other hand, the damaged part of the brain is left
in situ, it continues to function so that no other part usurps its role, but
it functions aberrantly so that normal development cannot take place.

Lenneberg [141] also believes that plasticity is a vital characteristic
of the human brain, and that the sheer length of time over which the brain
continues to develop maximizes the chance that it will come to function
as a unified whole even if parts are damaged or imperfect. He quotes
anatomical, histological, biochemical, and electrophysiological data all
showing that brain development continues at least until puberty.

While both the slow maturation and the plasticity of human brain
function can be taken as proven, their connection with the development
of language is not. But there is a good deal of evidence to support the
deduction.

Language develops in infants at widely varying rates, and therefore
at a range of ages, but it develops in an invariant sequence. The basic
learning may, under optimal conditions, be compressed into 2 or 3 years,

with only extensions of vocabulary, and the means of expressing complex abstract thought still remaining to be learned. Or the basic learning may stretch over the whole of childhood. At either extreme, the sequence is the same. There are, for example, experimental data demonstrating the identical language-learning sequence in first- and later-born children, in the children of deaf and hearing parents, in children from widely varying socioeconomic and cultural groups, in children from complete and attentive homes compared with those from broken and neglectful homes. Even children in extremely deprived institutional care develop language in the same sequence as family children, albeit far more slowly.

Mentally retarded children usually begin to acquire speech late, and improve slowly. But if they begin to use language at all they, like other deprived children, will continue to improve all through childhood. When they reach puberty language improvement tends to cease, presumably because brain maturation is then complete.

In practical terms it is unfortunate that this long-drawn-out language learning, within a normal, but usually much briefer, sequence, is not more widely recognized. All too often a child of six or seven whose language development is only equivalent to that of an 18-month infant is "written off" as being incapable of further language improvement. Even under ideal circumstances such a child would probably never catch up with his more fortunate peers. But if only he could continue to be given the kind of verbal help which is automatically offered to an 18-month infant, he would almost certainly continue to improve until he reached adolescence. And that might mean that he ended up with a "verbal age" equivalent to a normal 8- or 9-year-old, rather than equivalent to that of a toddler.

But even though language learning can continue throughout childhood, it is clear that the first 2 years comprise the optimum time for its foundation to be laid. It is far more difficult to teach an infant to use language if he is cured of congenital deafness at 2 years old, than it is to help one who heard normally in his first year or two, and *then* had a period of deafness. Similarly, children who become permanently deaf after about the age of two respond far better to language training for the deaf than do children who have been deaf from birth.

Normal infants begin to acquire real speech before they actually need it. They begin to use words at an age and stage when crying, sound-making, and gesture are still sufficient to ensure the meeting of their needs. Furthermore those first words, as we shall see (cf. also Chapter Thirty), are very seldom ones which have anything to do with the infant's needs in the physical sense. There is no obvious reason then why infants should bother to start acquiring speech. It seems that there must be an inbuilt propensity to develop language, just as there is an inbuilt propensity to babble.

Many people believe that the infant's basic motivation for making the effortful transition from babble to real language is social, that it is intimately tied up with his attachment to his mother or her surrogate, and with the pleasure and affection the infant gets from her. For example, O. H. Mowrer [165] put forward what he called the "autism theory" of language development. The word "autism" has psychopathological connotations in everyday speech but in Mowrer's terms the implications are simply "reinforcement of the self by the self." He believed that it is hearing his own sounds which stimulates a baby to make further sounds, and that the more affectionate the context in which his first sounds (from the outside world) are heard, the more he will make them himself, and be stimulated to make more. Mowrer cited research work on species of birds which are known to have the ability to reproduce human speech sounds. He pointed out that such birds only learn to "talk" if they are made into pets. Once they have learned to associate certain human sounds with loving care from their owners they become alert, hopeful, pleased, when they hear similar sounds from *themselves.* He summed up: "Words are reproduced if, and only if, they are first made to sound good in the context of affectionate care and attention."

Dorothea McCarthy [154] derived similar ideas from working with human infants. She believed that human infants came to associate the gentle speech sounds they heard with pleasure and the fulfillment of their needs. When the infant then heard his *own* sounds, they sounded to him like those gentle speech sounds from his caretakers and therefore they too made him feel contented and pleased. The pleasure of his own sounds stimulated the baby to make more. McCarthy cited the case of one little girl who, unknown to her parents, had a hearing loss such that she was cut off from gentle conversational tones yet able to hear the explosive sounds of anger or prohibition. She could hear when her parents spoke roughly to her but not when they spoke affectionately. This child developed no language of her own until the hearing loss was detected and a hearing aid enabled her to pick up the missing range of gentle speech.

Much recent research has confirmed and extended the idea that pleasure and affectionate relationships are vital in early speech development. Some workers, not content simply to prove that it is so, have arrived at theoretical formulations to account for it. Bruner, for example, sees language as an essential characteristic of human beings because their particular form of sociotechnical existence makes *agreement between them as to what they should or will do* at least as important as *what they do.* Our adaptation requires us to plan and to cooperate in order to manage our world and language is an essential tool for this. But young children do not learn language out of direct survival need any more than a baby tiger first learns to use its teeth to bring down a meal. Infants learn through play and pleasure and, for the human infant, Bruner [40] says

> The ambience of play is of central importance in providing the context for numerous joint activities between mother and child and in providing "tension-free" opportunities for exercising one's combinatorial abilities for dealing with the social and physical environment.

While this point of view cannot be said to be scientifically proved, it is well supported by observation. Early babbling, and the later inflected sound-making usually called "jargoning," almost always occur when an infant is pleased. When he is angry or distressed he does not "talk," he cries. It certainly seems that the precursors of language are related to pleasant emotions, not to unpleasant ones. Furthermore the idea that the infant talks because his own talk sounds to him like his mother talking is lent support by the fact that infants tend to talk to themselves in exactly the same way that they talk to their mothers. Babbling alone, in his crib, an infant will make a succession of sounds, pause, as if listening to those sounds, and then answer himself. In the same way when his mother talks to him, he listens to her and then talks back.

Infants who are in institutional care from birth often fail to develop the full range and frequency of sound-making which is normal in family infants. But if a baby is put into such care during the second half of his first year, after a pattern of self-reinforcing babble has established itself, then the pattern usually survives. It may be that the first infant has never had the chance to associate talk with loving care, and therefore does not develop it, while the second baby has already discovered the comforting, amusing aspect of talk, and therefore continues to direct it at himself even when he ceases to get much from his caretakers.

Finally, the first words acquired by infants themselves lend support to this idea that language development is a part of sharing pleasant experience or interest with a close partner. Infants very seldom begin their speech with need-fulfilling words such as "milk" or "up" or "sleep" or "want." The first words are almost always the names of deeply loved people or animals or of highly significant objects which give them pleasure. Such early words are almost always used in the context of calling the adult's attention to something, inviting her to share the experience.

At 6 months, most infants will carry on long babble conversations with the mother, listening intently to what she says, as long as she talks directly, face to face. A month later the baby will turn to the mother, definitely looking for her, if she calls to him when she is out of his sight. At this 7-month stage, too, his babble becomes enriched by two-syllable "words." At first these are linked repetitions of his first cooing sounds: "ala," "ama," "oogoo," "lala," and "looloo." A little later, linked repetitions of his later sounds come into play with "words" like "mimi," "ippi," "aja," and so forth. The syllables are quite distinct; they are not lifted subjectively out of a blur of sound, but can be written down, phonetically, as they are uttered, with a high degree of agreement between one listener and another. This new repertoire of sound will certainly be brought into play when the baby is being talked to; but it is also practiced when he is alone. A dawn chorus of babble often becomes the first thing parents hear each morning, rather than the crying which woke them in the earlier months.

By the eighth month most infants have learned to listen to—and try to join—conversations which are *not* directly aimed at them. If mother and father are talking, and the infant is sitting between them, his head will turn from one adult to the other and back again, as if the conversation was a tennis match he was closely following. Soon he learns how to interrupt. He develops a shout for attention. It may be jocular in tone, but it is a definite shout—not a yell, nor a squeal, but a shout. Some infants also learn their first singing tones about the time they learn to shout. Usually the "singing" is a few notes up or down a scale. It may be set off by the mother or some other adult singing to the infant, or it may be a reaction to music heard on the radio or phonograph, or even to a musical toy. When it happens it is unmistakably singing, quite unlike any of the infant's other sounds.

Toward the end of the eighth month, and in the ninth, the repetitive babbling syllables are strung together into long-drawn-out phrases of four or more syllables, such as "loo-loo-loo-loo-loo." Once this begins, very definite changes of emphasis and shifts of phrasing can be heard. Soon after, the first multi-syllable complex babbles can be heard. The infant no longer repeats the same sound over and over again, he combines different sounds, so that he says, for example, "ah-dee-dah-boo." Once this kind of combination is heard, the infant is on the verge of producing his first words. And his inflections become so marked and varied that he sounds as if he is talking, fluently, but in another language. Ruth Griffiths's English sample [99] produced, on average, one clear word during the ninth month, two clear words and a definite shake of the head for "no" during the tenth month, and three clear words by 1 year.

First words are difficult to identify or even to define. Infants' early vocabularies are often overestimated because when they reach the age at which parents begin to *expect* them to produce words, they tend to count as words babbling sounds which the infant has been making for months. Few mothers will maintain that her 6-month baby is addressing her when he says "mum-mum-mum." But when he repeats this sequence at 11 months she may stoutly maintain that he says "mummy."

A word cannot be counted as a true word until it is used consistently and exclusively to refer to one particular thing. "Mum-mum" becomes "mummy" when the child only says it to or about his mother. But there is an in-between stage which complicates matters. Some infants pass through a period during which they clearly understand the identity of a particular object and also clearly realize that a word for it will communicate to the mother. But they have not yet fixated one particular word-sound to that object. For a while they use different words for the same thing as if any old word would do. Mura Jun Ichi [167] gives the instance of a child who used the word "bon-bon" when asking for his ball. Later he used the word "dan-dan" for the same ball. To the infant these were clearly words. He meant his ball; he did not mean anything else. But he had not "decided" what to call that ball.

Even once an infant uses one and only one word-sound to mean always one and the same thing, it is not easy to say which of his words are true words. At this stage the sound the child uses may be an "own word" which is barely related to the correct word for the object. One child, for example, referred to the family dog as "gig." His name was "Tiger." It is possible that the little girl was trying to approximate the word "dog." Certainly she never referred to anything else as "gig" and would crawl around, looking for the dog, calling him and eventually greeting him by this name. Once such an "own word" is recognized by the adults around the child, it should certainly be counted as a true word. The very fact of the adults' recognition means that the sound the child makes is *functioning* as a word. The adults understand it. The word is communicating.

People of philosophical bent have often asked whether infants imitate words before they understand their meaning, or whether understanding must come before the child can imitate the word. As we shall see, the relevance of imitation to word acquisition is often exaggerated. The question itself is off-center. Anyone who observes infants finds that they understand a great many words months before they attempt to say any words at all, either spontaneously or in imitation. The mother says, "Listen, Daddy's coming," and the baby crawls, grinning, to the door. She says, "Let's put on your shoes," and he looks instantly at his own feet. Whether or not he *could* imitate a word whose meaning he did not know seems irrelevant when there are so many words he does understand just waiting to be said when he is ready.

Most infants who are approaching their first birthday are very ready to imitate adults: they copy gestures, reproduce grimaces, follow demonstrations. This general imitativeness, together with the very sociable context of the child's language learning, tends to make parents feel that they "teach" their children to talk. The mother discovers that if she engages the child in conversation, and makes a clear distinct sound, he will repeat it back to her. Once she has discovered this, she may spend long periods of time holding objects up for the child to see, saying their names, accepting or rejecting the child's response. While this sort of face-to-face conversation may help the child in his general language development, by giving him lengthy and enjoyable conversations with his mother, there is quite a lot of evidence that the actual teaching involved is so indirect as hardly to merit the name.

M. Bullowa, L. G. Jones, and A. Duckert [42] carried out an elegant study, using both film and tape recordings, of a mother trying to teach her infant to say the word "shoe." The teaching and the infant's responses followed the sequence shown in Table 9.

It seems clear from this fascinating case study that the mother's direct behavior had very little effect on the child. When she rejected the first imitation it nevertheless remained in the child's repertoire, unchanged, for some time. Later, when she accepted and understood, both in the presence and absence of the shoes, a further imitation, her reward-

TABLE 9. SEQUENCE OF ONE INFANT'S LEARNING OF THE WORD "SHOE"

	Mother	Infant	Comment
Stage 1	Said "shoe" in clear association with child's shoe →		
		Attempted imitation "tu"	
	← Rejected imitation →		
		Continued to use "tu" for all references to own shoes	Mother's rejection of imitation did not lead child to adapt or abandon her own word which had clear reference
Stage 2	Again links word "shoe" with child's shoes →		
		Imitated "tu-tu"	
	Accepted this imitation		"Tu-tu" is not linguistically closer to "shoe" than is "tu"
Stage 3	Understands when infant uses "tu-tu" in presence of shoe →		
		Modifies "tu-tu" to "tsu"	Mother's acceptance and understanding did not lead infant to continue using "tu-tu"
Stage 4	Understands when infant uses "tsu" in absence of shoe →		
		Modifies "tsu" to "chu"	Again the modification comes without need, since mother understood previous word
Stage 5	Continues to understand all infant's references to shoes		
		Modifies "chu" to adult "shu"	

ing behavior did not prevent the child from continuing to adapt the word until she finally arrived at the adult pronunciation. Furthermore the mother's accuracy as a teacher as well as her effectiveness is called into question. The imitation which she did understand and accept was no more accurate than the one she had rejected a few days earlier.

It seems likely, from this and from other evidence, that the infant's eventual production of words comes about more by watching the mother, and listening to her constant use of the word-related-to-the-object, than by her direct teaching. As daily life proceeds, the mother constantly says "Where are your shoes?" or "Let's put on your shoes" or "Oh, what muddy shoes" or "Off with your shoes." The mother uses the same noun in a variety of situations, and in combination with a variety of other speech forms. The noun "shoe" is the one consistent sound amid this complexity, and is always directed at those things that are put on and off feet. The infant may learn more from observing this than he does from having a shoe dangled in front of him while the mother says "shoe," "say 'shoe' " and so on.

Of course infants eventually learn to speak in the language which they hear, even if a tourist does find herself amazed at the fluency with which Greek 2-year-olds can speak that "difficult" language, Greek! But there are some research workers who believe that at this 9- to 12-months stage, infants are learning language in general rather than any one language in particular. Philosophically the idea is attractive. If human infants are innately programmed to learn language why should they not first use any or all of the sounds of *human* languages and only later refine that use to conform to their own family and nationality? Nakazima [168] believed that while babies, like older people, have different voices and therefore could usually be distinguished one from another by a listener, the nationality of the infants would be of no help: two American babies might sound as similar or as different as an American and a Japanese baby. He made a careful study of speech development in Japanese and American infants. Despite the marked linguistic differences between the two languages, he was able to find no differences whatsoever between the utterances of the two groups of infants, even with the use of spectrographic apparatus. When the infants began to produce their first "real words," there was still no difference.

More recent research has lent credence to this idea that infants start out ready to learn *any* language and only gradually narrow their learning down to their native tongue. Liberman [145] reported in 1976 on a study of adult listeners' ability to hear and perceive sounds which were not used in their native language. The Thai language, for example, makes no use of a differentiation between b and p; Thai listeners could not distinguish between the word-sounds ba and pa. Similarly, Japanese listeners were unable to hear the difference between r and l sounds although these were easily distinguished by American listeners. Out of these findings, Liberman devised 13 mock words; 7 were easy for Japanese and difficult for

American listeners to distinguish while the other six were difficult for Japanese and easy for American listeners. Peter Eimas [70] used these same synthetic speech sounds with 2- to 3-month-old American infants. Unlike their elders, the babies clearly showed (by their renewed interest in each new sound, see p. 273) that they could discriminate all the mock words.

If nationality, or the language he hears spoken around him, makes no difference to the sounds a baby can discriminate, neither does it appear to affect the readiness or difficulty with which he later learns to make different sounds. Certain speech sounds, such as s, z, th, r, and f appear to be "difficult" for all infants to learn. These sounds seldom appear in spontaneous babbling. They seem to be learned, slowly and with difficulty, only as children extend their actual vocabularies. Nakazima found that children whose native languages employed one or more of these sounds extensively were at no learning advantage when compared with children whose languages employed them comparatively little. The absence or inaccurate reproduction of these sounds accounted for much of the lisping and "baby talk" which is common in the second and third years of life in children from every studied language-group.

So do infants babble and jargon in a poly-language common to all nationalities and linguistic groups? It seems probable that they *could* but unlikely that they *would* do so because of the basically communicative and cooperative nature of speech. The infant is learning to communicate *with* one or more affectionate people. Communication is both the motive and the reward, and therefore the sounds which further that communication are the ones which the infant will gradually mold into language. At the Third Symposium on Child Language in 1975, many of the speakers were parent-researchers who had devoted themselves to studying their own children and their own effects on those children's language. The consensus from this naturalistic, home-based research was in complete agreement with Bruner that *joint understanding* was the key to word-learning. If a parent understood a child's sound and reflected it back to him with a meaningful expansion of what he had "said," that sound-word was confirmed for the child as meaningfully communicative and it was likely to enter his speech repertoire as soon as he was ready. A "Japanese sound" would be unlikely to receive this kind of understanding endorsement from a British or American parent. Such a sound would therefore be likely to slip rapidly into background noise, leaving "English sounds" in high relief.

BECOMING A TALKER
IN MORE THAN ONE LANGUAGE

Since this book was first published the author has frequently been asked about the advisability, or otherwise, of rearing infants to be bi-lingual.

There is surprisingly little research on this topic but there are, perhaps, some inferences which can be drawn from the kind of material discussed earlier.

Infants are clearly able to distinguish the speech sounds of all languages at least until they have discovered that certain sounds communicate and that others do not. It follows that any sounds, from any language-group, which *do* communicate, can be used by the child. An infant's language-learning is principally facilitated by the experience of effective communication in shared play with loved adults. Therefore if he experiences this kind of communication in two languages, from the beginning of his life, he will come to use them both. Parents who are truly bi-lingual themselves can therefore be assured that if they continue to use both their languages in whatever way is natural to them, their child will come to adopt a similar language-pattern. There is no evidence to suggest that under these circumstances it is more difficult for him to learn two languages than one. There is indeed no reason why it should be more difficult; the infant is selecting out effectively communicative sounds. If he learns only English, he will discover that the dog can be "dog," "puppy," or "Jack." If he is learning English and French, he will discover, in exactly the same way, that the dog can be "dog," "chien," "Jack," or "Jacques." Such a child may certainly go through phases during which his two languages are intermixed, but so does the single-language child go through phases in which "real" words are mixed with "own-words." The child in a bi-lingual family will sort them out for himself just as the single-language child does.

Complications sometimes set in, however, where the family is not "truly bi-lingual." If both languages are to be equally learned, both must give the child equal feedback and reward. For this to come about, parents usually need not only to be equally competent in both languages but to use both with equal spontaneity. Often this is not the case. As an example, consider an Italian family, long resident in America and long accustomed to conducting their lives and relationships in English. Both parents had retained total fluency in Italian and used it spontaneously on rare visits to their families in Naples. At such times both maintained that they "thought in Italian" but for the rest of the year only an Italian visitor or newspaper disturbed them from thinking in English. When their child was born, they decided to give her the benefit of their mother tongue. They decided, as a matter of policy, to talk to her in Italian some of the time and to encourage her to learn Italian as well as English words. Policy turned out to be the enemy of fluency. The parents stayed alert to Italian-sounding early words and fed these back to the baby in that language, but most of the time they spoke to her in English and, of course, that was the language she heard used between them and from other people. Around her first birthday, the parents began to insist that she produce Italian from time to time. She would comment excitedly to her mother about a bus that was passing. Instead of responding to her interest and enlarging on what she had said—by saying "yes, isn't it a big bus?" or words to that effect—her mother would ignore the content of the message of excitement and tell her to say "autobus." Over a period of months, the little girl became extremely confused. By the time she was two she was saying very little in any language except screaming tantrums. Language evolves under the stimulus of pleasurably shared communication. Attempts to teach it rather than simply to encourage and respond to it, usually, as in this case, involve more rejection than the infant can easily stand.

Complications of a different kind can set in where parents do not share a common tongue but talk with each other in an acquired second language for each of them. A Polish-speaking woman was married to a German-speaking man and they were struggling toward the English of their adopted country. They were fully aware of the possible complications for their child but pointed out to me that whichever language the child chose to communicate in, one parent was going to be actually unable to respond in kind. They eventually elected to forgo the advantages of multi-linguality for the child and rear him in, as they put it, "bad English"! Needless to say the child's language development was entirely normal and the few idiosyncratic phrases which he picked up at home soon vanished when he began to talk with other children. The parents maintain that their own fluency, now, largely comes from the child.

A more usual situation is that in which only one parent is "foreign" while the other is a native of the country in which the child is being reared. Sometimes such children seem able to acquire both languages but to do so not as a bi-lingual child does but by using the "foreign" tongue as a private second language, used in intimacy with that parent. Other children in this situation do not actually learn to speak the second language but nevertheless understand it, especially where it has been closely linked with affectionate situations such as nighttime lullabies, comfort rituals, and so forth. When they reach school age, such children may not be fully aware that they "know French" but may nevertheless find that language remarkably easy to learn.

At this stage of our knowledge it seems clear that a child will acquire whatever language brings him the rewards of effective communication with people he cares about, and that these rewards come from being readily understood and richly responded to. Truly bi-lingual parents who spontaneously interact with the infant in interchangeable languages certainly do not need to be concerned lest they muddle him. But all parents, single-language speakers as well as multi-linguists, who concern themselves with forms of speech rather than its content, with how the child talks rather than with what he is trying to say, should be concerned lest they spoil for their child what should be a joyous business: talking with someone.

ONE-YEAR SUMMARY

THE YEAR-OLD INFANT has made strides in his development which seem enormous to the adults around him. In fact, he has not changed his behavior as radically in this second half year as he did in the first. But now he is mobile (either as a biped or a quadruped); he talks (to some extent) and he uses objects. All these developments make him seem far more like a small human being than he did 6 months earlier.

The particular stage which any individual child will be at when he reaches his first birthday is dependent on the area to which he is devoting most of his time and energy. He is unlikely to forge ahead on all fronts simultaneously. If he is just beginning to acquire words, his motor progress may seem to be at a standstill. If he is concentrating on climbing the stairs and the chairs he may not seem to be learning words at the same time. If he is battling to stay on his own two feet, he may have no time for his toys.

As at 6 months, his relationship with his parents is critical too. If he has already joined some of the typical toddler battles with his mother, over eating, or going to bed, or using a potty, quite a lot of his behavior may be directed at getting back at her—at venting his frustration and demanding her attention.

While much of the slowness in development which arose from neonatal troubles has now been lost in the passage of time, the sequences of development remain almost invariable. Therefore it is useless to expect a child to pull himself to standing just because he is a year old, unless he sat alone between 7 and 10 months. It is useless to expect him to feed himself with a spoon if he only became adept at reaching out and picking objects up at 9 months. It is useless to expect him to begin to acquire real words, if his private "jargoning" is not yet heavily inflected and widely varied in content. As before, the infant's present development, and expectations of his immediate future development, are only meaningful in the light of the past.

Behavior	Likely stage reached at 1 year	Comments
Feeding	Three meals at ordinary family times. Snacks at mid-morning and afternoon.	Many infants will still be having a bottle, but at *their* bedtime, rather than the mother's. Some will have bottles more or less *ad lib.,* together with frequent snack foods. Their actual food intake may be more than twice as high as their "meals."
Food	Many will still be fed almost entirely on proprietary "convenience" foods. But all should have learned to chew by now, and should be having finger foods.	Infant *could* eat ordinary family diet, with meat minced, and other foods cut up, de-pitted, etc. Few are given the chance.
Feeding method	Infant is perfectly capable of taking all milk from a cup. If he still uses a bottle now, it will be as much a comfort habit as a nutritional tool and he is likely to continue through the second year. If given the chance earlier, the infant will feed himself from a spoon and with his fingers. He needs only minimal help.	Self-feeding now tends to avert feeding problems later. But it is rare. Most are still fed by the mother at this age.
Food preferences	As at 6 months, infant is likely to prefer soft or crisp foods, gagging on thick or sticky foods or those which, like meat, require lengthy chewing.	Infant is at height of imitative phase. Will wish to try same foods as mother. None are intrinsically unsuitable; anything he can digest

Behavior	Likely stage reached at 1 year	Comments
	May like far stronger tastes than mother expects, eating more enthusiastically if allowed some grated cheese, salad dressing, etc.	he can have. Drugs such as alcohol, caffeine, etc., should be avoided.
Weight	Gains roughly 2–3 oz. (60–90 g) per week from 6–12 months. An average birthweight baby (around 7 lb. [3.2 kg]), who has gained normally, will now weigh just over 20 lb. (9.1 kg).	Both food consumption and weight gain become less consistent around 1 year.
Sleep	Average sleep is around 13 1/2 hours with very wide scatter. Most will sleep a 12-hour night. Most will also need two "rests" but may sleep for only a few minutes at one or both of these.	After about 9 months, infant can keep himself awake if he wants to. Upsets may start problems over falling asleep. Cannot wake himself voluntarily, so night waking which is common can be dealt with only by comfort/reassurance. Comfort habits and the use of comfort objects are common at this age.
Crying	Crying from boredom or loneliness is largely replaced by tears of frustration when fails in self-imposed play task. Crying from anger is frequent. Cries when hurt—frequent when learning to walk—but may also cry from shock of bump which does not hurt. Cries when left by mother, and may cry when faced with strangers.	Infants vary in readiness with which they actually *cry* as opposed to using developing language ability to convey distress. By this age, there should be no crying for which the cause is not clear, even if the cause seems small to an adult.

Behavior	Likely stage reached at 1 year	Comments
Teeth	Will have cut two upper front and two lower front teeth. May have cut lower first molar, in which case upper first molar will be on the way.	Cutting of molars often causes some discomfort, relieved by biting hard foods or teething toys. First teeth should be cleaned.
Toilet training	A few infants will have been placed on the potty for some months. Some more will start around this time. A few infants begin now to "tell"—usually after the event.	Infants whose bowel movements are regular may become "clean." Few infants will tolerate regular frequent potting because their motor drive is so strong.
Sitting up	Sits independently on a hard surface. Leans forward or sideways and recovers balance. Gets himself unaided to sitting position from any other position.	Inability to sit alone by 1 year requires investigation.
Crawling	Crawls freely by some method. Usually hands and knees, but may be hands and feet, or, rarely, some version of shuffling on bottom.	Is unlikely to crawl well if sitting steadily has been late in developing. May skip crawling if advanced in standing and walking.
Standing	Pulls himself to standing by furniture.	May have trouble sitting down from standing.
Walking	May cruise around supporting furniture, or walk a step or two with both hands held. May momentarily stand unsupported.	
Manual play	Touches, strokes and picks up objects accurately. Can separate fingers from total hand grasp, to pick up tiny objects between finger and thumb. Can throw and push objects away.	Manual ability and desire to imitate means that infant will readily learn to feed himself with spoon, drink from cup, attempt to put on shoes, etc.

Behavior	*Likely stage reached at 1 year*	*Comments*
Manual play (*cont'd*)	Uses attached string to retrieve or pull toys. Fills and empties containers with small objects. May attempt to build with bricks, but inaccurate release still causes difficulty. Copies demonstrations: e.g., scribbling with pencil.	
Social responses	Typically highly emotionally attached to mother, to father if he is sufficiently seen, and to other adults who share personal interaction with him. Highly dependent on mother's constant presence, though better able to entertain himself, in her presence, than earlier. May be suspicious or actually fearful of strangers. Reacts to disapproval from mother.	Likely to be highly disturbed by separation from mother at this period. May react badly to any major change, such as house move, holiday, etc.
Language (spoken)	Typically accompanies own play with "jargoning"—highly inflected complex babble, with many different syllables strung together, containing exclamation marks, question marks, and paragraphs. Sounds like talk, but has no recognizable words in it. Most have three clear words, which may only be loose approximations to actual words, but are used consistently to indicate one particular person or object. Shakes	Language development is highly variable. Actual words will not be produced before expressive jargoning is established. Many normal infants will not say any words until the second year.

Behavior	Likely stage reached at 1 year	Comments
Language (spoken) (cont'd)	head for "no." Shouts for attention. Sings to music. Recognizes mother by voice alone.	
Language (understood)	Clearly understands many words and phrases. May obey simple commands to "bring" or "give," etc. May point to familiar objects in picture book, hold out foot at mention of "shoe."	Absence of expressive jargoning, together with failure to understand any words or phrases requires investigation of hearing.

PART V

THE SECOND YEAR
From Baby to Toddler

BEING A TODDLER

BETWEEN ABOUT 9 MONTHS and perhaps 15 months, infants become so diversified as human beings, and so clearly but variously affected by the environment in which they are being reared, that it becomes increasingly difficult to age-categorize their development. Most of the basic "milestones" are passed. Most of the special physiological features of early infancy have given way to more mature patterns. One can still give vague "norms" for both accomplishments and problems, but the range of variation around those norms becomes ever wider. That is why this last section makes no attempt to look at development by quarter or by half years. The developments to be discussed now will take place roughly during the second year. Infants who lagged in some or in all respects at the end of their first year will, in most fields, still develop later than others. Infants who were ahead at the end of the first year may stay ahead. Others will unexpectedly spurt forward or drop back in one or several fields. So for some people this section will appear to apply to any infant under 3 1/2; for others it will appear only to apply up to 20 months.

Being a toddler is a little like being an adolescent. The toddler is between babyhood and childhood, just as the adolescent is between childhood and adulthood. The adolescent is often stereotyped as a rebel —as one who fights against the upbringing, the background, the restrictions he has accepted as a child; in the same way the toddler is often stereotyped as likely to be a problem to his parents. He too reaches a stage where he resents and fights the absolute power and control which his mother had over him when he was a baby. He too looks for new fields in which to exercise a new sense of power, a new sense of self. But there the similarity has reached its limits. Many adolescents are ready for self-determination; toddlers are not.

Some families manage to integrate toddlers in such a way that this second year is smooth and easy. When this happens, mothers tend to remember it as a halcyon period, to remember two as their "favorite age." Looking through case records, and observations, this happy state of affairs seems to come down to both infant and parents being able to stay in step with themselves, and in step with each other. Innumerable chance factors—quite simple, practical ones—seem to play a vital part in this, perhaps a bigger part than many pediatricians or child psychologists allow for. For example, the infant who is concentrating on walking and the play activities associated with it, as summer begins, *and* has a garden, is likely to be happier, and therefore easier to handle, than one who reaches this stage in January, or while living in a cramped apartment at the top of a building with neighbors who object to noise.

Mothers who take pleasure in the infant's new mobility, longer waking hours and comparative independence, feeling that there are more and more nice things she can now do with him, are likely to ride through this year easily. Mothers who resent the loss of a comparatively controllable "baby," or feel that now the toddler has reached this stage he should hurry up and turn into a schoolchild, may enjoy it much less.

Some fathers find that it is only with the advent of toddlerhood that they can really come into their own. They may take great pleasure in doing things with the infant that were not possible before, and may therefore accept easily the concurrent tantrums and contrariness, seeing them as signs of growing up. Other fathers, often those who have basically resented the demands the infant made on their wives from the beginning, may find a mobile child who even interrupts conversations quite intolerable.

Even the exact "match" between the toddler and his brothers and sisters can have a major effect on this age period. An older sibling may be thrilled to find that the infant begins to join in games, begins to be company in the garden, begins to laugh at jokes. If a 3-year-old girl spends most of the winter playing versions of "house," "mother and father," and "hospital," the infant may be her constant companion, happily taking the role of baby or patient, comprehending little, but getting his own fun. But if that same 3-year-old is at the stage where she wants only to draw and paint and build block houses, the infant may be seen as the tiresome creature who grabs the pencils and spoils everything.

The importance of small practical details of daily life are well illustrated by the notes which the sensitive mother of an 18-month girl felt it necessary to make for her own mother, when she took charge of the infant for one whole day and night. They are reproduced verbatim because they give a very warm picture of the life of a toddler, of the issues which the mother felt were important to her, and of the extreme difficulty which any stranger, equipped with less information, or caring for the child in a strange place, would have had in keeping her happy and secure. Although the author has received many such accounts of daily life during the 7 years which have elapsed since this one was first published, it seems to have lost none of its relevance. Perhaps daily life with very small children has not changed quite as much as most people think.

NOTES ON ANNE!

Dear Mum,

 I know it seems ridiculous, when you know Anne so well, but the more I come to think about your managing with her for a whole day and night, the more I realize what a lot of things there are that you *don't* know, from visits, and which might cause trouble, especially if she is worried anyway because I am not there. So here is a sort of diary.

Before 7 A.M.	If she calls before this, it counts as still the night, and she does not have toys or anything; just resettle her as if it was 3 A.M. (I don't want to lose everything I've gained in getting her to sleep later in the morning!)
About 7:45	She will call. Has the lights on; a drink of diluted orange from her teacher-beaker; two rusks and all her cloth books, in her cot.
About 8 A.M.	She is got up, undressed, and cleaned with baby lotion. She likes to wipe her own face. Will insist on wearing a nappy and plastic pants, even though she will probably use the pot all day. I cannot persuade her that pants are more comfortable and I don't mind the odd puddle. *She* minds.
About 8:30	Goes in high chair and has slice of toast while her scrambled egg cooks. Then has both baby cereal and fruit. Will probably eat the lot and will not accept *any* help. Has milk from her teacher-beaker. If she tries to take the lid off, let her. She is just beginning to like to drink without the spout, and she is very cross if anyone implies that she can't manage.
Morning:	Plays around very self-containedly while housework etc. is done. But is always allowed to hide in our unmade bed before I make it, so don't imply that it's tiresome (it is!). Hates vacuum noise. Must be told when it's going on; will then go out of the room voluntarily until it is switched off. If she fetches her shoes, it means she wants to go in the garden.
	If she fetches her teapot she wants her teaset and the dolls. Keep her out of our bedroom, as my desk is a constant temptation to her.
Around 11 A.M.	Has diluted rosehip syrup in her teacher-beaker, and this is a signal that housework is over; expects more attention after this. Likes something like finger paints, or sand, or bricks, but expects to be helped or played *with* at this time. Don't shut the door on her if you go to the loo; being the wrong side of shut doors panics her.
	If she needs her pot she will probably announce, "Oh dear!"
	It doesn't mean you're too late, but only that she thinks you will be.

12:15 ish   Lunch in high chair. Prefers it if I eat mine at the same
                 time. Has sieved meat or liver (*not* fish which she loathes)
                 with mashed potato in with it, and carrots or peas left to
                 be picked up in her fingers. Then custard with a tin of
                 baby fruit. May not eat much; it is her worst meal, always.
                 Don't try to help her or she will get furious and bat the
                 whole dish on to the floor.

About 1 P.M.   Nap. Has a dry nappy if she needs it, her sleeping bag, the
                 curtains left open but the door shut. Must have white cat,
                 small teddy, red bear and mohair jersey. Will go to sleep
                 at once, and may wake again at 1:30 or not till 3 P.M. Never
                 goes off again once she is awake.

On waking: Always miserable and needs cuddling for at least 15 min-
                 utes. If you hurry her she will be grizzly for the rest of the
                 day. Likes to go out. Top treat is to push baby-walker
                 around in the park, but if you must shop will accept push-
                 chair if you let her push it some of the way. Very fright-
                 ened at the moment if running dogs come near. Always
                 visits the next-door cat on the way out and on the way
                 home again. If it is cold, put her pom-pom hat on; she
                 hates having the hood of her anorak up as it blocks her
                 side vision. May try to tell you about the squirrel we saw
                 in the big oak tree just across the fence. It seems to be
                 called "Cil." Don't take her to the playground; all the
                 equipment is too big and fierce for her. She insists on
                 going on the see-saw and then hates it.

About 3:30   Has fresh orange juice and squares of bread and butter
                 with honey. Likes to have it standing up at coffee table. If
                 you put her in her high-chair she'll think it is supper time.
                 Afterwards usually has stories or records. Will never play
                 on her own at this time. Will resent you even telephoning.
                 It is her most clingy period of the day.

Around 5 P.M.   Is ready for bath. Undress in nursery and take to bath in
                 a towel. Likes to "dance" and generally scruff while she is
                 naked. Adores the bath but is very scared if you try to lie
                 her down, or splash her. Is always allowed to play for at
                 least 20 minutes, with the plastic mugs and the duck and
                 the blue boat.
                 Take back to nursery in towel to get ready for bed. Wears
                 nappy padded with disposables, but no plastic pants. Pyja-
                 mas, and sleeping bag, but with her legs left out so that
                 she can stand up in her cot until she is ready to sleep.

Supper   Likes baby cereal with *cheese*, not sugar. Or yoghurt with
                 fruit stirred in. A cut-up apple or pear. All this in her
                 highchair, but then she has a full bottle, warm, which she
                 will drink on your lap.

6:15 ish   Into bed, with same animals as at nap time. May talk and
                 play for 30 minutes, but any crying is unusual and needs
                 investigation. Loud shouting means she wants her sleep-
                 ing bag zipped up and to be tucked up to go to sleep. But

sometimes she drops off without demanding this, so I just
do it when I go to bed.
Once asleep nothing will wake her except a bad dream. If
she does dream and cry, don't get her out of her cot, just
pat her and talk and she will go off again.
Leave the landing light on and the door ajar.

Large and small factors are peculiarly heightened during the toddler
phase because of the toddler's particular stage of understanding. The
toddler begins to move around as fast as an older child, but without the
older child's sense or memory. He does, of course, learn by experience,
but his learning seems slow, because he does not remember for more
than a minute. He cannot "bear in mind" that he always trips over that
step, or bangs his head on that table, nor can he remember prohibitions
at least until they have been repeated endlessly over weeks and months.
The fascination of the electric plug strikes him afresh several times a day.
If the last time he was removed from it and scolded was an hour ago, he
has probably genuinely forgotten—though he may remember, and stop
if he is reminded before he gets there.

If memory is lacking, so too is forethought. If the infant finds he can
climb up on to a chair, he is not going to be stopped from doing so by
considerations of how he is going to get down again. If he can shut
himself in a cupboard, he will not be stopped by thinking about how dark
and frightening it will be in there. However much he dislikes his mother
being cross, he will not think about her displeasure before he embarks
on a forbidden exploit.

Because he cannot think ahead, the toddler typically cannot defer
gratification for a minute, nor calmly accept its being deferred by anyone
else. What he wants, he wants *now.* If his mother said she would take him
for a walk, and then she is held up by the telephone, the wait is intolerable
to him. "In a minute" is a minute too late.

If the toddler cannot wait a minute for what he wants, neither can
he put up with a brief discomfort for the sake of subsequent comfort. He
may be desperately uncomfortable because his face and hands are sticky
with ice cream. He may weep and wail his misery, but he still cannot
accept the wash cloth without fuss, for the sake of the eventual comfort
it will bring.

The toddler is completely incapable of putting himself in anyone
else's shoes, however obvious and clear-cut the situation. He knows he
hates having his hair pulled, but that does not mean that he can understand that other children hate having *their* hair pulled too. To understand
that, he would have to imagine himself to be the other person; and this
he cannot do. Two toddlers together often illustrate this. One pushes the
other over, and watches while he cries and is comforted. The injured
party then takes identical revenge, and *both* are amazed when the second
child falls over, cries, and is comforted. The parallel between their experi-

ences is completely lost on them. Mothers who retaliate in kind against
their toddler's hitting or biting them often discover that it is useless for
this reason. As one ruefully put it: "He was smacking me quite hard, it
really hurt, so finally when he wouldn't stop I smacked him back. He was
amazed; really he was. You'd have thought he didn't know what smacking
was he was so taken aback."

Decisions, promises, and truth are all beyond the toddler too, however apparently sophisticated his verbal understanding of them. Offered
a simple choice, such as "Would you like to come and have dinner now?"
most toddlers will say or indicate "No!" Coming to have dinner involves
a change of activity; recognizing a desire for dinner means looking forward to the satisfaction of hunger. Put like that, the toddler will elect to
go dinnerless, even if he has been whiny with hunger for the past half
hour. The simple statement, "Dinnertime," will probably bring him
straight to his chair. Offered a choice between a red lollipop and a green
one, he will want both. In fact so much will he want both that his enjoyment of the one he is finally given will probably be spoiled. Offered the
chance to stay with Mummy or go with Daddy to buy a newspaper, he will
either go with Daddy and whine for Mummy all the way, or stay with
Mummy and cry for Daddy as soon as the door closes behind him. Again,
choice-making involves foresight and memory. Which will I enjoy most?
Which did I like last time?

The toddler cannot understand promises for another year or two. He
fusses at leaving the playground, clamoring for one more swing. Mother
says: "If I give you one more will you come home right away afterward?"
The child nods eagerly, but his mind is only on that swing. After one
swing, he clamors for another, and is surprised at his mother's moralistic
displeasure. Releasing him from a sit on his potty, his mother says: "Will
you come and tell me when you do need to go?" Interested only in being
allowed up, the child nods. He may or may not tell when he does need
to go, but if he does it will not be because he understood and remembered his promise. There is a very definite place for bargaining in handling small children. Later on, in the third and fourth years, the straightforward logic of "If I do this, will you do that?" appeals, and is
appropriate. At the toddler stage it has no meaning.

Much the same applies to truth. By the end of the second year many
toddlers talk fluently enough to issue frequent inaccurate denials of
wrongdoing and accusations against other children. The fact that what is
said is untrue still has no meaning for them. It might have been true. It
might have been the dog who broke the vase or made the puddle on the
floor; the child wishes it had been, so he says it was. There may even be
a psychological truth for him which happens to be quite different from
adult truth. He says his sister knocked him over, when in fact he fell. But
if he fell in the course of a squabble, he may well *feel* that she knocked
him over.

What this adds up to is the *appearance* of a human being, in a creature who rushes about, talks, understands what is said to him, and generally partakes of family life. But this appearance is superficial; inside the toddler there are not yet the controls and the socially inculcated beliefs and behaviors which we expect of people. As a full human being, the toddler is still an impostor.

In babyhood, the mother's role was to *be* the child, in the subtle sense of lending him identity and interpreting the world to him, and in the more obvious sense of using her brain and muscles to do for him what he could not do for himself. In toddlerhood she has to release him to be himself, allow him to be a separate, definite person: to want different things from her, to like different things, to like different people, to disagree with her, to pursue his own ends even when they conflict with hers. At the same time she has to continue to be the socialized bit of him, the righter of his inadvertent wrongs, the one who clears up his messes, rescues him from dilemmas, comforts the children he has hurt. She has to remain his safe haven, the platform from which he can set off on all his adventures, and to which he can always return.

While the mother's role as interpreter of the world is less continuous than it was—the toddler wanting and needing to explore it for himself—she is still the channel through which his experiences come. It is up to her to simplify what the child must discover, to make things manageable for him. For example, taken to an adventure playground intended for school-age children, the toddler will almost certainly get hurt, and is unlikely to get anything out of the experience to compensate. The other children are too big, the equipment is too complex; the whole setting is wrong for him. It is not explorable. At a toddlers' group or club for under-fives, the adventure becomes manageable. The scale, both physical and psychological, is right for the toddler. This is a sea he can chart. Similarly, taken to visit with a child of the same age, the toddler may enjoy himself, provided his own mother is there to keep his security, and to control for him the impulses to snatch, grab, and push which he cannot control for himself. Taken and left there alone, it will, unless the other mother is infinitely skillful, be an afternoon of misery. Many toddlers can get a great deal of fun and learning out of each other's company, but very few can avoid mutual misery unless their adult other-halves are there to help. This is why a parent-and-toddler group can be a joy to all where a nursery is seldom a treat for this age group. It is difficult to behave sociably when you are not yet 2, even when you have an adult to steer you. It is virtually impossible when five or six toddlers have to share one adult steering system. Adults have to arrange and control experiences within the home, too. The infant's potential—for destruction in adult terms, exploration in his—has to be recognized and allowed for. If he may not touch this, and this, and this, there must be many things he *can* touch. If he must not climb up on the sofa, what can he climb on? If he must not empty the trash basket, what can he empty?

Some mothers find it difficult to decide what they *really* mind the toddler doing, what they would rather he did not do, and what they mind him doing under certain circumstances and not under others. If one dare assume the toddler's skin—always a risky thing to do—one can see the fearful injustices to which this gives rise. It occurs vaguely to the mother that the child should not turn out the magazine rack. So she takes it from its usual place and puts it in the corner behind the armchair. The roving toddler finds it and empties it. This time mother puts it out of the way on the table. Using a chair the toddler gets to it again. By now, the mother feels he is doing it on purpose. But from the child's point of view if it is in reach at all it is fair game. If she had definitely decided, from the beginning, that he was not to have it, she would have removed it truly out of reach and the issue would never have arisen.

On another day, the rain pours down, the mother feels cheerful, the toddler is playful, and so she permits, even encourages, a long game with the sofa cushions on the floor. While the child is in his high chair having juice she restores the room to order. Released from his chair the toddler starts the game all over again, and this time the mother is cross. Her irritation is instantly understandable to any adult, but quite incomprehensible to the toddler.

Next morning the mother starts the child off playing with sand just outside the back door. Gleefully he squidges his hands in it, spreads it around, fills and empties his bucket. His mother is pleased. Brought in to lunch he does the same with his tapioca pudding and his mother is most *dis*pleased. Her temper does not improve when the toddler joins in the "game" with a bucket of soapy water, made necessary by the pudding on the floor.

The point, of course, is simply that in daily life we tend to attribute, unthinkingly, to toddlers far more understanding than they really have. The child does not *know* that mother put the magazines on the table so that he should not get them. He cannot understand that a messy room at 3 P.M. is all right, but that it must be tidy when Daddy comes home at 6 P.M. Far less can he see why squidging sand is to be encouraged and squidging tapioca pudding is not, nor why it is legitimate for his mother to play with water on the kitchen floor and not for him to do so. Most mothers recognize these things in conversation, but they are far more difficult to bear in mind throughout the day.

Toddlerhood can therefore be a time of almost continuous scolding and nagging from the adult world. Unfortunately, the more nagging there is, the more contra-suggestive and uncooperative the infant is likely to become. He cannot be "good." He cannot do what is wanted of him, or refrain from doing the opposite because that is what his mother wants. As we have seen, it is not developmentally his role to think yet about what anyone else wants or feels. He can only be "good" because he feels like doing what his mother happens to want, and because he does not happen to feel like doing what she would dislike. It is up to the mother, therefore, to organize life so that both of them want the same thing, as far as possible, most of the time.

Often the first step is to decide what objects or actions are truly outside the pale. They will vary from one family and situation to the next. Some of them may have to do with safety, the mother perhaps feeling that the toddler cannot be allowed on the stairs alone, or in the kitchen when the stove is in use. Some of them may be to prevent damage. Perhaps there are books that must not be bent and crumpled, records which must not be scratched, or ornaments that must not be broken. Once a mother has decided which particular issues are important to her, she can make it impossible for the child to go wrong. Removing him from the stairs time and again will make nothing but trouble; if the stairs are to be banned, a stair gate will ban them once and for all, and all fusses with them. Likewise the kitchen: a gate or "stable-type" door gives the toddler a view without access. Books and records may have to be concentrated in a room where the toddler does not play, or the precious books put on high shelves and his own left at the bottom. If ornaments are not to be broken, they will have to be completely out of reach, and furthermore *never* handed to the child "just for a treat." Somehow there has to be space where the child can do *most* of what he likes without being in danger of doing real wrong, or real damage.

Within that space there are lower-level decisions to make. There are drawers of spoons, table napkins, mats. He will empty them, and play with the contents. Does it really matter? Can he hurt them? Does it take any longer to put them away at the end of the day than to put away more conventional toys?

The more the mother can remain positive with the toddler, the more positive—and therefore manageable—he will be with her. He is no more capable of driving her around the bend on purpose than he is capable of being nice to her on purpose. Difficult he may be, but not, at this age, deliberately.

Being positive is easy in theory and often impossible at the end of a long hard day. It is worth considerable effort not just because it keeps the toddler happy, but because if he is happy following the mother's positive suggestions, she will not be driven mad. If she does not want him to turn out that drawer, can he be offered another one to turn out? If so, he will never notice that he has been manipulated, where if he is simply forbidden the first drawer there will be trouble. If he feels clingy, can the mother possibly leave the ironing, sit down and positively cuddle him? If she can, the ironing will not get done right away, but at least the toddler will do his clinging with smiles and talk rather than tears and whines. And the ironing would not have been very well or quickly done anyway, with small hands pulling at the mother's infuriated knees. If neither food nor feces is to be smeared around, can he have paint and Playdoh? If he can, he will certainly make a mess, but it will be an acceptable kind of mess and in a place chosen by the mother. Finally, where the toddler must do something that he does not want to do, almost anything tends to work better than a direct order. "Pick up your bricks" is usually hopeless, where "I bet you can't pick all those up before I've finished this" may actually get the bricks off the floor.

Some mothers feel that taking this sort of trouble to walk around conflict is a kind of spoiling. The infant ought to do what he is told, and desist when he is told not to, never mind why, nor whether he understands why. The trouble is that he won't. And, worse, the mother will have such a very unpleasant time trying to make him. Furthermore, if the mother does join in direct conflict with him, the infant can almost always win just because he has nothing else to do than play the fight-game. Suppose the mother gets into a quarrel over picking up those bricks. She has not a single chance of victory unless the infant decides to oblige. *She* is the one who wants the floor cleared; the infant does not care if the bricks stay there forever. So if it comes to waiting each other out, he will win. His memory, his forethought are not sufficiently developed for bribery to be very effective—if he is offered a bribe for when he has picked them up he will want it right now, and that will only complicate matters. The same applies to threats: "No ice cream" means nothing until he can actually see the ice-cream dish. Of course the mother can make him desperately unhappy. She can shout at him, smack him, put him out of the room, reduce him to a jelly, but none of that will get the bricks picked up.

Toddlers are not mature enough to be directly taught the kind of social responsibility, fairness, and consideration for others that is so essential to family life. At this stage the mother has to conduct the child's social behavior for him: not letting him have the bricks if she cannot bear to help him pick them up, avoiding the conflict of wills that arises from absolute orders resolutely refused, leading and guiding the infant into behaving acceptably because nothing has made him want to behave otherwise.

There is a pay-off, even for the most discipline-minded parents. If a child reaches the stage where he can begin to understand the feelings of others and the justice of their wants as well as his own, still feeling that his mother is basically well-meaning and on his side, then the chances are that most of the time he will want to please her. At this stage he *will* be able to behave well, or badly, on purpose. He *will* foresee the results of his actions, remember prohibitions, understand restrictions. And so, if he wants to please, he will, with lapses. On the other hand, if this second year has been characterized by trouble and rows, so that the infant feels that his mother is unpredictable, overwhelming, unfair, there is a good chance that the more he sees how she wants him to behave, the more he will be tempted to do the opposite. After all, once you are capable of being good on purpose, you are equally capable of being naughty on purpose.

This is why this last section of the book is so largely about the problems that can arise, and what is known about avoiding them. Troubles that arise inadvertently in the second year can, if they are wrongly handled from the child's point of view, become problems that continue throughout early childhood. This is the prime year for socialization; for making that toddler into the beginnings of a real person, rather than an impostor. If he finishes the year asocial, not wanting approval, not letting himself care whether people are cross or not, at odds with himself and his world, he will be infinitely more difficult to handle later. As for being spoiled, there is time later for making sure he is not that. At this age a happy child is an easy child, and a child who can be kept easy through this year will stay comparatively easy later on. He may clamor for his mother's attention at 18 months. Given it in full measure, he will understand, by two and one-half or three, that mother likes to talk to other people sometimes. He will begin to be able to withhold his demands for brief periods. But refused that attention at 18 months, he is likely to become more and more demanding; he will always be testing the mother's love and availability, playing with her irritation like an adult constantly testing a sore tooth with his tongue.

FEEDING IN
THE SECOND YEAR

THIS CHAPTER IS principally about feeding *problems*. An infant who accepts the diet of his family, in a family where that diet is adequate, needs no more special attention to his food than does any other member of his family. A few foods may be known to upset him, and these will obviously be avoided. Occasionally he may be offered an egg or some cheese in place of a main dish he is known to dislike. He will need help in cutting foods up, removing the bones from fish, knowing when foods are cool enough. But all this applies to older children too. If the infant is eating a good mixed diet, this chapter is irrelevant.

The point of the "good mixed diet" is that it is *mixed*. As Chapters Thirteen and Twenty should have made clear, working out the food values and the food needs for any individual is virtually impossible while working out the needs of whole groups of people is an extremely complex business, and one on which there remains considerable controversy among the experts. The simple way of ensuring, in a rich society, that every individual gets what he needs, is to feed him some of a wide range of foods. In this way, incomplete proteins complete each other; vitamin-deficient foods are made good by vitamin-rich ones; varying traces of minerals add up to a sufficiency, and natural hunger ensures that calorie needs are met. Such a mixed diet usually gives us *more* of many nutrients than we actually require. But where food is not scarce, this does not matter, provided the individual does not get too fat.

The pattern of our meals is culture-bound. There is no dietetic law which says that people require three square meals per day or two main meals and two subsidiary ones. From the nutritional point of view, the day's food intake can equally well be divided into six parts. Our assumptions about the content of a "proper meal" are cultural, too. A main dish with accompanying vegetables may be no richer in needed nutrients than the sandwich which we tend to think of as a mere snack. Some of these established attitudes to meals probably come from the elaborate food preparation which used to be typical of families in rich societies. Preparing the food took so long that meals were made into ceremonies so that whoever was doing the cooking could be sure that everyone would be gathered together at certain times of day so that all could be fed simultaneously. Changes in our social patterns may be altering all that. In many families it is impossible to timetable meals so that everyone can have them together. Many people leave for work before a "breakfast time" which makes sense for children attending local schools. Those schoolchildren may, or may not, have a "good meal" at midday, while some people at work eat a cooked meal in a restaurant and others eat a snack at their desks. Many children need an evening meal before all the adults are home from work, while adolescents may have to fit eating in before their evening activities, or go without. The vast range of convenience foods, available to and used by almost every family in the United States, makes it just possible to have food available for such varying numbers and at such idiosyncratic hours, but many families regret the changes which make these so useful. Some hang onto a ceremonious "Sunday dinner" as the one real family meal which is left in their week, but others find even this inequitable as it tends to burden a working mother's one "free" day as well as being more duty than pleasure for many older children. Individual regrets about changes in family living patterns are not the subject of this book. Nevertheless they are relevant if parents confuse such regrets with nutritional anxieties. All too often adults can be heard bemoaning the fact that a teenage daughter "doesn't eat properly from one Sunday to the next." Such statements often have more to do with worries about where she spends her time and the extent to which she is outside family control than to do with what she actually *eats* and whether that diet is adequate for her health.

A good breakfast is universally acknowledged to be important. It is not that we eat to prepare for energy expenditure—on the contrary, we eat to make good energy which has already been expended—it is that a whole night is a long period without food, even though sleeping is not very energetic. Unfortunately, because sleep is not energetic and because it often leaves people still feeling sleepy, many are not hungry when they wake up. It is when they start the school or work day that they find themselves feeling low and inefficient. The author made a small study of children who were being offered breakfast at school because they were known to have long journeys and often to embark on them with only a token meal. The school breakfasts were eaten with enthusiasm, much to the chagrin of some of their mothers: "It's not that there isn't a breakfast at home for her, it's just that she won't *eat* it. . . . half a piece of toast if I'm lucky."

There was no doubt that those children, formerly "low" by the middle of the morning, were far more alert and active when they received the extra school meal. But nor was there any doubt of the truth of their parents' complaints: there was no way they could persuade the children to eat heartily before catching a 7:30 A.M. bus. For such schoolchildren, that much-disputed school milk is probably far more useful if it is served at morning break than it is when served at lunchtime. Even the school "tuck shops" of which so many parents disapprove, may provide a valuable service if they enable children to buy a snack in the middle of the morning. Pre-school children customarily make up for a small breakfast by having "elevenses" while those who attend playgroups or nursery schools almost always have a morning snack. If a child is in circumstances where nothing will be available for him to eat between breakfast and lunch, it may be a kind cruelty to wake him up earlier than would otherwise be necessary. If he habitually has his bath first thing in the morning, or even goes out for a run or takes the dog for its first outing, he may find himself sufficiently awake to eat that breakfast after all.

While an adequate breakfast probably enhances everyone's efficiency, individuals vary tremendously in the directness of the relationship between their energy expenditure and their food intake. One child will be predictably hungrier after an afternoon's baseball than after an afternoon's lessons; another will be hungry irrespective of what he has been doing while yet another may, or may not be and probably will not. But however inaccurate an individual's energy balance may be, day by day, it will usually be extremely accurate over a longer period of time, unless outside pressures interfere with his ability to match what he eats to what his body needs.

All in all, it seems that just as a good mixed diet covers all possibilities of nutritional need, so regular meals several times a day cover all possible needs for stocking up on nutrients of which the body may have insufficient stores. Some of the combinations of foods which are traditional in Western societies make very good sense here. Hamburger and French fries, eaten together, make quite sure that the protein in the meat can be conserved for tissue building and repair, because the carbohydrates and fats in the potatoes will cover immediate energy needs. Eaten alone, the meat might be wastefully used by the body for energy. The same applies to a hot dog in a bun, to eggs with toast, to roast beef with yorkshire pudding. Combinations of this kind ensure that the protein is "spared." But where protein consumption is more than adequate—as it is in most Western families—the pattern of breakfast, lunch, and supper, each with its traditional dishes, is not necessary.

Unfortunately, a very great many infants between one and two refuse to eat what their mothers consider to be an adequate diet. Their mothers, anxious to give them every chance of optimal growth and development, and knowing that food is important, get worried. The toddlers, already searching for fields in which to assert their individuality and try out their independence (Chapter Twenty-four), soon discover the meal table as an excellent place to attract attention and get the parents running around them in circles. For many mothers, their young children's eating is a constant haunting worry, often for several years. The whole relationship between mother and child may be distorted by the food battle; the whole family may be disrupted by it. I have talked with mothers who regularly spent 4 or 5 hours every day trying to get a toddler to eat, mothers whose families were not allowed to accept invitations out to meals because the toddler would only eat at home, families where all mealtime conversation had to consist of nursery rhymes and stories to distract the toddler into eating. Not one of these toddlers showed the least signs of being under-nourished; often they were fat.

Sadly, the advice of pediatricians sometimes strengthens the anxiety of mothers. While being assured that the child is adequately nourished, they are often told that the child is "playing them up," that they should ignore him, offer him his meals, remove the uneaten food, say no more about it, and allow no snacks. If advice of this kind is not backed with hard nutritional information, few anxious mothers can possibly take it. If they try, the child may eat nothing for a whole day. That is the limit of most mothers' tolerance. Behind the advice, implicit in it, is a confirmation of the need, the rightness of the good mixed diet. The whole aim is to get the child back to eating "proper" meals at the "proper" times.

NUTRITIONAL NEEDS

I am not advocating the abandonment of "proper" meals and regular mealtimes. These are social considerations. I want, rather, to lay the basic anxieties about the child's *nutrition,* so that mothers can separate out, for themselves, their nutritional concern from their disciplinary one.

The infant whose birthweight was average, and who has gained weight at the average rate, will weigh around 26 lb. (11.4 kg) by the middle of his second year. But just as his food requirements, relative to his weight, dropped during the second half of the first year, so they drop even further during this year. He will now only need about 48 calories per pound of his bodyweight. So, if he is an average-sized baby, that 1000 calories a day which he needed at a year will creep up only to around 1200 by the time he weighs 25 lb. or thereabouts in the middle of his second year.

A mother who is anxious about her toddler's eating may find it useful to remember that the amounts of food which dietary authorities recommend should be made available to groups of toddlers are just about *half* the amounts they recommend for groups of 10-year-olds. Infants in this age group—newly promoted, perhaps, to family meals—are often expected to eat unrealistically large portions.

Recommended quantities of vital nutrients to be made available to groups of toddlers are given below (Table 10). They may be compared with data in Tables 3 and 6 concerning groups of younger infants but neither set of figures should, of course, be taken to suggest a required, or even an optimum, amount of anything for an individual child. A table of the average heights of girls of particular ages will give you some idea of your daughter's likely growth but it will not tell you how tall she ought to be now or will be in the future. In the same way these figures give you some idea of the nutrients toddlers need but cannot tell you that what he eats is inadequate for him nor what would constitute his perfect diet.

TABLE 10. NUTRIENTS RECOMMENDED FOR GROUPS OF TODDLERS;
PER TODDLER PER DAY

Total Calories kcal	Protein g	Minerals		Vitamins					
		Calcium mg	Iron mg	A μg	D μg	Thiamine mg	Riboflavin mg	Niacin mg	C mg
1250	31	600	7	300	10	0.5	0.6	7	40

Note. As pointed out in the notes to Table 3, American requirements for protein are set lower than those of most Western countries. The actual recommendation at this age would be 24 g. In this table it is set at the 30 g which allows an ample safety margin. This is because the calculations which follow are all designed to reassure parents. Set at this higher level, they can be sure that a child who is taking slightly less than the protein recommendation is taking slightly less than an optimum rather than of a minimum.

Infants who drink 1 pint (about 600 ml) of milk in the day already have an excellent start. The milk gives them more than half the recommendation for protein (18 g). It gives them all the B vitamins except thiamine. Their need for calcium is actually lower than it was in the first year, and the milk gives them plenty (680 mg). The need for vitamin A has dropped too, and the milk gives them almost three quarters of what is recommended (220 μg). The mother who worries about the infant's diet when he *is* drinking this much milk is almost certain to be worrying unnecessarily. The child will see to his total calorie intake, because he will get hungry. Almost whatever he eats to satisfy that hunger will fill whatever gap exists between his personal needs and that pint of milk.

If one considers the foods, or the groups of foods, which children refuse, and which therefore cause their mothers' anxiety, one is struck by the consistency from child to child, and also by the misconceived ideas of "necessary" foods. I have met no toddler who refused cookies and cakes, and remarkably few who refused bread and potatoes. If they did refuse them, their mothers would not worry. On the other hand I have met many who refused meat and greens, and their mothers regard these as vital to a good diet.

Protein Foods

As we have seen in earlier chapters, the first-class or animal proteins contain all the amino acids human beings need. They are therefore a convenient, if expensive, way of ensuring adequate protein intake. They also tend to be useful sources of fat-soluble vitamins and of minerals. But

TABLE 11. EXAMPLES OF FOODS WHICH WILL PROVIDE THE PROTEIN EQUIVALENT OF 1 OZ. (30 G) COOKED MINCED BEEF

Food	Quantity required to yield 8 g protein	Comment
White bread	3 slices	Not complete (first-class)
Whole wheat bread	2 1/2 slices	protein. But wheat protein has been shown to be excellent for children, maintaining good growth either in the presence of other second-class proteins, or limited first-class.
Potatoes	4 medium size 8 small new	Experiments have shown that potatoes can support life as the sole article of diet. Very small quantities of first-class protein render them complete.
Cookies (vanilla or chocolate)	8 cookies on average, according to brand	Will often amount to first-class protein, if milk or egg constituents are included in the recipe.
Plain pound cake	4 small slices	First-class combination
Baked beans in tomato sauce	6 level tablespoons	Not complete protein
Canned processed peas	4 level tablespoons	Not complete protein
Roast peanuts	1 heaped tablespoon	Contains all necessary amino acids but not complete, in sense that relative proportions of amino acids are at variance with body's needs.
Luncheon meat or "spam"	2 medium slices	Present food regulations in the U.S., including those concerned with the inclusion of textured soya protein, are such that all these can be regarded as first-class protein sources, not inferior to butcher's meat.
Frankfurters	1 1/2	
Fish sticks	2	
Bacon	2 normal slices	
Cooked ham	2 slices from vacuum pack	

they are by no means the only proteins available to us. A tablespoon of cooked minced stewing beef will yield about 8 grams of protein. Table 11 gives some examples of other, and less expected, foods which will provide the same amount.

From the table, it is clear that our ideas of which foods are protein sources and which are impoverished are often misguided. Of course protein is most *concentrated* in such foods as lean butcher's meat and cheese, but these are foods of which we eat comparatively little at one time. The concentration of protein in bread and potatoes is low, but we eat a lot of them, so that the protein they contain makes a useful contribution to the diet.

The Vexed Question of Vegetables

Vegetables are often regarded as essential to a good mixed diet. People seldom stop to ask themselves what makes them so valuable. If asked, they answer, "Vitamin C."

Although many vegetables contain a high concentration of vitamin C when they leave the ground, very few of them contain much by the time they reach the plate. Vitamin C is lost rapidly during storage, especially if there is exposure to sunlight. A green vegetable on display in front of the green-grocer's shop has probably lost half its vitamin C content even before it is purchased.

Since the vitamin is both water soluble and destroyed by heat, a great deal of what is left will vanish when it is cooked. At the worst, cabbage cooked for cafeteria meals and kept hot in a steam table has been shown to contain no vitamin C whatsoever. At best, bought fresh, cooked quickly in very little water and served immediately, it may contain as much as 6 mg in a serving.

If people enjoy green vegetables, fine. They will get a variable amount of vitamin C and some vitamin A and calcium. But if they do not —and most toddlers do not—they can hardly be regarded as essential dietary items.

Vitamin C is not a difficult essential to provide. Although the vitamin content of potatoes is variable, children will get some from this source. The juice of a single orange will provide three times the recommended daily intake. A single 3 1/2 oz. can of strained infant fruit juice will do the same. Or the child can be given the correct dose of a multi-vitamin preparation.

Root vegetables, particularly carrots, are usually preferred to green ones. One very small carrot provides the toddler with all the vitamin A he needs for the day, and a little calcium. But that is virtually all. Again, with the multi-vitamins available, and recommended, is the carotene content of the carrot worth a fuss?

In later life, of course, vegetables are valuable as roughage; but at this age the roughage content of cereal products, especially less refined ones, is usually sufficient.

Fresh Fruit

The citrus fruits are the most consistent of all dietary sources of vitamin C because they come in their own packaging, protected from light, and because they are almost always eaten raw, and thus the vitamin is protected from heat.

But the vitamin C in other fruits—highest in summer fruits such as strawberries—survives better than the vitamin C in vegetables even when the fruits are eaten cooked. This is because vitamin C is not broken down so rapidly by heat when it is in an acid solution, and most fruits are acid. It is also because the vitamin C which dissolves into the cooking water is commonly eaten as "juice," where the vegetable water is usually drained away. Canned fruits normally contain about half the amount of vitamin C which is found in the same fruit when fresh. But it may contain more than the "fresh" fruit which has been at the green-grocer's for several days. Dried fruits, such as prunes and raisins, contain virtually no vitamin C.

The protein content of dried fruits—apricots, prunes, and even raisins—looks high on a nutritional table. And it *is* high if the infant likes, and can digest, these fruits in dried form. But soaked back to the natural state, the protein is diluted. Where an ounce of dried apricots contains nearly 5 grams of protein, an ounce of soaked and stewed dried apricots will only contain about 1/2 gram.

Useful amounts of many vitamins and minerals are available in a variety of fresh fruits but, apart from vitamin C, the quantities are not sufficient to make fruit the most important source.

Fats

As far as we know, the only dietary *requirement* for fat is for minute quantities of three essential fatty acids, found both in animal and in vegetable fats.

The chances of an infant in the Western world lacking any of these three are minute. Even if the child appears to *eat* no fat, preferring his bread without butter or margarine, his ham, bacon, and other meat lean, his salad without dressing, sufficient fat will be used in food *preparation* to meet this biochemical need. And even where a mother is deliberately keeping her use of fats in the kitchen to a minimum—perhaps for the benefit of some other member of the family—there will be fats, animal or vegetable, in any commercially prepared cakes or cookies, and in other foods cooked outside the home.

The fat-soluble vitamins A and D are present in both butter and in margarine—which is fortified so as to contain more vitamin D than occurs naturally in butter. Since these "table fats" are also concentrated forms of calories, they are useful foods for the toddler who likes them. But the quantity of vitamins present is not enough to make these items *necessary* to the diet because even if the child eats a great deal of butter or margarine, he is still going to need supplementary vitamins. To meet his recom-mended intake of vitamin A from butter, he would need to eat only 4 slices of bread, spread to normal thickness. But to meet his vitamin D intake from this source, he would need the quantity one would spread on 60 slices. Using fortified margarine, 12 slices would meet his needs. Of course this is a frivolous calculation, and table fats are used in cooking as well as on bread. The point is that the concentration of vitamins is so low that enough to provide the vitamins from table fats alone would also provide a very high calorie intake. The toddler on a mixed diet will get some of his fat-soluble vitamins from table fats, some from meat, cheese, and eggs. The toddler who refuses a mixed diet needs vitamin supplementation.

The Egg Battle

Eggs are misunderstood. They, more than any other food except green vegetables, are drawn into moralistic (as opposed to nutritional) argu-ments at mealtimes. One egg contains just about the same amount of first-class complete protein as the tablespoonful of lean minced beef we postulated earlier. And each egg yolk provides about 1 mg of iron—one seventh of the amount recommended for this age group. So mothers tend, rightly, to regard them as an extremely valuable food; but they also tend, wrongly, to feel that the child is not "properly eating *eggs*" if he hates the sight of them.

Many toddlers intensely dislike boiled, poached, or fried eggs. Many more will eat them if they are made a little less recognizable in omelettes or scrambled egg dishes. Almost all eat them unknowingly in batter puddings, pancakes, cakes, and custards. A boiled egg is not better for the child than "apple snow" made with beaten egg white, or cheese pudding made with egg yolks and milk.

THE MYTHICAL "PROBLEM EATER"

It should by now be clear that while a mixed diet—with plenty of milk, eggs, cheese, meat, vegetables, and fruit, and ample bread and other carbohydrates to fill up with and provide energy—is an ideal, it is not a nutritional necessity. Much maternal anxiety about toddlers' eating is disciplinary and prejudiced. Two slices of bacon with bread and butter and an apple may not strike the mother as a "proper meal." Perhaps socially it is not. But it is not a bad meal nutritionally. The toddler who refuses all meat and vegetables, and nibbles cakes and fruit all day may be *behaving badly* but that does not necessarily mean that he is eating badly.

By way of illustration and light relief, Tables 12–15 analyze some of the socially peculiar ways in which a "difficult eater" might meet his nutritional needs if not his mother's expectations.

These tables require some explanation. The nutrient values ascribed to the different foods named are all derived from the *Manual of Nutrition* [158]. In this sense they are accurate values—the fruit of extremely painstaking research work. Nevertheless they cannot be treated as exact. The accurate nutrient content of "a piece of bread and butter" depends on the thickness of the slice, whether the crusts are removed, how thickly the butter is spread. Similarly, while the values given for "one sweet cookie" are average values for average plain sweet cookies, the exact content of any one cookie will, of course, depend on the manufacturer's recipe. In tables such as these one is therefore imposing a spurious appearance of accuracy on data which can really only be approximate.

For this reason, the figures are given only to two significant figures (except in the rare cases where three figures are justifiable). It is quite spurious enough to say that a cookie contains 70 calories; to state that it contains 68.21 calories is patently absurd. Some of the very small values, such as those for the B vitamins, may seem even more ridiculous. How can we be sure that a small banana contains 0.04 mg of riboflavin? The answer is that we cannot be sure, but we do know that it will contain more than 0.03 mg and less than 0.05. Furthermore, *if* it contains this amount of riboflavin, it will contain 0.02 of thiamine, or half the quantity. And the relationship between one nutrient and the next is vital.

The tables can therefore be used as a rough guide to the actual nutrient contents of the foods mentioned, and as a rather more accurate guide to the proportions of one nutrient to another. Other than that they are intended merely to illustrate the variety of ways in which widely differing food intakes can add up to a sufficiency of everything, or leave specific lacks which are easily filled. Nobody should be fooled by their apparent accuracy into searching for a food which provides 0.01 mg of a particular vitamin, or into criticizing a day's diet because it leaves a child 3 grams short of the recommended protein.

In each table, the day's total intake is compared with the recommended provision given in Table 10, to yield the difference between the quantity actually eaten by the child and the quantity which would have been made available to him if he had been resident in a group which was being catered for by a professional dietician. Nobody, of course, would assume that every child would eat everything.

During the years since this book was first published, these tables have been praised by parents as being "the only thing that really did convince me that she wasn't starving to death" *and* indicted by experts for suggesting that feeding a child is an exact science. They are intended to do the first but not the second. These are *real* diets, eaten, some time ago now, by real toddlers with very, very anxious parents. The figures were worked out to demonstrate to them that the scales did not lie: their children really were growing.

Table 12 describes a self-selected high carbohydrate diet. No tricks have been played with it. No portions of cheese have been slipped in; no

TABLE 12. TYPICAL DAY'S FOOD FOR A TODDLER "HOOKED" ON CARBOHYDRATES

| | Total Calories kcal | Protein g | Minerals | | Vitamins | | | | | |
			Calcium mg	Iron mg	A µg	D µg	Thiamine mg	Riboflavin mg	Niacin mg	C mg
On Waking										
2 sweet cookies	140	1.5	26	0.4	0	0	0.03	0.01	0.4	0
Drink Hawaiian Punch	65	0	4	0	0	0	0	0.01	0	58
Breakfast										
2 slices white bread and butter	250	4.8	60	1.0	280	0.36	0.1	0	1.4	0
During morning										
2 more cookies	140	1.5	26	0.4	0	0	0.03	0.01	0.4	0
Lunch										
French fries (1 medium potato)	270	4.4	16	1.6	0	0	0.12	0.04	2.4	4–16
1/2 fish stick	25	2	7	0.2	0	0	0.02	0.02	0.6	0
Slice cake	120	1.7	19	0.4	23	0.34	0.02	0.03	0.5	0
During afternoon										
Children's 1-oz. bar chocolate	165	2.5	70	0.5	2	0	0.01	0.1	0.7	0
Supper										
2 more slices bread and butter	250	4.8	60	1.0	280	0.36	0.1	0	1.4	0
Banana (small)	44	0.6	4	0.2	18	0	0.02	0.04	0.4	6
Cup (4 oz. [120 ml]) milk	70	4	130	0	44	1.25	0.04	0.16	1.2	0

Total intake rounded to 2 significant figures	1500	28	420	5.7	650	2.3	0.49	0.42	9.4	68–80†
Difference between intake and recommended group provision	+250	–3*	–180	–1.3	+350	–7.7	–0.01	–0.18	+2.4	+28–40
Comments	Too much: almost 1/4 in excess	Negligible: lacks 1/15	Too little: lacks 1/3	Too little: lacks 1/7	Ample	Too little: lacks 3/4	Negligible: lacks 1/50	Too little: lacks 1/3	Ample	Ample

*This protein intake is well above the minimum thought to be necessary to protect against protein deficiency, even though it is just below the "recommended intake" level.

†As we have seen, the vitamin C content of potatoes varies, especially with length of storage.

TABLE 13. TYPICAL DAY'S FOOD FOR A TODDLER WHO "EATS LIKE A BIRD"

	Total Calories kcal	Protein g	Minerals		Vitamins					
			Calcium mg	Iron mg	A µg	D µg	Thiamine mg	Riboflavin mg	Niacin mg	C mg
Breakfast										
1/2 portion (2 tablespoons) baby cereal	60	3	100	2	16	2	0.1	0.2	1.5	0
1/2 egg	25	1.7	8	0.4	45	0.2	0.1	0.05	0.5	0
Mug (8 oz. [250 ml]) milk	140	8	260	0	88	2.5	0.08	0.32	2.4	0
During morning										
Drink Hawaiian Punch	65	0	4	0	0	0	0	0.01	0	58
1 sweet cookie	70	0.75	13	0.2	0	0	0.01	0.005	0.2	0
Lunch										
2 teaspoons minced beef	30	4	1	0.7	0	0	0.005	0.03	1.5	0
1/4 medium boiled potato	23	0.4	1	0.1	0	0	0.02	0.01	0.3	1-4
2 teaspoons frozen peas	7	0.7	2	0.15	7	0	0.03	0.01	0.3	2
During afternoon										
Vanilla ice cream (small)	55	1.2	89	0.1	0	0	0.01	0.06	0.3	0
Supper										
1/2 jar toddler cheese entrée	110	6	110	0.1	60	0	0.1	0.01	1.5	0
Mug (8 oz. [250 ml]) milk	140	8	260	0	88	2.5	0.08	0.32	2.4	0

Total intake	730	33	800	3.8	300	7.2	0.54	1	11	61-64†
Difference between intake and recommended group provision	-520	+2	+200	-3.2	0	-2.8	+0.04	+0.04	+4	+21-24
Comments	Too little: lacks almost 2/5	Ample	Ample	Too little: lacks 1/2	Ample	Too little: lacks 1/4	Ample	Ample	Ample	Ample

†Vitamin C content of potatoes is variable.

TABLE 14. DAY'S FOOD TAKEN BY A TODDLER ACCEPTING ONLY MILK, BREAD, AND BUTTER

	Total Calories kcal	Protein g	Minerals		Vitamins					
			Calcium mg	Iron mg	A µg	D µg	Thiamine mg	Riboflavin mg	Niacin mg	C mg
During the day infant eats: 8 slices of bread spread with butter	1000	19	240	4	1100	1.4	0.4	0	5.6	0
1 pint (about 600 ml) milk	360	20	680	0	240	5	0.2	0.4	0	0
Total intake	1300	39	920	4	1300	6.4	0.6	0.4	5.6	0
Difference between intake and recommended group provision	+50	+8	+320	−3	+1000	−3.6	+0.1	−0.2	−1.4	−40
Comments	Ample	Ample	Ample	Too little: lacks almost 1/2	Ample	Too little: lacks 1/3	Ample	Too little: lacks 1/3	Too little: lacks 1/5	Too little: lacks total

TABLE 15. DAY'S FOOD TAKEN BY A TODDLER ACCEPTING ONLY PEANUTS, FRENCH-FRIED POTATOES, AND APPLES

	Total Calories kcal	Protein g	Minerals Calcium mg	Minerals Iron mg	Vitamins A μg	Vitamins D μg	Vitamins Thiamine mg	Vitamins Riboflavin mg	Vitamins Niacin mg	Vitamins C mg
During the day infant consumes:										
2 oz. (60 g) roast shelled peanuts (not recommended)	330	16	17	0.6	0	0	0.07	0.03	5.9	0
12 oz. French fries (3 medium potatoes)	800	13	36	4.8	0	0	0.36	0.12	7.2	24
3 apples, net weight 8 oz. (250 g)	100	0.8	8	0.8	8	0	0.08	0.08	0	8
Total intake	1200	30	61	6.2	8	0	0.51	0.23	13	32
Difference between intake and recommended group provision	−50	−1	−539	−0.8	−290	−10	+0.01	−0.37	+6	−8
Comments	Negligible	Negligible	Too little: lacks 9/10	Negligible: lacks 1/9	Too little: lacks almost total	Too little: lacks total	Ample	Too little: lacks almost 2/3	Ample	Ample

passion for cooked ham has been postulated. The child has taken only one food in the entire day which would be conventionally regarded as "good" for him—half a fish stick.

Yet there is remarkably little wrong with the diet, and what is wrong can easily be put right without altering the *kind* of food served, and therefore without risking putting the child off eating altogether.

The most striking point is that the child is having one quarter more calories than the average toddler would be thought to require. If he is a thin, active, tall child, or if he is catching up after illness, this may not matter. But most toddlers eating this diet regularly would become fat. We therefore must find ways of improving the quality of his diet without adding calories. And we must find ways of reducing the calorie intake for a fat child without him feeling deprived of his normal food.

The child must certainly have more vitamin D. This should be supplemented. A multi-vitamin preparation will do no harm, even though his vitamin A and C intakes are adequate. But vitamin D alone can be given. Such a large lack of the vitamin would be difficult to make up in any other way since he does not eat fatty fish or eggs. The use of a fortified margarine instead of butter would probably be the only other practical way of supplying it.

The child might need more calcium, iron, and riboflavin. These can be provided in a variety of ways. For example, if the juice of a fresh orange were substituted for the Hawaiian Punch, this would serve the dual purpose of increasing his iron intake while reducing his calories. Similarly the substitution of ice cream for cake at lunchtime would increase his calcium intake, leave his protein untouched and reduce his calories a little. Substitution of crispbread for ordinary bread at one meal would increase his iron intake and cut down his calories. A thin spreading of Marmite or some other yeast extract would ensure his riboflavin intake.

Finally, if his calorie intake is still too high and he is obviously getting fat, manipulation of the table fats he eats can reduce the calories without him noticing the change. One ounce of butter contains 211 calories and only 0.1 gram of protein. He needs some—this is the main source of his abundant vitamin A—but his intake could be cut by half without damaging the diet in any way.

To contrast with this diet, which contains quite a large quantity of carbohydrate relative to protein, Table 15 gives a diet which does not contain very much of *anything*. This is the child whose mother worries because he "eats like a bird."

This diet is basically excellent. But just as the first example was high in calories, so this one is very low. The child is having only two thirds of the calories that an "average" toddler is offered. Again, this may not matter. If he has always been small, is gaining weight steadily (even if slowly), is healthy, energetic, and wants no more of *any* kind of food, then it can be assumed that his appetite is correctly controlling his food intake. But if he is gaining weight more slowly than hitherto, seems listless or tired, or would like more of certain kinds of food though not of what his mother offers, then he should have it.

The child's only likely shortages—apart from calories—are vitamin D and iron. The first should be supplemented. His iron could be increased by substituting fresh orange juice for Hawaiian Punch, and perhaps by offering crispbread or bread and butter instead of his morning cookie. He might also accept a mixture of half-beef half-liver at dinnertime.

If the child wants, or will happily accept, some extra food, the mother does not have to worry about what it is. He needs the food only for fuel as he is getting plenty of all the vital nutrients. He can therefore have whatever he prefers that his mother is prepared to buy and serve. However "fattening" the additional food, he is unlikely to get fat because he probably has an actual gap between his energy expenditure and his food intake. Indeed, on this diet, he may be burning some of his protein foods for fuel, so that the addition of extra carbohydrates would actually improve the quality of the diet by sparing those proteins for tissue building and growth.

Perhaps he would like a sweet course at lunch and supper time. Perhaps he would eat a greater quantity of sausages or spam or bacon than he eats of pure minced beef. Perhaps he is bored with boiled potatoes, and would eat more if they were sautéed or baked. Any addition of cereal products, potatoes, or chocolate would, of course, give him extra iron.

Failing all this, if he does seem to need more food, but will not eagerly eat a bulkier diet, the answer lies in additional sugar and fats. Some butter could be used on his vegetables during the day, even if he will not eat it on bread. Sugar could go on his cereal, some on fruit; and he could be allowed some sweets.

Even further from the "good mixed diet" ideal are the really crazy diets (Tables 14 and 15) adopted by two healthy toddlers. Neither is recommended, but very little is needed to make the diets at least adequate, and they may therefore be comforting to desperate mothers!

Clearly the diet shown in Table 14 is not as "crazy" or as "impoverished" as most people would assume. The toddler lacks only iron and vitamins D and C. He is not getting the full recommendation for riboflavin and nicotinic acid, but in practice the difference is so small it would be unlikely to matter unless the child ate literally *nothing* else for a long period or happened to be one who needed more than most.

Obviously he, like most toddlers, should have a correct daily dosage of multi-vitamins. Apart from these, he may need more iron. Whole wheat bread tends to contain more than white bread, so substitution of some whole wheat for white would help. Other than this, if he will accept some of his milk flavored with cocoa, 2 heaped teaspoonfuls will give him sufficient iron. If he will not, every 2-oz. (60 g) bar of milk chocolate which he eats will give him 1 missing mg of iron. But if he has many, he will get fat—his calories are already on the high side.

This method of analysis is somewhat misleading when we come to the diet in Table 15. The toddler appears, from the figures, to be getting ample protein. But he is getting it entirely from peanuts and potatoes, with no first-class animal protein at all. While the amino acid composition of peanuts is such that they are an excellent source of vegetable protein, containing *some* of all the essential amino acids (see p. 146), the balance between these constituents is not ideal. And unfortunately the balance is not corrected by the amino acid composition of potatoes. The infant could maintain good health and growth on this protein mixture for some time. But he would be much better off if some form of animal protein could be added.

Since the diet is extremely low in calcium, the obvious addition to aim for would be milk. Even two thirds of a pint of milk would render the proteins complete, as well as giving adequate calcium intake. If he will not drink milk as milk, he might drink cocoa or milk shakes. If even these are refused, a good deal of milk can be slipped in by way of ice cream or even milk chocolate.

The toddler almost lacks vitamins A and D and some vitamin C. On such a restricted diet he almost certainly regularly must receive a multi-vitamin preparation.

IDIOSYNCRATIC DIETS

The lesson these examples teach is not that a good mixed diet is to be scorned. It is still the safe way to feed an infant: The way that ensures that he misses nothing, either among the food elements we recognize and can set recommendations for, or among the vitamins and minerals which year by year are being shown to be important, though levels cannot yet be set. The mixed diet is also, in our culture, the easy way to feed an infant. He can share in what is being prepared for everybody else. It is very tiresome to cook French fries three times every day. Again, it is psychologically the best way to feed him. Idiosyncratic diets mean that the child has become aware of what he eats as a focus of maternal attention. It has ceased to be a simple and pleasurable matter of satisfying hunger, and become an emotional issue. Later on, his social life will be affected—much of our social intercourse still focuses around meals.

But the examples do demonstrate how easy it is to meet a toddler's nutritional needs, how many enormously divergent diets will do this, and what comparatively tiny quantities are needed. After all, the packet of peanuts and the pint of milk which the children in our last examples are living on might well serve their fathers as an afternoon snack and a late night drink barely counted into their assessment of their daily diet.

The example of the child who is hooked on carbohydrates should allay the fears of those whose charges dislike meat, cheese, and eggs. There is a lot of protein in "carbohydrate" foods. The toddler who eats like a bird might teach us a little about the size of portion we serve to young children. Many would eat more, if they were not continually faced with three times the amount they actually want. While many toddlers choose—or insist upon—diets which their parents consider worrying or odd, a few toddlers have unusual diets thrust upon them. A good mixed diet is good just because it *is* mixed. It is not surprising then that deviations from the omnivorous diet which is still the norm in Western societies become increasingly risky as they become more restricted.

A vegetarian diet has no snags implicit within it; indeed many people consider that an excellent vegetarian diet is healthier than a comparable diet containing meat and fish. Many vegetarian families serve a diet which is more varied than that of the families who rely either on the conventional meat-and-two-vegetables meals or on packets and cans.

Vegan diets exclude eggs and dairy produce as well as meat and fish. Such a diet has been shown to produce children who are lighter for their height than children from vegetarian or omnivorous families. This is probably because plant foods contain a low concentration of calories for their bulk. The vegan child has to eat a large quantity of food to meet his immediate energy needs and his growth needs. He is unlikely to eat enough surplus calories to lay down much fat. There is no evidence that such a diet, with its associated light weight, leads to impaired growth or functioning. But parents wishing to feed a vegan diet to infants should be aware of the possibility of protein shortage. Lengthy breast-feeding will usually ensure adequate protein during the first year. Thereafter, if the child is to have adequate amino acids for growth, he will need a rich mixture of cereals, legumes, and nuts; starchy cereals, even with vegetables and fruits, might leave him short of protein. Many vegan families find that soya beans or products made from textured soya protein are a great help. Vitamins A and D both tend to be scarce in a vegan diet so these should be supplemented. Vitamin B-12 intake is also likely to be low. Vegan parents should consult a doctor or their health visitor about the advisability of supplementing this vitamin.

Fruitarian diets are gaining popularity among some vegetarians and vegans. Such a diet cannot be sufficiently mixed for good health and growth, even if sufficient money is available for the use of a wide range of fruits both in and out of season. Some fruitarian parents have attempted to get around the unsuitability of this diet for infants by permitting them to have some nuts and seeds. But even with this addition, the diet is unsuitable for the very young. Eating everything raw means that the proteins which are available are comparatively indigestible. Infants will not thrive.

Infants do not thrive on Zen macrobiotic diets, either. Various levels of these, together with various forms of fruitarian diet, are well described by Professor Dickerson [61]. He gives some interesting case histories of children offered these very restricted ranges of food. While the results were often alarming, the trouble taken by health professionals to find ways of improving the infants' health, without contravening the parents' principles, was impressive. Parents whose convictions lead them to offer a very restricted diet to their infant should consult such a professional at the earliest possible moment—certainly before any attempt is made to wean the child. Such early consultation will almost always mean that the child's healthy growth within the framework of his parents' beliefs can be ensured. It is when a child has already had his health impaired by an unsuitable diet that doctors and dieticians sometimes have to suggest dietary additions which the parents find unacceptable.

THE CHILD WHO IS FAT

The fat toddler, or the one who is gaining weight too fast and is clearly therefore going to get fat, is almost certainly eating a high carbohydrate diet. But this does not mean that the only way to give him fewer calories is to try putting him on a high protein diet—such as his slimming mother might adopt.

The first place to look for help is in the child's consumption of snacks. If he is a constant consumer of potato chips, sweets, ice cream, and cookies he may be getting more calories in his snacks than in his meals.

If so, some good can often be done by offering him his treat snack foods as part of his *meals,* and offering the mealtime foods he is less keen on as snacks. If he has ice cream at dinnertime, instead of rice pudding, that pudding can be available when he demands an afternoon snack. Of course he is then less likely to eat the rice pudding. Similarly, why not chips for supper, and then bread and butter if he demands more food before bedtime?

The easiest way to cut down an infant's calorie intake, without making him conscious of any change in his diet, is to limit his intake of fats. These are the most concentrated form of calories, and only sugar adds fewer valuable nutrients to the diet. To deprive the child of bread and potatoes is to deprive him of extremely nutritious food. To deprive him of butter is to take away only calories and vitamin A, and the vitamins should be supplemented anyway. Most people spread butter or margarine on bread at the rate of about 1 oz. (30 g) to 3 slices—more than 200 calories. It would take about the same amount to make fried bread, or sauté potatoes. French-fried potatoes have three times the calorie value of boiled ones, and twice the calorie value of roast potatoes.

If the child's milk intake is drastically cut, the balance of the rest of his diet may be upset—his protein and calcium intake may drop too far. But it is worth remembering that the food value of milk is in the *milk* not in the cream, which is almost entirely fat. Skim milk yields just as much protein and calcium for many fewer calories. If the child is drinking more than about 1 1/2 pints (860 ml) of milk per day, as well as eating too much in total, it is worth trying to cut him back to somewhere nearer a pint (about 600 ml)—although not below this. Unfortunately many mothers do this by offering the infant a proprietary vitamin C fruit syrup, suitably diluted, instead of the milk. This will not help the fat child. A glass of grape juice made with 1 oz. (30 ml) of the syrup to 4 oz. (115 ml) of water will give him exactly the same calories as the same size glass of milk. If the child's feelings are hurt by being offered plain water, a low-calorie fruit juice—provided he gets his ration of vitamin C in other ways—is a better alternative. Two birds can be killed with the one stone if fresh orange juice is used—half the calories and plenty of vitamin C.

FEEDING PROBLEMS

The easy way to deal with feeding problems is to avoid them. Perhaps the easiest way to avoid them is not only to read, but also to believe the kind of information contained earlier in this chapter. If mothers really *believe* that the package of chips the infant consumed in his stroller on the way to the store, together with the milk he drank at breakfast, and the apple he is eating now, will nourish him adequately for much of the day, they are far less likely to convey anxiety to that child when he does not eat his next proper "meal."

Accepting, indeed encouraging, the infant's dawning desire for independence will usually help in avoiding feeding problems too. The child who feels that his mother is overbearing and smothering is more likely than most to be on the lookout for battlegrounds. And he may choose the meal table. Even if he does not feel generally oppressed, he may well come to resent being fed by his mother. Being fed with a spoon is an uncomfortable business. Perhaps parents should feed each other a few spoonfuls and discover this for themselves. The food does not come at the right rate; the feeder does not select exactly the right combination on each spoonful, and it all makes one feel very helpless. Of course infants have to be fed during the months when they cannot feed themselves. But usually these months are over by the first birthday, yet very few babies are allowed to feed themselves at this age. Perhaps the mother wants to avoid the mess of self-feeding, or speed up the child's meal, or give him sloppy canned foods which are difficult to manage. As long as she ladles in the food, the child does not eat, he is fed. Eating is not something active which he does but something which he must passively accept. If he can be allowed to feed himself, his eating can become his business, and can be kept separate from the vagaries of his relationship with his mother.

Toddlers will not, of course, feed themselves to adult standards. The child will use his fingers most of the time, a spoon some of the time. He will eat in idiosyncratic orders and combinations, alternating peas with stewed fruit and dipping cheese in his pudding. But if he is allowed this degree of self-determination, he is likely to eat the amount he needs of what he likes and his nutrition is unlikely to become bedeviled with discipline. If he cannot have his pudding until he has finished his first course it will not take him long to realize that his mother minds more

about him eating the entrée foods. By the laws of toddler contra-sugges-
tiveness such a realization may quickly make him want the meat less and
the pudding more. If he cannot have his food at all unless he eats it
"nicely" he may well decide that he does not want it that much anyway.
Parents who can be deliberately easygoing about meal-table behavior
may find it useful not only to relax the rules but even to introduce some
fun. Some toddlers, perhaps especially those whose own plateful has
become something to be faced with distress, are interested in what is on
other people's plates. While I am not suggesting that toddlers should be
encouraged to snatch handfuls of food from their neighbors, I am suggesting that "would you like to try a bit?" can be a friendly and reasonable
encouragement to a child to be interested in food. Some very young
children acquire the most surprising tastes in this way; they may even ask
to be served next time with a portion of those fried onions. Being allowed
to serve himself from a dish rather than having his food pre-served on
his plate can be encouraging too. Of course oven-to-table dishes are a
problem and so may be the mess on the tablecloth, but with a little tactful
assistance a 2-year-old can probably choose—and may therefore also eat
—his own particular potato. In some families toddlers who were being
"difficult" about eating have been transformed by being allowed not just
to serve themselves but to *taste* what was in the dish before doing so. After
all, we say politely to adult guests "would you like some spinach?" but
if we say the same to a 2-year-old he may not know the answer. "Try a
bit and see" can remove the horror of having a spoonful dumped on his
plate and then being expected to eat it.

If the infant is to be allowed to eat what he wants from what is
available on the table, and to eat it in the way he finds easiest, the
corollary is that if he does *not* want to eat, that is his business too. The
whole idea is ruined if the mother lets him feed himself the amount he
wants and then tries to push a bit more in, or if she lets him eat the bits
he likes and then tries to give him the bits he has rejected.

Sometimes it is weaning from the bottle that makes trouble at mealtimes at around a year. If the infant has been allowed a bottle for this
long, he has usually built it into his bedtime routine and made it part of
his comfort rituals. Mothers who in conversation express horror at the
idea of allowing a baby to suck himself to sleep with a bottle, find themselves doing so. The infant *might* choke. His teeth will certainly suffer, but
peaceful naptimes and evenings are so desirable that the infant gets his
bottle all the same. If it is taken away from him at this sort of age, he may
refuse adamantly to touch milk from a cup. Water and fruit juice he will
drink competently, but if he cannot have milk in a bottle he will not have
it at all. Those rejected cups of milk can start a cycle of pressure from the
mother and refusal from the child which rapidly spreads to include other
foods too. It seems that this may be the most difficult stage for weaning
from the bottle. If the mother does not want to allow the infant to have
his bottle through most of the second year at least, she would probably

do better to wean him much earlier—at 8–9 months. Weaned at a year, both his nutrition and his eating patterns are likely to suffer.

Often it is not the food itself which starts feeding problems, but the social conventions of the family dining table. Sitting up to table and being reasonably still and quiet go against the infant's every instinct at this age. His attention span is still very limited. When he plays freely he wanders from position to position, from object to object. He never voluntarily sits still for the length of time a family meal is likely to take. Furthermore he cannot join in general conversation, nor easily keep quiet while other people talk to each other and ignore him. He likes conversation, but he likes it to be directed exclusively at him! So if he is forced to join in social eating, forced to sit still, he will probably make the mealtime extremely uncomfortable for everyone else and end up by being scolded or banished. Over many days, such an atmosphere at mealtimes does not make for enthusiastic eating. Parents who feel they must demand conventional table manners from anyone who eats at their table may do better to feed the infant on his own for a few more months. After all he *is* still an impostor in human shape. Parents who feel that it is good for the infant to feel himself part of a family group around the dinner table might try sitting him up with them, but allowing him to get down as soon as he has finished what he wants to eat. Gradually he can be taught that once he has elected to leave the table his meal is over, that he cannot return every 2 minutes for another mouthful. He can later learn not to bother the others who are enjoying their leisurely meal. At three or four he will regard it as a privilege to sit up with the adults and be able to join their talk. At one or two he regards it as torment and will make it torment for all.

Once feeding problems form they are difficult to deal with. But they are usually best handled by exactly the same methods which hopefully avoid their formation.

Parents who find themselves trying to feed a toddler food which he refuses need to ask themselves, honestly, whether he appears in any way malnourished. If he is healthy, growing, energetic, and cheerful (except at mealtimes!) they have to try and accept that the worry is not rational, or at least that it is not really about the child's nutrition. Possibly a few days of actually making a note of what the child eats, and comparing it with the information earlier in this chapter may help. If, having worked out exactly what the child is eating and having compared it with the kind of amount he is likely to need, they still find themselves worried, a checkup of the infant's general health by his doctor may reassure them. Somehow or other they have to become convinced that the child will not starve himself into illness. Without that conviction the parents are bound to go on worrying. And if they go on worrying they will have to be superhuman to conceal the anxiety from the already sensitized child.

If the mother can reduce her own anxiety, the next step is to consider how much effect her present policy is actually having on what the child eats. How much extra food does he take because of those hours of persuasion and scolding? Usually the answer is very little. Making a person eat is impossible. So trying is doomed to failure and bound to make the situation worse.

It is not easy to stop trying to make a contrary child eat good food, expensively bought and lovingly prepared. The more one tries to find things the child will like, and make them delicious and attractive, the more hurtful and maddening it is when he rejects them. So it often helps to simplify the whole performance. There is no point in cooking minced liver and three vegetables if he is not going to eat them, so what is he likely to eat? If sandwiches are a possibility he can be given those instead. If he eats them, well and good. If he does not, at least the mother has not wasted so much money or time.

Even when mothers make the effort to get themselves into this new, less emotional state of mind over the infant's eating, he is often very slow to respond. If he has come to regard meals as horrible or as a challenge to his independence, or as a battleground with his mother, or indeed as anything except opportunities to satisfy his hunger with food, it will take him quite a long time to come to regard them differently. Sometimes a radical change of scene speeds things up. If the rows have always been associated with a high chair at the living room table, a low table-chair combination (which can probably be borrowed) in the kitchen may strike him as quite different. If he has always wanted to get down from his chair, to get away from the meal, then giving it to him on a stool while he sits on the floor may work. He is not confined or tied down, so he may stay voluntarily. However it is done, the infant has somehow got to be made to feel that things have changed. He has to be helped to see practical evidence of his mother's determined change of attitude.

But it will not happen very quickly. And all too often a mother starts out with the explicit intention of adopting this kind of line, and then finds that she has ruined it all for herself because her nerve or her patience failed her at a critical moment. She gives him what he likes and leaves him to get on with it, but then she cannot resist the temptation to feed him the last few bits "because he really seemed to be enjoying it." Or she brings him in from a long walk and finds herself ladling in his supper "because he is so tired." She puts him in the borrowed low chair, with much emphasis on how nice and different it all is, and he gets out again without eating anything. Before she can stop herself his mother has swooped him up and dumped him in the hated high chair after all. Hardest to bear of all is the day when, unforced, the child goes from waking to bedtime without eating anything. Probably there were really some snacks that the mother has forgotten, but it is not easy to hang on to the fact that the infant will just be hungry tomorrow; that letting him not eat is good mothering, not bad; and that he will not starve himself.

The infant who has really got his mother and the rest of his family involved in his non-eating may have come to feel that food is his principal means of getting attention. When his mother decides not to fuss about it any more, he may actually miss the attention that used to center on him at mealtimes, even though most of it was cross attention. If this is the case, the child may adamantly refuse to feed himself.

Such a refusal does not mean that the resolving-eating-problems policy needs changing. The child will feed himself when he is both really hungry and really sure that his mother will not change her mind and revert to the old ways. But it does make it even more difficult for the mother to stick to her chosen guns. If he positively asks the mother to feed him it seems brutal to refuse, and difficult to remember that if she consents he will at once reject her attempts.

If the infant has to be faced out in this way the mother needs to make it very clear to him that she has not stopped bothering about what he eats because she does not *care* about him any more. He has to be helped toward feeling that the fuss has only stopped because his mother now flatteringly regards him as old enough to decide for himself about food. At mealtimes she may be able to emphasize this by eating her own food with the child, saying, and conveying, that eating is something they do together, she enjoying her food, he enjoying his. But outside mealtimes the infant will probably need to have made up to him the amount of attention and fuss he used to get over food. If he is to be left to get on with eating in his own way, he needs to feel that his mother is just as involved (or temporarily even more involved) as she ever was in all other aspects of his life. She will not feed him, but she will play with him. She will not interest herself in the state of his plate, but she will look at his toy car.

If the mother manages to remain adamant in her refusal to fuss over food any longer, some infants will do their best to get a fuss started in some other area of life. Often, having ceased to be able to involve the mother in a food fuss the infant will try a toilet-training fuss. Mothers who want to stay sane will keep an eye out for this maneuver and resolutely refuse to be trapped into it. The months when one is dealing with an eating problem are not the months for toilet training. One emotionally charged issue at a time is quite enough.

26

SLEEP

AND ITS PROBLEMS

PROBLEMS CONCERNING SLEEP bedevil many families from the time of the first baby's birth. But parental anxiety often seems to peak as the child enters his second year and becomes able—and often all too willing—to stay awake on purpose. Informal study by the author over the past four years suggests that there is a genuine time factor involved: the longer troubled evenings and broken nights go on, the more intolerable they seem. But I believe that there is another factor, too. Parents seem to find it easier to tolerate their *own* lack of sleep during the months when the baby can be seen to be making up *his* rest in daytime naps. Once short and broken nights combine with brief or non-existent naps, the problem comes to seem overwhelming and parents find themselves afraid that the baby may actually be doing himself harm.

During these past few years the frequency with which parents express worries over sleep has overtaken the frequency with which they express worries over eating. Sleep is now the most likely topic to be raised during any lecture question period, radio phone-in, or invited correspondence. Worries over sleeping and eating share many features in common. Food, as we have seen, is a simple biological necessity which we have made complex and problematical by hedging the business of eating it with social and disciplinary considerations. Sleep is also a simple biological necessity and, like food, human beings will take it, in varying amounts which are adequate for them, if they are left to "help themselves." Just as every dieter knows that it is really difficult to eat less than the body requires for its energy, so anyone who has ever tried to finish an exciting novel in the middle of the night knows how difficult it is to stay awake when sleep is truly needed. Experiments have been carried out in which volunteers have been deliberately deprived of sleep. Increasingly strong stimuli are needed to keep them awake as their need to sleep increases.

Stimuli can, of course, come from inside a person as well as from outside. A toddler who is extremely anxious, angry, or upset may keep himself awake for longer than he would have remained awake had he been relaxed and ready to drift off. But there will come a point at which self-stimulation is not enough to counter-balance his need for sleep. It is on this basis that miserable, homesick, frightened children eventually "cry themselves to sleep."

There are no known circumstances under which a child could keep himself awake for long enough to do himself harm. Being forcefully kept awake is extremely unpleasant and, if it is continued over long periods, as in forcible interrogations or "brain-washing" techniques, it can lead to very peculiar and alarming experiences. But even these extreme results of extreme sleep deprivation are temporary. As soon as volunteers are allowed to sleep, they do so. As soon as they awaken from that sleep they find themselves back to normal [36].

Sleep problems with this age group are not therefore really about ensuring that *children* get "enough sleep"; they are about whether *parents* can get enough sleep, peace, and privacy. Just as the parents of a "fussy eater" tend to confuse the nutritional with the social desirability of eating cabbage, so the parents of a "poor sleeper" tend to confuse the health with the convenience aspects of an afternoon nap or a ten-hour night. Devoted parents in child-centered households may bristle at the suggestion that they want their toddlers to sleep primarily in order that they should be safely and legitimately out of the way. But I have never met a parent whose concern with a child's sleeping takes the opposite form: "It's such a pity she can't stay awake to enjoy the evenings with us," or "How can I teach him to wake early enough to enjoy the dawn?," or "It's such a waste of time for her to sleep half the afternoon."

People who really are concerned for children know that adults who are caring for toddlers need both time off to recharge their batteries during the day and a predictable end to that day, too. The more parents are putting in to the child's lively life, the more they need opportunities to recoup their energy and rediscover their adult selves. I have come to believe that parents who can recognize this need *of their own* without any guilt are the ones who are most likely to be able to arrange for it to be met, to the benefit of everyone concerned and especially to the benefit of that wakeful child. At 10 P.M. one evening, a mother whom I know well announced to her 15-year-old daughter, "I'm so tired that you must go to bed." A 15-*month* infant will not greet such startling honesty with the laughing understanding that mother received. The attitude is nevertheless a healthy one.

Parents who do accept that their infant will sleep just exactly the amount he needs to sleep and that the very worst that will happen to him if he stays awake longer than usual is that he will sleep sooner and/or for longer next time, will be able to see that what matters to the rest of the family is *when* he does his sleeping. If his pattern can fit with everyone else's then his actual hours will probably be adequate for all. But if he does his brief sleeping when others can make no use of the break, every-one but him may get ragged around their edges.

Families vary, of course, both in their patterns of living and in the importance which they attach to having a pattern at all. Most small chil-dren will adapt themselves to any pattern or lack of pattern in which they find themselves, but it does need to be reasonably consistent. For exam-ple, a family which steadfastly sets itself against any kind of routine for anyone will not harm an infant by letting him play around the adults every night until he finally falls asleep on the floor. But they may produce unnecessary difficulties if they make occasional and half-hearted attempts to put him to bed; they will clearly be being unfair if having allowed him a very late night, their do-as-you-please ideas do not carry over into letting him sleep on in the morning and they will be doomed to failure if one night they suddenly want him in bed by 6 P.M. because the boss is coming to dinner. At the other extreme, a family which has "bedtime" as a rigid rule will not harm an infant. But such a family may produce unnecessary difficulties if, slightly guilty about banishing a wakeful child, they easily and frequently allow him downstairs again. Between such extremes, families have to make decisions about their way of life and find compromises between their own accepted and acceptable need for the toddler's absence and his equally accepted and acceptable desire to be with them most of the time that he is awake.

Somewhere between one and two most babies go through a phase over daytime naps which is awkward for them and for their mothers. They reach a point where one nap in the day is not enough, and two naps is too many. The infant who used to rest between 10 A.M. and 11:30, and between 2 P.M. and 3:30, and sleep for some of both those periods, is now not ready to be put to bed in the morning, but if allowed to stay up cannot last until after lunch. By midday, just when his meal is cooking, he is exhausted, whiny, and may even drop off to sleep on the floor. If the mother, trying to avoid this, puts him to bed at 11:30 A.M. and gives him a late lunch, the same thing happens in the afternoon. He does not want to go to bed after lunch, but cannot stay awake happily until bedtime. By the end of the second year, this awkwardness usually resolves itself into a single nap, taken either before a late lunch, or after an early one. But in the meantime the mother may find herself giving the infant his midday meal at 11:30 A.M. or putting him to bed for the night at 5 P.M.

By soon after a year, most infants bitterly resent being woken up from their naps. Many are quite unable to eat or play or do anything but moan for as much as an hour after such an awakening. The timing of naps therefore has to be calculated carefully around the mother's other com-mitments. If she wakes him just in time for lunch, he is unlikely to eat any. If she leaves him to sleep during the afternoon, and then has to wake him to go and meet other children from school, he is likely to make it impossible for her to give the older ones proper attention. But if she lets him sleep as long as he likes during the afternoon, he may not wake himself until 5 P.M. and will not then be ready to go to bed at his usual time.

Physical exhaustion often plays a part in this sort of minor difficulty. The infant is likely to be pushing himself to the limits of his strength in learning to walk and climb. He is also likely to be hurting and surprising himself several times a day with the falls that go with this physical activity. As with an older child, the more tired he gets, the less well he manages his body: coordination becomes increasingly effortful. The more his coordination fails him, the more physical effort he has to put into everything he does, and the more times he will fail and fall. He may therefore need ways of resting physically, which are different from actual naps. Being taken out in his stroller in the second half of the morning or afternoon may rest him sufficiently to last without a sleep until after lunch or until bedtime. A period of sitting-down play, with the mother showing him books or helping him build, or teaching him nursery rhymes, may have the same effect.

Getting overtired is a common problem in the second year, and one which mothers sometimes unwittingly encourage. If the infant is difficult to put to bed at night, mothers sometimes feel that the more energetic he is during the day, the more likely he is to sleep well. Often the exact reverse is the truth. The newly mobile infant is bombarded with stimuli. Much of this he provides for himself, as he crawls, and walks; much more is provided by other people and other children, and all the places he is taken to. A public sandbox may be an idyllic place for him to play if it is comparatively empty. But that same sandbox in high summer, seething with bigger children, noisy, alarming, and incomprehensible, may well be too much for him to take in. He may be far too tired, too excited, too strung up to sleep when bedtime comes.

Trouble in settling children down for the night in the second year is so general we ought almost to consider it normal. Unfortunately many advice handbooks are misleading. They tend to imply that the infant should be affectionately but firmly put to bed at the time decided by the mother, and that that should be that. Mothers, reading this sort of advice, often believe that this is what happens in every house but their own, and that it is only their own mishandling of the situation which has led their infant to cause such trouble every evening. In fact when survey workers give mothers the chance to say, in an uncritical atmosphere, what actually happens when they put their toddlers to bed, it becomes clear that somewhere around 50 percent of all infants between 1 and 2 years regularly make a major fuss about bedtime [66, 170]. The Newson survey gives detailed accounts, in the mothers' own words, of the lengths to which families went, every night, to get 1-year-olds settled. It is clear that every practice scorned by the advice books is in fact *common* practice. Infants are sat with, rocked, sung to, cuddled, taken back downstairs, allowed to stay up until all hours, cuddled to sleep on the parents' bed, walked up and down, fed, and re-fed.

Such extreme nightly measures seem absurd to the fortunate families whose toddlers settle happily. But nightly settling problems are very disrupting, so much so that parents will do virtually anything to avoid or cut them short. The mother wants to get the infant settled so that she can give her attention to older children, to her husband, and to supper— which may well be the main meal for husbands who eat sandwiches on the job, or children who dislike their school lunches. Furthermore many women cannot properly relax and enjoy adult company until they know that the infant is settled. And they are very conscious that they *are* bad company until they stop listening to their husbands with one ear—with the other ear halfway up the stairs.

Many (43 percent in the Newson survey) solve the problem by giving the infant a bottle to take to bed with him. In discussion, they know full well that the infant could choke if he goes to sleep with milk dripping into his mouth; they know that nothing, except a bottle of fruit juice, could be worse for his new teeth. But getting the infant settled seems worth almost anything.

Much the same applies to bringing the baby back downstairs again. Mothers realize that they are inviting bad habits when they do this; that the infant cannot be expected to regard bedtime as final if he can get another hour of sociability by crying. But if the infant will not let the mother out of his bedroom, and the potatoes are burning, the older child has news and the husband is hungry, the situation tends to resolve into "I'll break the bad habit tomorrow, if I can just get through tonight." Many authorities believe that none of these problems would arise if parents would be firm from the very first time the infant cries on being left for the night. Illingworth [111] for example says that once the child has been settled he should not see his mother or father again until morning; he should just be left to cry himself to sleep. But at least Illingworth suggests that unseen parents should peep in from time to time to make sure the baby has not actually howled himself sick. Not so Dr. Spock. In his most recent edition of *Baby and Child Care* [208] he suggests that vomiting is a weapon used by spoiled babies and that if parents show sympathy or concern the child will use the vomiting more and more often, to bully them: "I think it essential that parents should harden their hearts to the vomiting. . . . They should stick to their program and not go in. They can clean up later after the baby has gone to sleep." I would consider it somewhat dangerous to leave a near-hysterical child in a pool of vomit which could, possibly, be inhaled. I would also find it quite impossible to "clean up" a crib without waking the occupant. It is difficult to see the feasibility or the logic of the "leave him to cry" view. Its possibility is limited by the fact that infants at this age can keep themselves awake, and cry if they feel like it, literally for hours. Few people's housing is so isolated that they could leave the child for long without complaints from neighbors. And even if neighbors do not complain, older children will certainly be kept awake as well as the parents' nerves shattered.

Logically, if the infant is crying because he cannot, for the moment, bear to see his mother go, it is difficult to see why her refusal to return should make him feel more able to relinquish her. Indeed, leaving him to cry alone is only likely to make him feel more sure that letting her go in the first place is dangerous. One is working, after all, toward the child being *content* to be left to sleep, not toward him going to sleep in abandoned despair.

There is, however, a "testing cry." Almost every infant in this age group will begin to cry when he is left for the night—and often when he is left for a nap too. If his cry is a test, a simple statement that he would prefer the mother to stay with him, and an attempt to see whether she will, then it will only last for a couple of minutes. If the infant does not really feel abandoned, or unable to be alone, he will then stop crying, fall asleep if he is ready, or start to play or talk if he is not. But if it was not a testing cry, the crying will build up. If the mother then stays away, what message is she conveying? "Don't bother to cry, because I shall not come back, however sad you are." It hardly seems a message likely to lead to easier bedtimes on subsequent nights.

There is a middle road between leaving the child desperately alone, and allowing him victory in terms of getting him up again, or sitting with him. The sort of message this middle road is supposed to convey is, "There is no need to cry. You are not deserted, we will always come if you need us, but it is the end of today and time to go to sleep." Such a message seems most likely to get through to the child if one of his parents goes back, every 5 minutes or so, for as long as he continues to fuss, but stays on each visit only long enough to smile, tuck him in, repeat his usual good-night, and leave again. If the house happens to be so arranged that the infant's sleeping room is close to the family quarters, the mother may be able to have the same effect by calling to the infant. Or he may never begin to fuss if he can hear her moving around, tidying up, bathing the next child and so on. The point is that the infant should feel that there is no *need* to cry, because his mother is available, and that there is no *point* in crying, because she will not let him start his day again.

Sometimes this kind of policy can be made easier on the parents and the child if a mild sedative is prescribed by a doctor for the infant. Many people are shocked at this idea. They are convinced that the problem is due to the mother's mishandling, convinced that it could be put right with a little firmness, and revolted at the idea of "sleeping pills for babies." In fact such sedation can act as a much kinder version of the "leaving the baby to cry" policy, and a much briefer and less exhausting version of the "visit him for 2 minutes every 5 minutes" policy. The whole point is that if such a drug is prescribed, it is given well before bedtime, so that the infant makes no connection between the medicine and sleep, and so that he reaches his bed already relaxed and sleepy. Left alone, he cries and his mother visits him. A few minutes later, he finds himself too sleepy and comfortable to be bothered to grumble any more; he finds himself asleep. Over a few nights, the infant ceases to connect being put to bed with crying and misery, and a cross, harassed mother. He begins to expect to go to sleep. In this way a problem pattern can be reversed.

Not all doctors will prescribe such sedation. And it does not always work. Sedative drugs are notoriously difficult to prescribe for the very young, because they can excite rather than calm a child, and so have the reverse of the desired effect. But they are certainly worth considering before the parents reach the screaming (or slapping) point.

By the middle of the second year, a new reason for visiting the crying child, rather than leaving him alone, often emerges. Infants who are left often start to learn to get out of their cribs. If mother will not come to them, they go to find her. This is a development which has to be avoided at almost any cost, because once it has begun it is extraordinarily difficult to deal with. While he is learning to climb out, the infant may hurt himself —crib sides are high for a child who is only just learning to climb. Once he has succeeded in getting out, he may find himself on dangerous stairs in search of his mother. But above all, once it has occurred to him that he *can* get out of bed at will, only the most medieval methods will actually stop him. Of course he can be physically imprisoned, by stretching netting over the top of his crib, strapping him in, or locking his door. But once being put to bed does literally mean being put into prison, all hope of peaceful bedtimes and peaceful nights is gone. Very few mothers actually go to these lengths. But thousands are driven wild by their toddlers appearing downstairs or in the parents' bedroom, several times during the evening and night.

If the infant is always visited when he cries and is never taken out of his crib or taken downstairs, he is unlikely to think of getting out for himself. He is even less likely to think of it if he has always been accustomed to wearing a sleeping bag. Once the child has begun to wander at night it is too late for this solution. He will either climb out despite the bag, and fall and hurt himself, or he will regard the bag as a trap and refuse to wear it. But if he has always worn one, he will know he cannot get out and walk until his mother comes and takes it off. A simple piece of mother upwomanship, but very effective.

Waking in the night can be a very serious problem. It seems that about 20 percent of children up to the age of two wake one or more times in almost every night *and wake their parents.* I stress this last phrase because *every* child—and every adult too—wakes in the night. The difference between that 20 percent and everyone else is that they insist on other people knowing about their awakenings. Infants who wake their parents —and possibly other children and the neighbors too—place the family under extremely heavy stress. Some parents become so tired and desperate that they are conscious of being irritable with the child and with each other during the day. A few fear that if the constant disruption of their own sleep patterns goes on for long, they will eventually lose their tempers and hurt the child. There are parents who regularly park the baby with somebody else one night a week in order to have a rest; alternate night and day shifts so that one of them can sleep through or resort to ear-plugs in an attempt to ignore the whole problem. While every desperate family must work out its own survival methods, all these are desperate measures and all can be counter-productive. Banishing the baby to another house and caretaker does not help parents to feel that their family life and child care are going smoothly. Taking turns does not make for a companionable or sexually fulfilling life, while those ear-plugs can make caring parents feel distressingly guilty.

Until recently, many parents have been reluctant to consult health professionals about this kind of sleeping problem because, if they did so, they were usually told that the problem was of their own making: that they had permitted the child to "get into the habit of waking up" and that they must "break the habit with firmness." Gradually this attitude is changing. Research on the natural history and physiology of sleep [176] has provided a new basis for thinking about night waking and some doctors are beginning to do so [17]. There is still no overall panacea for exhausted families, but there is beginning to be some sensible thinking on which many can base a new approach.

In all human beings, periods of deep sleep alternate with periods of much lighter sleep during which there are frequent moments of "surfacing" when the person comes toward wakefulness and then usually turns over and resettles himself. Although the infantile pattern of very rapid alternation between the two types of sleep is gradually settling toward the adult pattern by this age period, toddlers still have more light-sleep periods than older people. Their number of "surfacings" is therefore greater too and each "surfacing" is a *potential* awakening. Children who do not demand attention in the night either come to the surface without fully becoming conscious, or are able to make themselves comfortable and sink down again without help. Children who do demand attention are not waking themselves on purpose (none of us can do that) but are finding themselves fully conscious at these times and/or are unable to keep themselves comfortable during the transition back into deeper sleep.

Attentive parents may unwittingly encourage their infants to full consciousness during these light-sleep periods. Drillien [66], for example, found that a number of problem-wakers had parents who were alert to the least sound from the infant's room and went in to check on him at the least snuffle or murmur. A murmuring, snuffling, restless child may *have been going* to subside back into deep sleep. But if a parent arrives, unsummoned, at his crib, he will obviously be stimulated into wakefulness. A useful first-line strategy for exhausted parents is simply to decide never to go into their baby's room until he actually *cries*. If they want to check that he is warm enough, comfortable, and so forth, it is better to choose a time when he is deeply asleep than a moment when they can hear him moving. If the child sleeps in his parents' bedroom, such a policy is difficult to adopt. They will hear every sound the infant makes and, furthermore, the parent who is woken by his little grunts and half-waking sounds may well be inclined to hurry to soothe him before the other parent is also awoken. But the soothing is more likely to cause than to avert full disturbance. If the parents really cannot train themselves to stay out of sight and touch until the infant makes it clear that he is fully awake and needs something, they may find life easier if he can sleep in another room. Many parents find that an intercom between two rooms is a great help. These gadgets can have their volume control adjusted so that any real cry will reliably awaken the parents but so that the baby's private murmurings will not.

Once it is accepted that the child *will* almost-wake several times each night and that the aim therefore is to prevent him from being uncomfortably conscious of being awake, it is clear that disturbance or stimulation of every kind should be kept to a minimum. Noise, lost in the general background sound of a city during the day, can be sharply disturbing in the night-quiet. Airplanes, heavy trucks, squawling tom-cats can all jerk awake the child who was poised in light sleep. Similarly, the child who shares a room, whether with his parents or with a brother or sister, can be brought awake at these times by their sleeping noises, trips to the bathroom, and so forth. Sudden changes in lighting, such as may come about when the adults come upstairs to bed, can disturb the child who was almost awake already; so can the dazzle of headlights across his ceiling, not to mention the arrival of the family cat.

But if parents can do a great deal to guard a child's sleep and prevent him, so to speak, from realizing that he has awoken from time to time, different strategies are needed when he makes his awareness loudly clear.

A sudden scream or sudden crying almost always means fear or discomfort. And there is never any purpose in leaving the child. Indeed the longer he is left, the longer it will probably take to resettle him. J. W. Macfarlane, L. Allen, and M. P. Honzik [151], in a careful statistical study of behavior problems in normal children, found that nearly 30 percent of girls and nearly 40 percent of boys woke frequently in the night at 21 months. Often the cause was bad dreams; often it was unknown. In the Newson study [170] 35 percent of mothers of 1-year-old babies had had to get up for them at least once during the night immediately preceding the interview.

In the majority of night-waking incidents, all the child needs is a reassuring glimpse of a parent. Whatever fear has beset him in his sleep is dispelled by this reassurance. But if the comforting is not quickly forthcoming, the distress can build up to panic proportions, and the child may be shaky and tense for a long time after the parent finally arrives.

A child of this age who wakes afraid probably must have the comfort of an adult visit so parents with a child who is having nightmares are bound to have disturbed nights. There is no immediate way to prevent the nightmares. The drugs which sometimes prove useful in helping the child relax into sleep at the beginning of his night will not keep him asleep throughout it. Indeed one of their unfortunate effects can be to make any nightmare very much worse. Sedated, the child may be confused and difficult to reassure. But while there is no immediate solution to nightmares, parents may be able to find long-term solutions. Nightmares are usually worst and most frequent when the infant is under stress in his daily life. Many parents report, for example, that nightmares began to be a problem soon after the birth of the next child, whether this took place when the older child was 12 months or 2 1/2 years. Some relate the problem to a stay in the hospital or some other obviously distressing experience, while others notice that it relates to a period when the child himself is making extra-determined efforts to be independent and/or engaging his parents in a battle about food or toilet training. If parents can identify a stress area, they may be able to relieve it. The new baby cannot be sent back, but the toddler may be able to be helped with his feelings about her.

A great deal of problem-waking comes into a gray zone between these two extremes. The child wakes fully; there is no question of guarding him through light-sleep, hoping that he will not "notice" that he is awake. He is awake; he knows it and he wants his parents to know it too and come to him. Yet he does not appear to be afraid; sometimes he is extremely chatty and sociable, as if he had completed a nap and was ready to get on with life. Some parents deal with this kind of waking by having the infant sleep in their own bed with them. To some this seems entirely natural and obvious; after all in many parts of the world every child sleeps with the comfort of a huddle of bodies. But to others it seems inconvenient, if marginally better than having to get up several times each night, while to yet others it is intolerable. Every family has to work out the pros and cons for itself. The principal pro is that the method does seem to work in the sense that the baby will almost certainly remain peaceful *himself* all through the night. He will sleep, half-wake and wake, but he will seldom make any direct demands which impinge on the adults; he will help himself to a snuggle or a suck. The cons, though, can be many. Sometimes one parent does not mind the infant being there but the other parent does. It can be a pity if father is driven from what is, after all, supposed to be the marital bed. Often one or both parents find that while the infant may feel peaceful, they do not. Flailing arms and legs, mutterings and sucking noises constantly disturb them. The baby's wakings are replaced by their own insomnia. If neither parent minds the infant's presence, other children may mind it very much indeed. I know of several families where soon after the year-old baby joined the parents in their bed, the 4-year-old insisted on sleeping there too while the new baby was never expected to sleep anywhere else. If everybody likes it that way, fine, but it is a pity to start something and then regret it. Certainly a toddler who does sleep with his parents is unlikely readily to accept a return to his own bed, much less replacement in the parents' bed by a new baby.

If parents do not want to have the child in with them, there are some practical aids to being awake but staying contented. Each of them works sometimes for some people. Nightlights, for example, are far more generally used that most advice books suggest. A very low-wattage electric bulb can make it possible for a toddler to stay calm when he finds himself awake. Such a bulb does not flicker, or throw worrying shadows, as the old-fashioned wax nightlight tends to do. It simply banishes darkness so that the child can orientate himself.

Getting cold in the small hours may encourage an infant to come fully to uncomfortable consciousness during his otherwise momentary wakings. Most toddlers kick off their bedding, produce a large gap between pyjama top and bottom, and make the whole lot fairly damp. The whole muddle can be covered with yet another blanket when the parents go to bed, but a sleeping suit covered by a sleeping bag is a far more certain remedy.

Some children who are deeply attached to pacifiers or to the transitional comfort objects which are usually called "cuddlies," cry in the night because they cannot instantly find them when they surface. Tying the beloved object to the crib bars helps some families, but the string needs to be short and weak to obviate any risk of the child strangling himself and some infants resent it anyway because it restricts their use of the object while they are going to sleep. It may be more useful simply to unearth it from the bedding and place it beside the sleeping child's head just before the adults go to sleep themselves.

My own observations suggest that children who do use cuddlies are more able to comfort themselves both when left for the night and when they wake in the night, than children who have no such emotionally important object in their lives. A cuddly is thought to "stand in" for the mother as a comfort object which the infant can use when her comfort is not available to him. The logical explanation for these observations would therefore be that the child comes up to wakefulness (or begins to get sleepy), finds his cuddly safely wound around his head, threaded through his crooked arm or wherever he habitually puts it, and goes to sleep in its benign presence without needing to demand his mother's. While more research into the whole subject of cuddlies would be extremely welcome, a recent paper concerning 3-year-olds certainly suggests that children who do use cuddlies benefit from them and that there is no evidence whatsoever that their use suggests disturbance in the child or that it can do harm to his adjustment [25]. In this study, 16 percent of 700 children were attached to a cuddly. Parents whose children wake in the night in this younger age group might like to try the harmless experiment of actually encouraging and facilitating such an attachment.

If an already-appreciated soft toy, diaper, or small cellular blanket (or the scarf, hat, or underpants the child has already "borrowed" for holding and stroking) is regularly offered, along with the mother's comforting arms, at times of stress, and regularly put into his crib at nap and sleep times, the child who is cuddly-prone may gradually invest it with emotional importance, to good effect. If he is one of those to whom cuddlies mean nothing, no harm will have been done.

Otherwise the phase has to be lived through. Mothers, partly in order to feel they are doing *something* about it, will probably try every solution they can find in books or the experiences of friends. But what helps one child sleep through the night may make another worse. Cutting out the daytime nap may make one sleep longer at night; but another will simply be too tired to settle, and then too tense to sleep soundly. A larger supper will help one, and give another indigestion. Gleaning through the sparse available evidence, only one factor seems at all general, and that is the whole emotional tenor of the infant's daily life. It does seem clear that *both* settling to sleep, and sleeping through the night, are associated with overall calm and happiness.

The calm and the happiness apply both to the infant and to his parents as Martin Bax [17] so clearly shows. If a tense, anxious child can be helped to be happier and more relaxed, his parents will relax, at least a little, too, because whatever is happening in other areas of their lives, their child care will be easier and more fun. Where it is the parents who are obviously under stress, it is easy, and usually accurate, to say that they are conveying tension to their infant. But it is far more difficult to say whether the infant is waking at night because his parents are tense or whether in fact they are tense primarily because the infant keeps on waking. There are no easy, general answers, but if professionals can do nothing else for the parents of a night-waking child, they can at least offer an investment of time and patience in discussion with them which is commensurate with the time and patience the parents are having to give the child.

Early waking in the morning is very general during this year. The infant is tired enough to begin his sleep at 6 P.M., but by 5:30 A.M. he has had plenty of night. He is awake, hungry, and usually very cheerful. How much this matters to the parents depends on many practical factors. Some families get up by 6 A.M. anyway. Others go to bed late and would like to sleep until 8 A.M. There may be an older child who also wakes early, and is delighted with the toddler's company. Or there may be a younger baby whom the mother does not want awakened.

Between 1 and 2, early waking is not usually as difficult to live with as it is in earlier months. The infant is at his best first thing in the morning, and can usually be persuaded to occupy himself very happily if toys, books, and perhaps a zwieback or two are left within his reach. At worst his mother may have to come to him, change his diaper and open his curtains or switch on his light. But after that he will probably give her another hour or two of peace and song. Often, too, this is the time of day when the 3- or 4-year-old most likes the infant. They may amuse each other, talk to each other, in a way they do at no other time. There are no adults around so the two of them are not vying for adult attention. The infant is in his crib, so the older child can escape his attentions if they move in a hair-pulling direction; the infant has no one else to pass him toys or help him with things, so he is likely to give the older one the benefit of the kind of charm he usually reserves for his mother.

Toward 2 years, many infants will accept the mother's desire for morning peace to a point where they will wait for a given signal before shouting for attention. They may learn to wait until they hear her alarm clock go off, or until the radio is switched on. In the winter, early waking is an excellent argument for providing infants with low wattage night-lights. No child can be expected to occupy itself for an hour or more in total darkness.

Common sleep problems in the second year do add up to a very great deal of fatigue for parents. With bedtime problems, night waking, and early morning waking, the parents may never get a peaceful evening and a solid 8-hour night. If there is also a new baby needing night feedings, or an older child having occasional nightmares, sleep may become the parents' chief treat in life. Yet the exhaustion which comes from months of broken nights is often overlooked, by husbands who cannot understand why their wives are so grumpy, or doctors who prescribe tranquilizers for the "bored housewives' syndrome."

TOILET TRAINING

AT 1 YEAR, some babies will be thoroughly experienced in sitting on potties, while most will never have met a potty in their lives. As we saw in Chapter Twenty, it does not seem to make any difference to the child's eventual acquisition of control. True toilet *training,* as opposed to conditioning or catching, starts in this second year.

For reasons already discussed, it is extremely difficult to find out how mothers actually go about toilet training. We know much more about the ages at which success is, or is not, achieved than we do about training methods. Our "knowledge" of the process of toilet training must come more from the informal observations of doctors and nurses who see infants while training is in progress, than from formal statistical surveys, where the mother's lack of memory and her desire to show up well may seriously distort the results.

Toilet training is unique among infant-socialization processes in that it offers only intellectual satisfaction to the child. When we set out to socialize a child's eating, or even his sleeping patterns, we are only attempting to steer or deflect things he positively wants to do anyway. Hunger is a positive feeling, and eating satisfies it. However overlaid with emotional problems the eating process may become, that physiological need-fulfillment pattern remains, working on the parents' side. The same is true of sleep. However great a fight the child may put up, eventually he wants to sleep; at the end of the battle letting go into sleep fulfills a need.

Elimination is a physiological need, too, but when we toilet train a child we are not trying to persuade him to void (as we try to persuade him to eat or to sleep), we are trying to persuade him *not* to void in his pants or on the floor, but to save it for a potty or bathroom. There is nothing in this for the child except eventually, and if all goes smoothly, a satisfaction in being grown up, in being like the parents, and in pleasing them. The strength of adults' early training is shown by the difficulty which they often have in believing that wet pants are not uncomfortable for an infant, that bowel movements do not smell disgusting to them. Many adults cannot understand why an infant does not prefer to be clean. Eventually he will so prefer, but only when he has absorbed the message, however gently it is conveyed, that wet pants are babyish; that soiled ones are "dirty."

True toilet training cannot even begin until the infant shows, by word or gesture, that he is aware when he has wet or soiled himself. At around a year, everyone in the house may know when the infant passes a movement—except him. He may turn scarlet, strain as if constipated although he is not, grunt and generally make his performance clear. But he may still appear quite unconscious of having produced anything. When he urinates the child may become motionless on the floor, then pull himself to his feet leaving a puddle behind him. But he does not even glance back at it; he still does not connect the bodily sensations with the product.

Most infants begin to make this vital connection somewhere between 1 year and 15 months [7]. When the child urinates, he will point out the puddle to his mother, or clutch his wet diaper with an exclamation. Placed on a potty when a bowel action is obviously imminent, he may look in the potty to see what came out.

Once the child connects his bodily sensations with a product, things become both easier and more difficult for the training mother. They are easier in that the infant is on the way toward learning to tell her *before* the event rather than after. But they are more difficult in that the child becomes aware that what he produces is his, comes out of his body, is part of him and therefore does not belong to the mother, should not necessarily be in her power.

This is the basic toilet-training conflict. The infant is being asked to treat what he rightly regards as part of himself as if it belonged to the mother. He is being asked to give it to her, where she says, when she says. It is his gift to bestow, yet he is not allowed to decide not to give it.

The more capable of being trained the child becomes, the less he may wish to be trained. The more able he is to withhold his urine or feces, the more he may decide to withhold them from the mother, not from the diaper. The more valuable she makes the gift seem, the more may he decide that today she shall not have it.

Against that, the mother can set only the child's desire to grow up, together with any flattering acknowledgments of being grown up that she can think of for a particular child—like wearing ordinary pants instead of diapers, or being allowed to take his own toilet paper.

Bowel training almost always precedes bladder training. Indeed bowel training may, in infants who have been placed on the potty well before a year, simply progress from catching. Bowel control is far easier for infants. Most only move their bowels once or at most twice a day by this age and many not that often. Many are naturally quite regular in their timing, the movement almost always occurring at the same time in the day. The signs of an impending movement are often clear for the mother to see, but the urgency is not nearly as great as it is for urination. The mother therefore has time calmly to take the child to the lavatory or potty when she knows a movement is coming, and the infant is not bored by frequent unsuccessful visits. Gradually, at around 15 months, he becomes interested in what he produces. Very shortly after that, he may attract his mother's attention when he is about to perform, although he would still carry on in his pants if she ignored him. By 18 months he may actually ask for the potty, and by 20 months—the average in Ruth Griffiths's sample [99]—his bowel training may be complete so that he only soils his pants during rare episodes of diarrhea, and is horrified if he does so.

But that smooth and easy picture is an ideal, and it is entirely dependent on the infant remaining happy to be taken to the lavatory when he is going to have a movement. Often the 18-month baby is at just the stage of emotional development when he least wishes to fall in with any urgent suggestion of the mother. If she tries to rush him in to lunch or hurry him into his clothes, he fusses. So he is equally likely to refuse if she tries to hustle him to the lavatory.

When he realizes how important it is to her that they get there in time, his negativism is likely to increase. He is contra-suggestive. At least when she hurries him to lunch, he knows he is going to get the lunch. When she hurries him to the lavatory he is only going to have a movement, and he was going to have that anyway—only she cares where. If mild negativism is met with increased pressure, accidents with scoldings, successes with triumph, the infant often begins to see his movement as an area of great power over the mother. He can really make her care. If this stage is reached, the infant may actually refuse to sit on the potty at all; or, even more cleverly, may sit there quite goodly, but use his new power to withhold the movement until he is allowed to get up. The mother *knows* he needs to go, but she cannot make him. In extreme instances, the infant will perform anywhere but in the lavatory or potty, and any time except when his mother suggests it. Worse still, he may learn to withhold until his movements have become so dry and hard and his colon so distended that it loses sensation, and he becomes actually unable to go, truly constipated.

Most families experience something in between these two extremes. The infant remains reasonably cooperative, but has days when he will not use the potty or indeed pass a movement at all; on other days he will have accidents, or refuse to go when his mother first places him on the potty and then relent a little later on but rather too late. Most mothers manage to avoid extremes of concern, though few fail to get irritated once soiling is obviously calculated. The hope, in bowel training, is to prevent the infant seeing it as a weapon in the power game, by keeping the emotional temperature of the whole process down. J. W. Macfarlane, L. Allen, and M. P. Honzik [151] found that by 21 months only 32 percent of boys and 20 percent of girls in their sample still regularly soiled.

Urine training is a far more difficult problem for the infant—and therefore for the mother. The physiological difficulty is well explained by S. R. Muellner [166]. He points out that the infant's first method of holding up the passing of urine comes through learning to prevent the destrusor muscle from contracting, and simultaneously holding in the levator ani muscle. As an older child would put it, he "clenches his bottom" and, as the older child would certainly explain, you cannot do that for long. The intra-abdominal pressure has already reached a high level, and the urgency to urinate is extreme. Only later does the child learn to take charge of matters at an earlier stage, by using the diaphragm and the abdominal muscles to control intra-abdominal pressure. Once he can do this, he can delay much longer. But it is later still before he can void voluntarily when the bladder is not full. Furthermore, his bladder capacity at the age of 2 years is normally only half that of a 4-year-old.

Urine training is practically difficult too. In this second year of life the infant may need to urinate 8 or more times during the day, depending on how much he drinks, the temperature, whether he has any fever and so on. The problem is therefore not one which can be dealt with for the day in one successful potting. The mother has to be alert all day to help the infant. The infant has to be alert, or at least prepared to have his activities interrupted, all day, too. Obviously discouraging accidents are far more likely than they are with bowel training. Obviously too the infant is the more likely to get fed up with the whole business. Less obviously, the mother may find herself being very inconsistent in her handling of the infant's urination. At home she may keep an eye on the child or the clock or both, and place him on the potty consistently, congratulating him on being a big boy who does not need diapers in the daytime any more. But as soon as she takes him out she may find herself having to put those diapers back on. She knows she will not get him to a public lavatory on a busy street in time.

Time is of the essence early in urine training. At around 15 months, the infant may tell his mother he has wet himself. At 16 months he may announce, often with a loud scream, that he is about to do so. A month or so later, he learns the first bottom-clenching control, but it is momentary only, and furthermore it roots him to the spot. He cannot run for his potty because if he moves he will urinate. Only if the mother gets to him like greased lightning can she help him to be in time. At 18–20 months, that more timely intra-abdominal control may have begun, so that the infant does have time to tell and then go. But his waiting time is still not very long, and he cannot yet urinate in advance of needing to. It is no use, at this age, asking him to go to the lavatory now, so that he will not need to go later at the store. He cannot go until he does need to, and then it must still be quickly. Hardly surprising, then, far more children still regularly wet themselves by day at 21 months than soil themselves. In Macfarlane's sample [151] 62 percent of boys and 43 percent of girls still did so at this age. Daytime control for the whole sample was not certain until the children were 3 1/2.

Clearly there is a delicate balance to be struck in toilet training. It has to be made clear to infants that their parents would prefer them to use a lavatory or a potty, and that older people always do so. Very occasionally mothers are so concerned not to put pressure on a child, but to "leave him to train himself," that they forget to communicate this preference. R. S. Illingworth [112] quotes one such mother of a 4-year-old girl, who had attempted no training of any kind because she "did not mind washing diapers." Many children, neglected in this way, would in fact copy other members of the family and train themselves before 4 years. But it is no kindness to leave them to do so. By 3, most children will experience some scorn from other children if they are still in diapers. There are no severer critics of toilet-training deficiencies than those who have only just completed their own.

At the same time, there must be no temptation to the child to use toileting as a battleground. The mother's apparent emotions about the matter have to be kept at low key. Wet or soiled pants are not wicked; clean or dry ones are not superb accomplishments. It is just a nuisance or a pity when they are wet or dirty, clever and grown up when they are dry or clean.

The constant interference of daily activities which urine training involves needs to be kept to a minimum. Unless the infant prefers to use the lavatory, a potty is useful because it is portable; it can be brought to the playing child rather than his needing to be taken out of the room and away from what he was doing. Clothes also need to be easy. It is seldom any use trying to urine train a child who wears diapers in the day. He may fail to notice a small urination. And the pins and general difficulty of getting him undressed will certainly be too much for his precarious early control. The boredom of being redressed will also irritate him. Once the mother decides she is seriously trying to help him stay dry, it has got to be pants and puddles.

Once any trouble starts over toileting, no authority any longer suggests that the mother should join battle. Trouble usually starts with the infant not wanting to sit on the potty. Often in the first instance this is only because he was busy with something else. But if the mother tries to insist, it becomes a physical battle. Unless she holds him down, he gets off. If she holds him down she is overpowering him in just the way he finds most objectionable. It is as if she tried to force-feed him, or tied him in his crib in a lying down position. She cannot win—she cannot force him to void any more than she can force him to eat or sleep—but she can very easily turn what started as an objection of the moment into a real problem. While momentary objections, leading to a couple of puddles a day, can be simply ignored—the mother reckoning that she and the toddler are still basically making a joint effort—consistent potty refusal over several days probably means that the child is not ready to play his part. It will be easier on both him and his mother if he is put back in diapers and the whole business forgotten for a few weeks.

Some infants do become toilet-training problems, however sensitively they appear to have been handled. A study of the very many theories put forward by different workers, both theoreticians and research workers, does not produce any one reason or even any convincing group of reasons.

Immaturity is probably often a factor. The infant may be less physiologically ready for training than he appears, and attempts to train him make him anxious and resentful. He is socially mature enough to realize what the mother wants, and even—with part of him—to want to do what she wants, but he cannot manage.

Sometimes small practical considerations have a disproportionate effect. The child may feel insecure and wobbly sitting on a potty instead of a supporting chair, or the solid floor. Or he may feel afraid sitting high up on the hollow lavatory. Occasionally he may pass a hard movement which hurts, or which even makes a tiny anal tear which is sore for several days. A girl may be sore from fingering herself, so that urine stings. Mishaps of this kind can put the infant off for a day or two. Then if the objections are tactlessly handled by the mother, the whole business may become an issue between them.

The real issue probably centers around the new sense of independent self which is a vital part of being a toddler; of growing away from babyhood toward childhood. The child sees his movements as a part of himself. Passing them is physically pleasurable and the mother receives them with pleasure, as if they were a gift. Yet they are not a gift which the child is allowed to bestow as he pleases. Nor are they a part of himself which he is easily permitted to play with or to keep. They are quickly flushed down the lavatory.

Sometimes objections to toilet training become confused with the child's feelings about genital play. As far as we know all children eventually discover the particular pleasure of genital play as opposed to play with other parts of the body. The casual clutching of earlier months gives way to a more deliberate, obviously pleasurable rhythmical handling. And this discovery of masturbation often takes place during the toilet-training months. If the parents have made it clear to the baby that they disapprove of genital play this new pleasure will already be a guilty one. The parents angrily remove the child's hand from his own body just as they remove his feces if he tries to play with them. They try to control his giving of genital pleasure to himself just as they try to control his passing of his own movements. The toddler tends to see such control as intrusive and overpowering. He is at a developmental stage when he must assert himself by taking issue with the mother on anything that comes up. And, as we have seen, toileting comes up more frequently than most issues;

counting in urination, more frequently even than those other prime areas for conflict, meals and sleep.

As with feeding problems, the two most useful pieces of avoiding action do seem to be for the mother to be prepared to leave things alone at the very first sign of trouble, never allowing herself to be trapped into insisting that the child use the potty when he cannot be persuaded to want to. And to hand the responsibility primarily to him at the very first possible moment. If the potty is on the floor in the room where the child plays, and he has pants he can pull down (or even none if it is warm enough) he is far more likely to go and do it for himself than he is to submit to being done to. And if he empties the potty himself and flushes the toilet, he may actually feel that disposing of his waste products is fun—rather than mother hurtfully rejecting a gift.

This kind of child-paced approach to toilet training is probably more widely accepted now than it has ever been. Helped, perhaps, by the widespread availability of disposable diapers, plastic pants, and easy-care bedding, and perhaps by less criticism and comment from outside the family, most parents do seem able to delay the start of training until children are ready, and to accept realistic time-goals for its completion.

There is, however, a diametrically opposed approach which has received sufficient publicity to confuse some parents. This is the approach to training which relies on behavior modification techniques. Its use in toilet training is described in *Toilet Training in Less Than a Day* [12]. Its use in teaching toddlers to read is described in *Teach Your Baby to Read* [65]. The fact that a child can be taught almost anything an adult wants him to learn if the right teaching methods are used is excellently put across in a recent book by Janet Carr called *Helping Your Handicapped Child* [46]. Behavior modification techniques, as the last-mentioned book makes clear, were developed by psychologists to help individuals with particular learning difficulties to acquire important skills. The techniques depend on rewarding desirable behavior while carefully avoiding rewards (or giving mild "punishments") for undesirable behavior. A massive concentration of attention and effort is usually required of the teacher, with endless repetition from the pupil.

The principles behind these techniques can give parents interesting food for thought. Many of us, for example, unwittingly "reward" (with our reluctant and irritable attention) behavior, such as whining, which we should like to extinguish. When the child does not whine (and is therefore behaving in the way we prefer) we do not reward him with attention; we get on thankfully with whatever else we want to do. But while thinking in this way can be refreshing and useful, direct attempts to apply behavior modification techniques to toddlers' learning is a very different matter.

The techniques have been used to help mentally retarded adults to acquire the socially acceptable lavatory habits which enabled them to be discharged from institutions. They have also been used to train autistic children to communicate in speech, thus making further social and educational contact with them possible. In both these instances—and in many others—the progress of the patients themselves was being blocked by a specific learning disability. Overcoming that disability improved the whole quality of their lives. The toddler who is not yet clean or dry or does not yet recognize or use many words does *not* have a specific learning disability nor is the quality of his life being lowered by his lack of these skills. He is simply immature and his learning in all these areas will, and should, be part and parcel of his growing up. Perhaps the quality of his *parents'* lives would be improved by having a 3-year-old who could read, but singling out one developmental skill for forced-teaching will not assist the child's overall development.

While few parents will choose to devote the time and energy required by the reading program, the toilet-training system could prove tempting, especially with its advertised success in " . . . less than a day." If a particular babysitter will not accept the child until he is out of diapers, a nursery group offers a place "as soon as he is dry," or a holiday abroad is looming, why should a parent not give it a try? The author believes that the parent should not because a child under two will probably be incapable of doing what is asked of him so that the method cannot work and both he and his teacher-parent must inevitably experience disappointment and failure. If the method does appear to work, as promised, the child's immaturity will probably ensure that it does not last. The experience of disappointment and failure will be no easier for being delayed. If the method both works and lasts then the child was probably ready to become dry anyway and would have done so, with ordinary parental assistance, very shortly. Finally, whether it works or not, the essence of this method of training is the focusing of the child's attention on that one particular skill and its rewards. We surely do not want toddlers to believe that using a potty is the pinnacle of achievement and the one accomplishment of which his parents truly approve.

28

MOBILITY

LEARNING TO WALK ALONE is regarded as a major landmark in an infant's development. But often, what he *does* with his ability to walk is ignored. Once he can walk alone, mothers and other observers lose interest in his mobility. This is a pity. Just as the infant learns to get hold of objects first, and then only gradually learns what to do with them, how to use them, so he learns to walk first, and then only gradually learns to use his walking in such a way as to approximate mature patterns of mobility.

As we saw in Chapter Twenty-one, the majority of infants can make some form of progress on their own two feet by the first birthday. Some will only pull themselves to standing by furniture, crib, or playpen bars, and then cruise around the support. Others will hand themselves from one support to another, thus getting around a conveniently arranged room; others will actually relinquish their hold on one support to cross a gap to the next. A few will walk without any support at all.

Almost all infants will pass through these stages on their way to independent walking. There is little purpose in trying to persuade the child who does not yet hand himself from one support to another, to toddle two steps across the room toward his mother. This is asking him to leave out two stages. And he will not. If he did he would almost certainly fall; and as we have seen, falls at this age are to be discouraged. They can do damage to both skull and confidence.

This kind of premature "encouragement" from parents and caretakers is very common. It often arises because the infant's mobility does not increase at a consistent pace. He passes from one stage to the next, but often there is a long period between two specific stages, during which he appears to have got stuck. He has learned a certain degree of walking competence, and progresses no further, often for several months. Illingworth [109] points out that once the child has become a biped to *any degree*

347

a delay in actual independent walking is very seldom a cause for concern. Any spasticity, or other disease affecting neuromuscular control, will already have manifested itself during the first stages of learning to walk.

Such delay, after reaching a certain level of competence, is usually a simple reflection of the fact that the infant does not have enough hours of waking time, enough energy and concentration available, to progress at an equal rate in all developmental fields. As early as 1946, A. Gesell [95] put it thus: "The course of development turns upon itself in a manner to suggest a spiral kind of neuromotor organization, characteristic of reciprocal interweaving. . . ."

Having reached a certain point in his walking development, the child turns his developmental attention to other matters. His bipedal achievements have given him some added mobility, an interesting new view of the world, and extra height so that he can reach more objects. He may be happy to rest upon that, and *use* the new view, the new interest and the new objects. He may enter a phase where he concentrates for the moment on play with toys, or on learning to talk, or on a high level of social interaction with adults.

Getting stuck in this way in walking development may also reflect a lack of confidence. In such a child, the point where development stops is usually the point between walking competently with any form of support, even one finger from an adult, and actually taking off across the room alone. A particular fall may shake his confidence, so that he decides to abandon independent walking for the moment. Slippery floors or shoes may make independent walking feel impossibly difficult. The rowdy presence of older pre-school children may make the middle of the floor on his own two feet feel a very vulnerable place to be. Such children continue to develop their ability to walk even while they continue to insist on token support. When they do finally gain the confidence to set out alone, they usually do so with great competence, as if they had been practicing for weeks.

A child who stops progressing in his walking is therefore seldom a cause for concern. Regression is a different matter. If an infant's balance and muscular control appear to slip back, so that he is actually less competent at, say, 18 months than he was at 15 months, there has to be a reason. If the reason is not obvious, advice should be sought.

But usually the reason is obvious, and the prognosis excellent. Severe illness, even of quite unimportant etiology, such as an acute infection of any kind, with high fever and some days of comparative immobility, will reduce both the infant's energy and his muscle tone to a point where he has to regress a little and then catch himself up. He may revert to crawling, and then repeat all the stages of learning to walk, all over again. Only this time he "re-learns" them in a few days instead of over months. Parents whose children suffer an illness known to be serious, and known to be occasionally followed by brain damage, such as meningitis or encephalitis, often go through days of needless agony because this natural regression is not recognized. The doctors may assure them that the infant has come through his experience undamaged, but they watch the child who could walk three steps alone before he was ill, crawl uncertainly around the room, barely able to pull himself up to stand at the crib bars, and they cannot believe he is not permanently damaged. They fail to allow for the effects of confinement, drugs, trauma, and little food. And they panic.

Any severe emotional upset may have much the same effect. Separation from the mother often leads to a general regression to more babyish ways, and this will include more babyish locomotion. Just as recovery from illness will start the infant back to progressing again, so the end of the emotional upset will give him the confidence, the heart, to catch himself up again.

R. Griffiths [99] had 150 infants between 10 and 15 months of age in her sample. At 12 months, most of them could side-step confidently around the furniture and could walk at least one or two steps with their hands held. At 13 months most could stand alone for at least a few seconds: they would release their grasp on the furniture before sitting down, for example, or remain erect for a few moments if the mother gently disengaged her hands. Once this stage was reached, the babies tended to progress rapidly to independent walking, so that most were taking one or two steps between supports, quite alone, by the end of the 14th month. By 16 months most of the infants were toddling competently, and had largely abandoned crawling as their ordinary means of getting around. While these very approximate norms still seem valid for British children and are, indeed, confirmed for an American sample by work reported by the Gesell Institute in 1980 [7], some researchers predict greatly accelerated motor progress. White, for example, whose book *The First Three Years of Life* [222] first appeared in Britain in 1978, expects unaided walking by one year of age and skillful running at 14 months. This variation in reported "norms" is a salutary reminder that in any large group of children there will be many individuals whose behavior, in any field, and at any given age-point, is "atypical." Such norms need to be interpreted cautiously both by parents who think their child gives cause for concern and by those who think him advanced.

Infants tend to remain partly dependent on supporting furniture or adult hands for some weeks after they can first walk alone because they cannot yet get up alone. Few infants learn to get to their feet without support until 15–16 months. Just as the baby who can sit on the floor and play, still, for some weeks, has to be put in sitting position by his mother, so the baby who can toddle has to have help in getting into toddling position in the first place. The infant's actual mobility can therefore often be pleasurably increased by giving him what is commonly known, in England, as a baby-walker. This British version is quite different from the American baby-walker. Personally I regard the American version, in which the baby is seated within a frame on castors, and can push himself around the room, as extremely dangerous. It teaches the baby nothing useful and can, and indeed often does, lead to bad falls and bumps. The British version is simply a small truck, or cart, carefully designed so that the handle can be used by the baby to pull himself upright, without it tipping, and so that as he walks with it, it does not run away from him. Obviously the design is vital. A doll's carriage or other stroller designed for older children can be disastrous. It tips backward when the child pulls himself up, and once he starts it rolling it goes too fast for him. Given a true baby-walker, a child can use a garden or park, taking his pull-up support and toddling support with him across the grass. With years of use ahead as a brick truck or doll's carriage, such a walker is an excellent investment. While handy fathers could no doubt make such a walker, the exactly balanced design is so important that I would not advise this. But an excellent version, most carefully tested for safety and durability, is manufactured by Galt.

The first competent toddling, around the sixteenth month, has many limitations. The two most unnerving are that the infant can neither stop suddenly, nor change direction. Collisions, painful meetings with door-posts, and falls down garden steps are the frequent result. Such accidents are most common out of doors. It is usually there that the infant has space to get up the speed which leads to disaster due to absence of brakes and steering.

By the seventeenth month, most infants are so steady on their feet that the mere process of walking need not take up all their energy and attention; they can do other things at the same time. The infant will probably be able to stoop from standing posture and pick a toy up off the floor, rather than sitting down to get the toy, and then having to get up again. Having got the toy he will be able to walk and carry it at the same time. He can look over his shoulder as he walks, and will therefore probably enjoy pulling a toy along behind him on a string. Very shortly afterward he learns to retreat by walking backward.

By 20 months he will probably be able to run, rather than merely toddling fast; and he may be able to jump so that both his feet leave the ground together. Few infants will be able to balance on one leg, however, until the third year, even though by two they will be able to kick a football after a shuffling fashion.

The actual use the infant makes of his increasing mobility does not depend only on his ability; it also depends very largely on his attachment to his mother, and therefore on her behavior.

Infants are most mobile and most exploratory when their mothers are present in a familiar setting. In these circumstances the infant walks about, exploring, playing, conscious always of his mother's presence, using her as a secure base. Some of the earliest observations and thoughts upon mother as an explorer's base were made by William Blatz [22]. Since then many studies have demonstrated that the infant's willingness to move around and to explore are largely dependent on his mother's presence. The human child and the infant rhesus monkey need the mother to give them the courage to face the insecurity of the wider world, to refer to for reassurance as they explore it and to return to in haste if it proves alarming. The kind of behavior which demonstrates this need has been well shown in a study of 1-year-olds placed in a strange play-room environment and observed with their mothers, with mother plus a stranger, with just a stranger, and quite alone [6].

All the infants played most actively and covered most ground when they were alone with their mothers. The addition of a stranger slightly diminished their activity, but most were prepared to accept the stranger's advances. Left alone with the stranger, the infants became immobilized. If they had failed to notice the mother leaving, their play tailed off as soon as they did notice. Those who became actually distressed could often be somewhat comforted by the stranger, but none could regain his former mobility and activity with only her presence for support. Left quite alone most of the infants did not move at all.

The disruptive effect on play of being left by the mother seemed also to be cumulative. Where the mother's first reappearance usually cued active, pleased greeting-behavior by the infant, her second departure and return evoked miserable clinging. Had the research design demanded a third departure, few of the mothers would have been able to interest the child in a toy sufficiently to escape yet again.

In 1978 [4] Ainsworth reported that these experiences were not only cumulative in their effects on the infants' play but also remembered. She repeated the procedures with 1-year-olds, 2 weeks after their first session. It was clear, from the moment they entered the playroom, that this time they anticipated the mother's departure and did so with distress.

The parallel with a normal situation with the mother and child to-gether at home is not perfect, of course, because the experimental play-room was strange to the infants. Nevertheless it remains generally true, from observations made in homes, that the more sure the infant is that the mother is there, and will remain there, the more independent activity he will indulge in. Sometimes mothers will say, in frustration, "This morning I was busy, trying to clean around the house and so on, and he wouldn't let me alone for a minute, whining and clinging around my legs. Now I sit down to play with him and he doesn't want to know—he's all over the place and busy as a bee."

Although such behavior may sometimes be inconvenient for busy parents, preventing them, for example, from leaving the infant for a few minutes in the "play area" of an exhibition hall or a crowded store, there is some evidence that the behavior is developmentally desirable. Children who do *not* react in this way to brief separations in strange circumstances may be children who are insecure about their mother's feelings for them and uncertain of a kindly response from her. Main [152], for example, found that where the secure infant between 12 and 18 months always greeted his mother's return with heartbreaking relief and enthusiasm, insecure infants tended to turn away and busy themselves with a toy as soon as they saw their mothers. If the mother of such a child decided that he was "happily occupied" and slipped away again, he would usually maintain his careful detachment although his play with the chosen toy could be seen to become increasingly stereotyped. Bowlby [33] points out that this kind of studied indifference to the mother's comings and goings may be easily misconstrued as healthy, if early, independence. Far from feeling independent, the child who behaves in this way is "effectively excluding any sensory inflow that would elicit his attachment behavior and thus avoiding any risk of being rebuffed. . . . There is much evidence that the strategy is no more than second best and to be adopted only when a mother's attitude is adverse."

The independent locomotion of slightly older children, from around 15 months to 2 years, has been beautifully observed by J. W. Anderson [8]. He studied 35 children whose mothers were sitting peacefully in the sunshine in a secluded corner of a familiar park.

Of the 35 children, 24 remained within 200 feet of the mother in any direction, without her taking any action whatsoever to retain contact with the child. Eight infants set off to go farther afield, attracted by seeing swings in the distance. All the mothers of these infants got up to follow as escorts, with the infants still remaining within their self-prescribed distance limit. Only 3 children had to be retrieved by the mothers because they wandered too far or got out of immediate sight.

The behavior of the infants was highly consistent. All tended to move away from the mother in a direct line, and in short bursts punctuated by brief stops on the way. Their original foray was not caused by seeing something interesting. It was simply a moving away for its own sake. When the infants started to return, they often did so without ever looking at the mother, as if they were so aware of her exact position that a visual check on how far away they had got was unnecessary. The return journey was never instigated by an alarming external event, simply by it being "time to return to base" by the infant's own internal clock. Once the infants had started back toward their mothers, they tended to progress in longer stretches, stopping less often than on the outward journey. But as they got closer to the mother, so the halts became longer, until finally that journey was over altogether.

Half of the children finished the journey still out of physical reach of the mother. They made their next outward sortie without physical, verbal, or eye-to-eye contact having been made. It was as if it was enough for these children to have been briefly in the mother's orbit. Another quarter of the children rested close to the mother before setting out again; the remaining quarter made actual contact, leaning against the mother or climbing onto her lap. Mothers and infants spoke to each other only when they were in close contact. Very few mothers attempted to keep in contact with their exploring infants by calling to them. Those who did were totally unsuccessful—the infants behaved as if they were outside the maternal aura, and therefore not reachable by voice alone.

If the mother got up from her seat, and moved to retrieve something, or into a new patch of sunlight, without first signaling her intention to the infant, he at once became rooted to the spot. His natural coming and going pattern was broken by her shift, and usually no amount of patient calling would induce him to join her in her new position. The mother had first to retrieve the infant, and then let him start going and coming again from the new base.

We regard walking as a means of moving along, and getting from one place to another. But toddlers do not. Not only do they naturally tend to go and come to a seated mother, they are quite incapable of following, or moving along with, a *moving* mother. The infants observed by Anderson tended to ask for transport as soon as the mother signaled her intention of moving on. If a stroller was offered, they climbed willingly into it. If there was no stroller, they at once held up their arms to be carried. When mothers tried to make the toddlers walk along with them, there was invariably trouble. Holding the mother's hand, and with her walking extremely slowly, the infant might manage for a few yards. But after that either the mother would lose her patience and drag the child by the arm, or he would move deliberately and directly in front of her, and stand holding up his arms, demanding to be carried.

J. Bowlby [32] calls on data from a further 12 children studied by J. W. Anderson, to confirm their complete inefficiency in remaining oriented to a moving figure. The mothers of these 12 children were each moving very slowly through the park with their infants following them. Each child stopped repeatedly at varying distances from the mother, so that each mother spent more time waiting for the child than walking. Frequently the children wandered off course, and were then distressed because the mother was not where they had expected her to be, even though she was still in close, full view.

Bowlby believes, on the basis of these and other data, that following behavior does not develop in human infants before about 3 years. Until that time it is instinctive for the child to seek transport whenever the mother moves, even though he is fully capable of covering great distances when she is still. After 3 years the infant can use newly developed goal-corrected systems to keep with a moving object, but for a further year or two most will prefer to be attached to that object, by holding hands, clutching clothes, or holding on to the carriage handle.

Observations of animals tend to confirm this view. Many herd-animal young run and frolic while their mothers graze, orienting their excursions around the herd. But as soon as the herd begins to move off, the young return to their mothers, to move close against their sides, or under their bellies. Similar behavior can be seen among apes even by casual observation in a zoo. As long as the mother ape sits grooming herself on a branch, her infant will play and explore all over the available cage space. But if the mother moves to another branch, the baby will freeze and cry until she fetches it. If the mother indicates that she is moving across to the eating place, the infant at once clings to her belly fur for transport, even though he had made eight independent journeys across the intervening space in the previous ten minutes.

An understanding of these peculiarities of early walking helps mother-child harmony. All too often mothers are highly irritated by their infant's refusal to walk home, when they are clearly not tired, having been toddling all over the place two minutes before. All too often the infant's refusal to hold the mother's hand and walk nicely beside her is seen as a willful desire to escape and play, rather than an actual inability to stay oriented to her moving thigh. And all too often those constant stops and wanderings off in the wrong direction are seen as a desire to explore, a refusal to come home, rather than an inability to follow.

Handbooks of advice on child rearing commonly advise mothers to deal with this kind of lagging behavior in the second year by keeping moving slowly ahead, on the grounds that the child will catch up when he sees mother getting further away. He may, but he may not. Mother's self-removal may leave him totally disoriented. If the following ability of toddlers was as good as these books suggest, there would not be so many lost and terrified infants in parks, streets and stores. Using a stroller should not be seen as a sour reflection on the child's ability to walk, but as a means of keeping him where he wants to be while his mother is in motion—close.

LEARNING TO THINK

By HIS FIRST BIRTHDAY the infant's perceptions, through his five senses, have largely become organized into meaningful wholes. He recognizes objects, even when their lighting or their position or their context is unusual. He will know that his bottle is his bottle, even if it is presented endways on. He will know that his big beachball is itself, even if it is so far away across the grass that it looks small. He will recognize his mother's voice even when he cannot see her, and the ice cream van's chimes even if ice cream has not been mentioned.

But the infant has still got a good deal of perceptual sophistication to acquire by experience. He tends to see wholes, rather than the component parts of wholes, so that he will not notice the flowers that make up the pattern on the wallpaper unless they are pointed out to him; he will not be the one to notice the blood on the family dog's cut leg. He is still more readily fooled than an older person by tricks of environmental lighting, exclaiming at the "pretty stone" when a piece of coal is turned into gleaming glass by a shaft of sunlight. Even more than an adult, he may be amazed at the lightness of a large parcel, or the heaviness of a small piece of lead. And much of his perceptual recognition is dependent on context. He may still greet his mother with a blank stare when she returns from the hairdresser with a new style, fail to recognize his father if he arrives home in a strange car, be unable to realize that it is his mother speaking if she talks to him on the telephone.

But all in all, the 1-year-old's perceptions are ready for the very beginning of the fresh and more complex organization we call concept formation.

If a perception is the organization of simple sense impressions into meaningful wholes, concepts are the groupings and categories into which such perceptions fall. Before he can form a concept, the infant must

355

discover and define for himself the critical features common to a group of objects or a group of events.

Concepts therefore depend crucially on the development of language. Indeed whether they can exist at all without language being at least understood, if not spoken, is a subject of hot philosophical dispute. The nature of a child's concepts also depends on his culture. A Western infant may have, say, three different impressions which he must learn to recognize as "rice": dry rice in the packet or jar, rice pudding, and the boiled rice that sometimes accompanies meat dishes. An Indonesian infant may have as many as a dozen rice impressions of far greater variability and subtlety—for instance, rice growing in the paddy, which is dramatically different from rice prepared for eating, and refined rice, which is only a little different from rice left with the outer husk.

The infant begins the developments which will lead to concept formation through play. He has learned to see and hear and feel things more or less as adults do, and he has learned to get hold of things and manipulate them. By seeing, getting and manipulating, he finds out more and more about the nature of things: how they work, what they do, how they resemble each other and differ. During this year he will learn about up and down, about few and many, about in and out, about big and small, heavy and light, loud and soft. He will learn that what is round rolls, that what is square does not; that paper crumples where thin wood will not; that water is wet and will wet him.

We know that infants learn all these things. As we shall see, we can watch them doing it, and by the end of the year, we shall be able to hear their growing understanding in their early speech. But how these cognitive processes take place remains largely a mystery.

The most systematic and comprehensive theory of cognitive development is probably that of Jean Piaget. A Swiss psychologist, Piaget began to study his own children and others during the thirties. He wrote copious, brilliant, difficult papers which, perhaps because they were an unfamiliar mixture of personal, small-scale, observational research with mondially applicable theory, made little impact on the English-speaking world until the fifties. Since then Piaget's work has generated a vast literature and stimulated the thinking of an extraordinarily wide range of professionals. Many of his illustrative experiments have been repeated. Some have proved impossible to replicate on large, random samples of children. A few have been discredited. Nevertheless both his theories and his findings are now basic to the study of development. Since a book of this size cannot hope to do justice to this giant, readers may like to know that Flavell's book *The Developmental Psychology of Jean Piaget* [82] is widely regarded as giving a fair and accurate picture. Readers who want a book which enables them to apply Piagetian ideas to their own individual infant may prefer Mary Sime's *Read Your Child's Thoughts: Pre-School Learning Piaget's Way* [202] although the text is patronizingly divided into material considered suitable for parents and "for the more serious student." The best possible view of how Piaget's ideas are being built upon by the next generation of serious researchers in the field is given in the chapter called "The Enigma of Development" in Kagan's book *Infancy: Its Place in Human Development* [120].

Piaget regards intelligence as a form of adaptive behavior, a means of coping with the environment, and organizing and reorganizing thought and action—adapting these to changes in the outside world. He believes that this process of adaptation starts with the random, diffuse, instinctive behavior of the newborn baby and progresses, by definable stages, to the formal abstract logical reasoning of the adult. The child passes from one stage in this development to the next through his own continuous creative activity and his continuous interaction with his environment. At each stage, the child's knowledge and understanding of the world (his "schemata" as Piaget's words are best translated) expand. New information coming in from the environment makes the old schemata gradually inappropriate. Accommodation takes place, letting in the new stimuli, and causing each particular schema to be restructured.

Piaget labels the first stage of intellectual development the "sensorimotor" stage and sees it as lasting from birth until about 2 years, moving in this period through six phases. In the first month of life the infant's only schemata are his reflexes. These he exercises (the first phase). Through exercising them, he gradually learns to coordinate them with appropriate responses, so that by the fourth month, or thereabouts, hand and eye, ear and eye are operating together (the second phase). In the third phase the infant, between roughly 4 and 8 months, begins to anticipate the results of his own actions, and to repeat, intentionally, those that are pleasurable in their results. He begins to be interested in the world of objects, and to know objects as separate from himself, and as existing even when they are not seen. In the fourth phase, he begins to differentiate means from ends, repeating actions which make others laugh, searching for toys which he has dropped. At around 1 year, he enters the fifth phase, a phase of extreme curiosity, experimentation, and varied behavior. Through this phase, he reaches the vital sixth phase, during which, around the middle of his second year, he becomes able to respond to or to think about objects and happenings which are not presently in view, and to invent for himself new mental combinations of objects or ideas. At this stage the infant becomes capable of imagination, of originality, of primitive symbolism.

Once this stage is reached, one can clearly see problem-solving, planning, remembering, and pretending going on in the child's activities. Although he has years of speech development, of experience, and of maturation ahead of him, the foundations of his human intelligence are clearly seen.

The infant's very first concepts are broad, vague, overgeneralized, and always attached to concrete objects. As we shall see in the next chapter, the *child's* ability to make the concepts in the first place, and the *observer's* ability to know that he has done so, are both intimately tied up with language. The child may learn the word "dog" among his first labels. But his use of the word, simply as a label for the family pet, cannot be taken to imply that he has formed a concept of "dogs" as one class of animal. Indeed, without other evidence, it cannot be assumed that he even classes a dog *as* an animal. He can use the *name* "dog" without knowing anything at all about the nature of the species. To reach a real concept of "dogs" the child must first separate them, in his mind, from people and from all inanimate objects. Since concepts move from the general to the particular, he will probably start by classing *all* furry animals as dogs. We shall only realize that he has done so when every animal he sees, real, toy, and pictured, is called "dog."

The idea of all furry creatures as "dogs" is both overgeneralized, and concrete. The child is applying one very broad concept to a large variety of specific objects. The concept will, during the second year, become less vague, while still remaining concrete. By the time he reaches 2 years, the infant may have "dogs" and "horses" as mutually exclusive concepts, clearly knowing the differences between the two, and able to sort equines and canines into suitable groupings. But his concepts will remain concrete for some further time. He will at this stage find his mother all the dogs on a sheet of pictures, but he will not find her all the "nice things" or all the "heavy things."

Some people would maintain that these very early, general, concrete concepts are not true concepts at all—that they do not become so until the child can do more with them than attach them to concrete realities. But here again language is critical. When an infant makes it clear that he differentiates dogs and horses, we cannot know, until he can use language to tell us, whether he merely *perceives* them visually as different, accepting that the different appearances of different dogs are less various than the difference between any dog and any horse, or whether he can in fact compare and describe them in terms of other characteristics. Eventually he may say, "Doggie bow-wow, horsie neieieigh!" Then we shall know that he is demonstrating true concepts. He has abstracted characteristics (the sounds the animals make), generalized them (all dogs bark, all horses neigh), and compared them (dogs do not neigh, horses do not bark). But he may have known all this before he could say it.

More abstract concepts are probably only beginning to form during this second year. Number concepts, for example, remain extremely primitive. By the time he is two he may understand more and less and bigger and smaller, but any number of objects more than one is likely to be regarded as two or many.

Time concepts remain very simple too. In so far as they exist at all, they usually relate—because at this stage thinking is concrete—to the infant's own daily pattern. For example, the infant learns that when he wakes up it is morning, and that the meal he then receives is called breakfast. But he may then go right through toddlerhood believing that there are 2 days in every 24 hours, because when he wakes up from his afternoon nap it must be morning, and supper must therefore be breakfast.

Interesting information on the understanding of such abstract words among children of 29 months is given in a study by Jerome Kagan published in 1978 [120]. The procedure used did not require the children to *express* concepts in speech, but it did require them to *understand* the speech labels for the concepts. Although called a test of "concept formation" the procedure did therefore have a heavy speech component which was reflected in the positive correlation between individual children's results on this test and on a language test. To test a child's understanding of the concept "in," for example, the examiner seated the child at a table containing an empty, open box and a closed, upside-down box. She then produced two little dogs and asked the child to "put the dogs in the box." Thirty-one different concept-words were tested in 77 children; "in," "on," "up," and "open" were understood by more than 80 percent, while "around," "in front of," "behind," and "over" were understood by only about 30 percent. Some interesting and as yet ill-explained findings included a better understanding of "empty" than of "full" and of "top" than of "bottom," as well as more frequent recognition of "white" than of "black."

Perhaps the most vital aspects of concept formation during this second year are concerned with the new ways in which the infant's new thinking allows him to deal with objects—to play. In the 12–18 month period, he is a scientist and an explorer. He deliberately sets out to separate means from ends, and causes from effects. Where at 9 months he might manage to put cubes in a box, and at 1 year enjoyed putting them in and out, now he decides that he wants the cubes and can hold that end in view while he fetches a stool and clambers onto it in order to reach them. His behavior is purposive. He did not climb on the stool just for the sake of climbing, but in order to get those cubes.

By around 18 months, his behavior is not only purposive, goal-directed, he has also reached the vital stage of being able to think about and respond to objects and events that are not immediately, concretely present. He can have a goal in his mind, and make a long-term plan for getting there. For example, released from his high chair after lunch, he may go straight to the closed garden door, struggle to open it, return to the garden where he was playing before lunch, and retrieve his ball from where he left it. He had that ball clearly in his mind, could remember where it was, could plan to play with it some more, and could execute that plan through obstacles and time-elapse. This dawning ability to think about what is not there enables him also to anticipate events better than before. A few months ago, he might cover his face with his hands when he saw his mother coming toward him with the wash cloth. Now he may cover his face as soon as his mother leads him toward the bathroom. He has a mental image of that wash cloth, a concept of face-washing.

Once the infant has reached this stage, he becomes capable of making new "mental combinations." He does not have to see two things together before he can think about combining them. Out of the blue, without ever having seen anyone do it before, he may fetch his toy walking stick, and use it to hook toward him a toy that has rolled under the fence out of reach. Imagination blossoms in other ways too. Familiar toys begin to be used in truly original ways. His saucepan is put on his teddy bear's head for a hat. This may not look very original to his mother, who has often seen children use saucepans for hats. But it is original for the infant, who has not seen it done, but simply "thought of it." Symbolic play begins to come into its own at this stage. Again the importance of symbolic play is often missed by mothers, because they do not recognize the difference between an infant doing "housework" in direct imitation of his mother, and the child doing "housework" at his own instigation in an area he has mentally designated as his own "house." A 15-month infant may want to be given a cloth, and allowed to help Daddy clean the car. But a 2-year-old infant who takes a pair of pants off the clothes horse, dips it in the dog's water bowl, and cleans his pedal car with it, is involved in play that is conceptually far more advanced. It is but a short step from this kind of imaginative play to full-scale symbolism in which the objects the child uses are not only transformed to fit his purposes (as that pair of pants became a car-cleaning cloth) but have their real attributes ignored or distorted in order to fit his fantasy. At 2, or soon after, the child whose present fantasy concerns fathers, mothers, and babies will unhesitatingly people it with large, medium, and small blocks from his recently constructed castle.

Sensorimotor development is the principal criterion, in the Western world, for infant intelligence. Developmental tests for pre-verbal infants are based upon sensorimotor achievements, on what the infant will do with objects, the nature of his exploration, his persistence in solving tasks with objects, his understanding of the relationship between what he does and how the object behaves. Unfortunately a confusion of long standing exists about the use of such tests. It is a confusion based upon our difficulty in deciding what we mean by "intelligence" either in the infant or in the older person, and upon our desire to predict later intelligence from earlier performance.

Psychologists used to believe that however difficult it might be to find the exact words with which to define intelligence, it was, in the end, an entity: a separate factor from specific abilities, a factor not open to influence from the environment, not modified by teaching or opportunity, nor by the drive or motivation of the person being studied. Such external influences might affect what the individual *did* with his intelligence, but not that intelligence itself. Sir Cyril Burt, for example, wrote in 1934 [43]: "Of all our mental qualities it is the most far reaching; fortunately it can be measured with accuracy and ease. . . . It is inherited, or at least innate, not due to teaching or training; it is intellectual, not emotional or moral, and remains uninfluenced by industry or zeal."

If such a view of intelligence were correct, it should be possible to devise intelligence tests which could be repeated, over and over again, on the same individual, over a period of years, and yield similar results each time. And it should be possible to devise tests for children, and from their results predict accurately the adult level of intelligence to be expected for each child.

Neither has yet proved possible. There are still some psychologists who believe that this is because we have not yet devised the best possible battery of tests, but most now believe that it is because looking for such a battery is like looking for gold at the end of a rainbow. The idea of "intelligence" as an entirely separate, measurable-if-only-we-knew-how entity within each individual, is dying. Research workers are increasingly aware of the difficulty of trying to separate such a variable from the use which the individual makes of his abilities. That use—his performance, whether in life or in a test situation—also depends on dozens of other variables such as his motivation to succeed, his industry, his reaction to challenge or frustration, his ability to concentrate, his mood and state while being tested, and so forth. All this makes it difficult to be sure what we measure in a particular IQ test or battery of tests and difficult to know what it is that we say about an individual when we assign him an Intelligence Quotient. The uncertainty does not necessarily make IQ testing useless. If the Pentagon, for example, finds that people who do well on a particular battery of tests are likely to repay the investment made by training them as officers, the *army* will not care that the variables concerned are less than clear. All the army requires is a selection procedure which works. The problem with the uncertainty is that the *individual* may care very much indeed when his "failure" on that test battery leads to his rejection. The difficulty is the ethical one of people's life-chances and amour propre being damaged by a "score" which sounds objective but is largely pragmatic.

Western societies have gone some way toward resolving the ethical problems of IQ testing. In many areas—assignment to secondary education in Britain, for example—group rather than individual performance ratings are used and account is taken of long-term assessments by teachers. With comprehensive schooling, attempts are also made to ensure that no individual is permanently categorized in a way which may limit his opportunities later on. But ours is an achievement-oriented society which still tends to equate "success" with "being clever" and "being clever" with having a "high IQ." People's interest in their own IQ scores is demonstrated by the sales of popular books of tests for self-administration. Their desire to claim possession of a high IQ is shown by the number of applicants for societies, like Mensa, which select their members on the basis of "outstanding intelligence" measured, in the first place, by self-administered IQ tests. Television panel games pander to the same narcissistic streak, and there are many schools, including two *nursery* schools known to the author, in which children can be heard discussing their relative IQ's. Parents want their children to "do well" and therefore will tend to want them to excel at whatever their society deems admirable. Chinese infants are taught to work for the good of their group from an extremely early age and parents take more pride in their 2-year-old's contribution to the nursery vegetable crop than in his cognitive abilities. Western infants are pushed toward cognitive achievement and the potential for sales of "puzzle books" and "work sheets" seems unlimited.

With this degree of concern about "intelligence," it is not surprising that people should want to know, at the earliest possible moment, whether or not their child is "bright." IQ tests have to use symbols—words, pictures, shapes, numbers—and are therefore manifestly unsuitable for babies. But there are developmental tests, often scored to yield a Developmental Quotient or DQ, which are invaluable when rightly used, but which are too often seen as "baby IQ tests."

Developmental tests assess the infant's current capabilities and activities and relate them to the capabilities and activities which have been found to be typical of children of his chronological age. Testing covers several areas. It will include, for example, the "motor milestones" which are familiar to all parents; it will include the stage the child appears to have reached in understanding and/or use of language; it will include aspects of his social development such as smiling or talking back in the first year and aspects of self-care later on. It will also include an assessment of the cognitive stage he shows himself to have reached in play with standardized toys in a test situation.

A score is assigned to the child's performance in each area so that a profile of the various aspects of his development can be compared with the standardized age-norms for that particular battery of items. A 10-month infant might therefore be shown to be performing at the 13-month level on motor items, the 11-month level on verbal items and the 9-month level on social items. The vital point, as we shall see, is that in almost any infant there will be a scatter of scores around the age-norm.

The value of this kind of profile picture can clearly be seen in the case material from her pilot work which Griffiths [99] describes. The profiles give the reader a "feel" for the child they describe which cannot easily be obtained from an ordinary written description. Her relating of the peaks and valleys of a given profile to "norms" or "averages" adds depth too. It seems a pity that with all her first-hand evidence of the value of the profile procedure, and the invalidity of using it to assign an overall "quotient," Griffiths devotes the remainder of her book to recommending and describing the derivation of "general quotients" from her test items.

As we have seen, infants do not forge ahead steadily in all fields.

They may spurt for a while in motor progress, leaving sensorimotor activities almost abandoned. Having reached a given point in, say, learning to walk, they may then rest on their motor laurels, and put all their energies into learning words. So at any given point in time there is little logical relationship between the infant's measured abilities in one area and another. The fact that his motor score is high tells us nothing about his verbal score.

In order to arrive at a quotient of any kind, these natural peaks and lags, the differences between the infant's advanced and retarded areas, must be smoothed out and forgotten in favor of an average or weighted score. A particular score could therefore be arrived at in a number of different ways. In one child a given score may indicate high verbal ability, average motor ability, and low sensorimotor ability. In another child of the same age, the identical score may represent low verbal ability, average sensor motor ability, and high motor ability. To call the two children "the same" in any sense is patently unreal.

Again, attempts to relate the child's profile and quotient at one age to his scores at a later age are also doomed. His advancement in motor abilities at 1 year does not predict a similar advancement a year later. Nor does an above average overall quotient predict overall superiority a year later. The natural peaks and valleys of his development see to that.

M. Lewis and H. McGurk [144] carried out a small-scale but intensive study of 20 infants which nicely proves these points. At 3, 6, 9, 12, 18, and 24 months they gave the infants the Object-Permanence Scale from a test of sensorimotor development [79], and the Mental Index from the Bayley Scales of Infant Development [19]. At 24 months they added an adaptation of the Peabody Picture Vocabulary Test. They found no positive correlations whatsoever between the scores, for an individual infant, on any of the tests at the earlier ages, and his scores on any of the tests at 24 months. Looking only at the results achieved at the 24-month testing, there was no relationship between an infant's sensorimotor scores and his verbal scores. There was, on the other hand, a positive relationship between his Mental-Development Index score at 24 months and his Peabody verbal test, reflecting the fact that at this age the Mental-Development Index is heavily verbally loaded, and was therefore measuring much the same achievement as the Peabody test.

With findings such as these, it should not be surprising to find that developmental tests carried out before a child is at least 3, and probably 5 years old, are virtually useless in predicting his later intelligence, however that intelligence is defined or tested. Bayley [18], who devised one of the most widely used infant development tests, known as the "Bayley Mental-Development Index," wrote in 1970: "The findings of these early studies of mental growth of infants have been repeated sufficiently often so that it is now well established that test scores earned in the first year or two have relatively little predictive validity." Most of the tests in current use in the Western world have been exhaustively reviewed and critically evaluated by Stott and Ball [211], who reached much the same conclusion.

Yet still there lingers a belief that the infant who develops rapidly, especially if he does so in all spheres, must be an intelligent child and/or one who will come to do well in IQ tests and in school learning. It lingers because it is based on facts but on *different* facts from those cited by the believers.

Infants with high developmental quotients, especially if those quotients are derived from profiles showing rapid development in most areas, do become "bright" children *more often than could happen by chance.* Furthermore, such an infant becomes a child of less than average intelligence (however that is measured) *less often than could happen by chance.* But this does not mean that DQ *predicts* later IQ. The explanation appears to be that high DQ's and high IQ's both tend to go with certain kinds of environment and upbringing.

With his colleagues, Jerome Kagan has contributed an impressive corpus of findings to our knowledge in this area during the past few years. In the course of his work he has searched for consistencies in the characteristics of individual children followed up from earliest infancy well into secondary school age. He has also searched for relationships between early characteristics and later IQ and school performance. Justice cannot be done to this work in a few sentences and interested readers are therefore recommended to Kagan's own review of it in *Infancy: Its Place in Human Development* [120]. Some of the findings which are most vitally relevant to this area are these: 13-month babies varied widely in their "attentiveness." Babies who were highly "attentive" at that age were likely to be highly "attentive" when they were tested at 27 months. "Attentive" infants were also likely to become children who, at the age of 10 years, obtained high scores on IQ and reading tests. Thus far the findings could suggest that these 13-month infants were simply bright children who were going to go on showing their brightness. But the next pieces of the puzzle are vital. "Attentiveness" at all ages, and high IQ and high reading scores were all highly correlated with the educational level of the family. If that social-class variable was statistically controlled (so that the child data could be analyzed without being affected by it), that infant "attentiveness" ceased to bear any marked relation to the later IQ and reading scores. This strongly suggests that, far from measuring intrinsic qualities in the *children,* the infant and child tests were all related to that family background.

Some psychologists, favorably inclined toward genetic explanations for observed differences in IQ, might suggest that these findings simply reflected the fact that the children of middle-class parents were born brighter-than-average and stayed that way. But Kagan has later data which dismisses that interpretation. He found that high scores on the various measures, infant and child, were not dependent merely on *being of* middle-class background but on *staying in* that ambience. He puts it like this:

Thus we suspect the relation between infant attentiveness and later reading score or IQ is due to the fact that middle-class infants and children are exposed daily to experiences different from those of working-class families. If a highly attentive upper-middle-class 2 year old were to have been transferred to a working-class home he might not have become a highly skilled reader and if a minimally attentive young child from a working-class home had been transferred to a professional family he would have both attained a higher IQ and become a more skilled reader.

Kagan's argument suggests that little is fixed in the cognitive development of very young children, by genes, by the intrauterine environment, by the birth experiences, by very first relationships with people or by anything else. A "good start" is just that: a *start*. Such a start may produce excellent early development, but the development will only continue to be excellent as long as the good conditions last. Such an argument does not, of course, exclude the possibility of a genetic contribution to the eventual differences between people's IQ's or any other variable used to describe or differentiate them. But it puts the genetic contribution into place alongside every other factor which may contribute to a child's development.

The argument is two-way of course. If a "good start" is only a start, a "poor start" is also only a start. If the development of the early months can be slowed up by a worsening of the infant's conditions so can it be improved if those conditions improve. While it is inevitable that parents should regret anything which they feel is less than ideal in their children's very early lives, it is never "too late" for this age group. Kagan himself describes several infants who seriously worried his staff during their 8-month test sessions but who were entirely normal when re-tested at 27 months [121].

If we can accept that the results of developmental tests do not predict later results on intelligence tests—or success at school work—then we shall be able to use them as an extremely useful descriptive tool. Such tests are a poor way of telling us what a child *will be* like but they are an excellent way of describing what he *is* like. If we can avoid the temptation to wrap all his varying abilities up together into one overall developmental score, we shall be able to use the profile of his different sub-scores, at any one point in time, to see how those abilities relate to each other, how widely different they are, whether this is an infant who *does* tend to develop steadily over all fields or an infant who has marked spurts and lags.

Developmental testing of large groups of infants, representative of whole populations or of defined sub-groups within populations, has done much to show us the usual sequences in infant development and the ages (and the range of ages) at which most infants become able to do a variety of things. This research work is vital. Without it parents could have no background of knowledge and expectation against which to rear their own children and societies could make no use of individual experience in planning or changing their policies for child care—for families or for education. And the need for research continues because fashions in child-rearing change, society changes, children themselves change. The American 2-year-old of today is capable of many things his father could not have done at the same age because he would not have been given the chance to try. Kagan argues that an infant's development is affected by the social-class background in which he lives with his parents, but social class is, of course, only one way of differentiating or classifying people's total environment. There is evidence that children's development is affected by far more sweeping and less tendentious environmental changes, too. The Gesell Institute, for example, has always been dedicated to the idea that infant development is a process which is almost entirely *biologically* determined and paced. Yet when they compared the groups of infants which had been tested in the thirties with those tested in the seventies, they found that in almost half the measurements made, the new generation of children were as much as six months ahead of the earlier generation [7].

But this is developmental testing for research purposes. The observers are not attempting to say anything about the individual children they study, simply to study them and count them. Developmental testing can be a useful tool in the hands of those who seek social improvement for deprived groups of children. Suppose, for example, that an organization wants to set up playgroups for children confined to high-rise apartments, or slum streets, with little opportunity for exploratory play. Developmental testing can both lend credence to the need—by demonstrating that the children are generally behind the norms—and can identify the optimum nature of the help to be offered—by showing the areas of development in which the deprivation is taking the greatest toll. Later testing can then serve as part of an evaluation of the program's success. But even here, a lack of understanding of the nature of development and developmental testing sometimes leads to unfortunate errors. Suppose that there is evidence that the children lack opportunities for sensorimotor play, and are behind the norms for their ages in such achievements as the understanding of object-permanence and cause and effect. Having carried out the program, the testing which is intended to evaluate that program must use the same criteria. To give a general test, such as the Mental-Development Index, for such a purpose would be as foolish as to give 10-year-olds an intelligence test to evaluate a course in history. The 10-year-olds need a history test, the infants a test of sensorimotor development.

As M. Lewis and H. McGurk put it [144]:

> It cannot be emphasized too strongly that the success of specific intervention programs must be assessed according to specific criteria related to the content of the program. By focusing attention upon the criteria for evaluating programs, the necessity for careful specification of the program's goals will be emphasized . . . the failure to specify goals has been a contributing factor in the confusion over means of evaluating intervention programs.

It is when developmental tests are carried out on individual children for the purposes of advising their parents that the most caution has to be used. This kind of testing can be extremely useful in many situations. Used within the normal population of infants attending well-baby clinics, for example, routine developmental tests can help to identify the child with a physical or mental defect. Most such defects will eventually show themselves unmistakably, but the child who is being kept under this kind of surveillance will probably have his problem spotted earlier. Early diagnosis is often critical to prognosis, so this alone would probably justify a developmental screening program. But such a program—or special sessions arranged outside it—can also be invaluable when parents are concerned about a child but no specific handicap can be found. The "profile" may help to pinpoint areas in which the infant is having difficulty and suggest ways in which he can be helped. Where an infant is known to have had inadequate care and/or poor health in his early months, testing can similarly help the parents or the foster or adoptive parents who are now in charge of him. His test profile will help the pediatrician to see in which ways the infant's development appears to have suffered so far and therefore in which areas special trouble should be taken. Careful, informed handling of such a child now may prevent him from being assessed as "backward" when he is 2. Again, where a child does appear to be "backward" in some way, developmental testing may enable the parents to be reassured that he is within the normal range for his age. It may also show that, although in their concern about the child's walking they had not noticed it, his verbal ability or his sensorimotor performance is in fact advanced. Parents can leave such a session not only freed from a specific anxiety but with a new determination to consider their whole child and not to be over-affected by comparisons between him and his cousins. If in fact such a child's ability does not prove to be within the normal range for his age but no specific disability is shown, parents can be offered the opportunity to bring him back for re-testing and re-assessment.

But it is important for parents who seek, or are offered, a developmental assessment of their infant to understand that it is neither easy nor entirely objective. Faced with an individual child, we cannot say, from available tests alone, that this child *is* behind for his age, highly gifted, mentally retarded, or anything else. To yield useful information, the tests have to be administered as part of a clinical and history-taking situation. They are merely a tool for the examiner to use in assessing the child; their results alone are meaningless.

The subjectivity of such tests arises out of the fact that *how* the infant approaches the task items is at least as important as what he manages to accomplish. His general interest, his alertness, his ability to concentrate are all vitally important—especially in sensorimotor tests. Such variables can be seen and felt by the examiner but they are not *measured* in a routine battery of tests. Furthermore they are dependent in their turn on other immeasurable variables such as the infant's mood, his physiological state, and the extent to which the set task is similar to or different from games he is used to at home. As a frivolous but nonetheless telling example, I was disconcerted by the total inability of a very bright 18-month girl to come to grips with the simplest type of formboard. Offered the board, with its big round holes, its square, and its triangular holes, she appeared quite uninterested in the matching blocks; quite incapable of grasping the *idea* of fitting them in, much less of actually doing so. If I had been attempting to use the test completely objectively, I should have scored a failure, and should not have progressed with this girl to the more difficult items later in the test. But it turned out that she had an older sister whose current passion was jigsaw puzzles. This infant was accustomed to doing lift-out board puzzles of up to ten pieces. The task I set her was as unchallenging as it would be to ask a 10-year-old to write his name. The task was simply beneath her notice.

Even in apparently simpler motor items, an objective pass-or-fail scoring system can be very misleading. It sounds simple to assess whether or not an infant can sit alone for up to 1 minute. But at 7 months the infant may be unable to sit alone, and, from the state of his head and neck control, be clearly some weeks or months away from independent sitting. Or he may be on the verge of sitting, but not quite able to manage a full minute today, in this strange setting. Or he may be able to sit, not only for a minute but all afternoon, playing freely. Subjective assessment of the infant must therefore play some part in helping the examiner to decide at what age level he should begin to test the infant, how far forward, beyond the infant's chronological age, he should continue, and how much belief he should put in the mother's statements that "he can usually do that. . . ." At the same time, the examiner has to decide how much allowance to make for the almost right, the nearly there performances. The infant is usually being tested in a strange setting, and always by a strange examiner. Could he sit alone, if intelligent interest in the strange room did not make him crane his head around so? Does he know the little cubes are in that closed box, and merely refuse to look because he is worried by the stranger? Does the way he *looks* at the pictures suggest that his mother is correct in saying he can name six objects, even though he chooses to be silent here, today?

Background information is needed too, if developmental-test results are to be useful—or if they are to avoid being downright misleading [109]. A. Gesell's tests [93, 96], which form the basis of most of those in use today, were originally designed to be used in conjunction with a home visit by a trained social worker, a complete physical examination of the child, a careful history from the mother and a full staff conference of all those involved with the family. Today few can work under such ideal and leisured conditions. But any attempt to use developmental tests without *some* background data can be disastrous. That 18-month child who "could not do" the first formboard managed all the sensorimotor items up to the age-norm for 3-year-olds. If I had not chatted to her mother about her preferred activities at home, and thus found out about the jigsaw puzzles, I should have stopped the test after two attempts at the formboard, and scored her somewhat below average for her age. Similarly, if a child is brought for testing because of lateness in walking, only patient inquiry can discover that late walking runs in the infant's family. With that information the examiner, if all other aspects of development are normal, can safely reassure the parents; without it he might instigate all kinds of medical tests designed to exclude motor handicaps. Finally, if the examiner does not find out, in detail, about the child's recent experiences, he may totally misread the developmental level. One mother, for example, was given an appointment for her infant to be tested some weeks ahead. In the interim he had measles, badly. Not realizing this could make any difference, she kept the appointment, and was horrified to be told that her baby was "lagging behind rather badly at present." She worried for 3 months, and then brought her bright, cheerful, forward infant to another clinic. Once the misunderstanding was cleared up she could not understand how *she* had been so silly as not to mention the illness: "But he seemed so grim and certain; he said, 'The tests show . . .'!"

People who accept all these limitations and shortcomings of developmental testing in infancy still tend to believe that at the extremes of intelligence such tests must be more accurate than not. Yet it is at the extremes that a misinterpretation by parents, nursery-school teachers, or even doctors can be most tragic.

An infant whose development is accelerated in all fields, and remains so over a year or more, may be highly gifted. Certainly highly gifted adults often turn out to have been rapid developers in infancy. But he may not be highly gifted. Plenty of "average" adults were also rapid developers. Such a child may simply go through many stages of development more rapidly than most infants, and then settle on a plateau, to consolidate everything he has learned. He is most unlikely to be of below average intelligence when he grows up, but average he may well be. And it is a tragedy if his perfectly normal abilities, by the time he reaches school, seem disappointing to parents who were convinced they had a prodigy. At best, very early signs of rapid development should be taken only to mean that the child is not retarded, and that he is receiving care of a kind which is excellent for him. Parents can take such results as a good report for them in a parenthood examination, but not as a prediction that they have reared the new Einstein.

The infant whose actual development is not particularly accelerated, but who *seems* very bright, very alive, interested and intense, is somewhat more likely than the first infant to turn out to be highly intelligent. A. Gesell [96] said that it was not excellent performance in one or all fields which indicated a highly gifted child, but the *manner* of his performance: ". . . intensification and diversification of behavior rather than conspicuous acceleration. The maturity level is less affected than the vividness and vitality of reaction . . . the infant with superior equipment exploits his physical surroundings in a more varied manner, and is more sensitive and responsive to his social environment." Nothing we have learned since upsets Gesell's judgment, which he summarized thus: "The scorable end-products may not be far in advance, but the manner of performance is superior."

The infant whose development lags behind in all fields certainly needs investigation, because there are numerous handicaps from which he may suffer. But he may not. Once careful examination and testing has excluded obvious problems, such a child may well simply be a "slow starter." Such infants often get off to a difficult start, being premature, or excessively jumpy or sleepy babies. Others seem perfectly normal in early infancy, but go through the normal phases of development more slowly than most. Some workers believe this to be due to a delay in maturation of the nervous system. Some believe it to be due to minor damage during birth, to a brain which was normal *in utero*, and which gradually heals and adapts itself. Yet others, notably H. F. R. Prechtl [181], believe that many such children have actual minimal brain damage, which increasing maturity enables them to overcome.

Whatever the causes—and no doubt they are various, and variously combined—if there is no discernible handicap, by 1 year, either a slow but steady improvement, or a sudden acceleration in development is highly likely. Just as it is tragic if early advancement leads parents to expect too much of their eventually average infants, so it is tragic if early slowness leads parents to label a child as "retarded," or at least to decide that his intellectual potential is low. Where some parents might be spurred to offer all the extra help, stimulation, and affection they could muster to such a child, many would give up. As we have seen in earlier chapters, it is the alert, highly responsive, and therefore highly rewarding and enjoyable babies who tend to get the most attention from the adult world. Yet it may be the slower, less responsive, less rewarding ones who need and will benefit from that attention most.

30

LANGUAGE

THE HIGHER THE LEVEL OF an individual's intelligence, the better one expects his language ability to be, and vice versa. In very young children, language development is probably the best single indicator of later intelligence; though, as we have seen, that is saying little as all infant abilities are unreliable predictors. But the relationship between intelligence and language is not one-way. We need intelligence to learn to understand and to use language, fluently and richly; we also need fluent rich language for our intelligence to work with. If high intelligence helps us to find the words to say what we think, so the words we know help us to decide what to think.

What do we, of a temperate climate, think about snow? Probably not very much. There is deep snow and powdery snow and wet snow; snow is fun for the kids, inconvenient for the adults—clean, dirty, frozen, mushy. That is about all. But the Eskimo language is rich in snow concepts; it has snow words which are not only difficult for us to understand, but are uncommonly difficult for us to learn. We cannot translate them into words we use about snow. While the differences between them are too subtle for us, all those words mean something to the Eskimo. For him "snow" is hardly a unitary concept. He does not think about snow as we do.

More surprisingly, some languages handle relative concepts, such as size, in ways which materially affect the thinking of those who speak them. The African language Kpelle *has* words which translate as "big" and "small," but the word for "big" is *used* very much more frequently. A group of children reared speaking Kpelle was compared with a group of American children on a test of size discrimination [157]. During a preliminary phase, the children were asked to guess whether the experimenter was "thinking about" the larger block or the smaller one. American children guessed equally between the two, but the Kpelle children almost always guessed that he was thinking about the larger. Later in the experiment, it was shown that they could be *taught* to discriminate accurately between the two blocks—they could *perceive* that one was larger than the other—but even after this, on a return to the guessing game, they returned to their bias toward the concept that came naturally to them from their language: "big" not "small."

Peculiarities of environment may therefore affect language and through it, thought. And peculiarities of language may affect concept formation and spontaneous thought.

An experiment by N. O'Connor and B. Hermelin [171] shows that the mere presence, or absence, of verbal labeling ability may affect ability on a "practical task." They found that while mentally retarded children can be taught to discriminate one shape from another with a fair degree of accuracy, those who do not spontaneously *label* the different shapes with words perform less well than those who do, and furthermore the non-labelers do not remember their own classification system. On each trial they have to rediscover the classification principles all over again. If such children are directly taught appropriate verbal labels, so that they can think "This is the *square* one, that is the *round* one," their performance improves, and they remember it, so that the shape discrimination remains intact over time. It is as if they are, from the beginning, capable of *seeing* the difference between a square and a circle, but can only make these differences into meaningful, consistent, lasting concepts with the help of words.

Environmental factors may therefore affect the language which an individual uses. The language available to the individual may affect his thinking while his cognitive abilities, overall, may affect the language which *is* available to him. We must therefore expect that a child's language development will be related to his background, just as we have already established that his developmental-test performance is related to his background (see pp. 364–65).

In the late fifties and early sixties Bernstein put early knowledge of these interrelationships into a wide sociological context [21]. He studied the speech, language, and communication patterns of British families and found what he termed a "restricted verbal code" to be typical of families from lower socioeconomic groups. Bernstein argued that children reared within this restricted code were limited in the kinds of thinking which were easily available to them. Furthermore they found it difficult to communicate with, or learn from, professionals and other middle-class people whose "verbal code" was different. Bernstein's social concern was that these differences in communication patterns, implicit in different levels of social privilege, might effectively block potential social mobility. If a working-class child necessarily found it difficult to communicate with, or understand, a middle-class teacher, for example, he would tend to be shut off from the very educational experiences which might have extended his language and thinking, so that poor school attendance/performance became, so to speak, a self-fulfilling prophecy. In the same way, an underprivileged pregnant woman would be unlikely to learn from her middle-class attendants the different ways of thinking and communicating which might have extended the experience of her coming child.

Although Bernstein's work did receive a good deal of attention, studies based on social-class differentiations were unacceptable to many people and have become increasingly unfashionable. Many people find it distasteful to categorize groups on the basis of their social class and intolerable to have it suggested that members of one social class may actually *be different* (rather than just having different experiences) from members of another. But while political and philosophical egalitarianism may be highly desirable, a blind insistence that ours is a "classless society" and that research based on social class should therefore be disregarded, is not. If social class does, in some way, affect the cognitive development of young children and the use which they can eventually make of the opportunities society offers, we need to understand the facts. Nothing can be changed by burying our heads in the sand.

A very wide variety of research studies has demonstrated a positive correlation between language development (and other aspects of cognitive functioning) in young children and the social class of the family in which they live. Studies have been carried out by different research workers, in different countries and cultures, and using a range of samples of infants and toddlers, sometimes followed up well into childhood. Much of the work is American and can be found excellently summarized in Kagan's *Infancy: Its Place in Human Development* [120]. Some of the work is cross-cultural, demonstrating, for example, a similar correlation between social class and infant developmental achievement in urban America and rural Guatemala [128]. Some of the work is British, including the ongoing follow-up study by the National Children's Bureau [55].

What do such studies mean us to understand by the term "social class"? Different workers use different definitions but the common factor is usually the father's occupation, assigned to a pre-determined classification. In Britain, for example, the Registrar General uses, for census purposes, a five-fold classification: I–higher professional occupations; II–other professional and technical occupations; III–all other non-manual occupations (this is often subdivided so that the lower half of III includes skilled manual occupations); IV–semi-skilled manual occupations; V–unskilled manual occupations. Within this framework, research workers use coarser or finer divisions.

The value of such a classification in the study of families is well expressed by Davie and his colleagues [55]:

> In our society a man's occupation tends to be related to the way he lives outside his work situation. At the most obvious level it will be linked to his income and hence to the kind of house he can afford and often to the kind

of neighbourhood in which he chooses—or has—to live. The classification
of occupations is directly related to qualifications, training and skill; and
therefore it is often linked to level of education. A less direct but still quite
marked association can be shown between social class—as we shall now term
it—and attitudes, most obviously to education but also to child-rearing.
. . . In short, social class is a convenient and useful indirect measure of many
aspects of children's environment which will to some extent shape the way
they develop.

Of course this, or any other, type of classification is open to criticism on
the grounds that its criteria will not accurately apply to everyone thus
classified. There are many families, for example, in which the mother's
occupation and/or educational level would "place" the family differently
and is therefore ignored at the researcher's peril. There are others which
would be classified as "working class" on the grounds that the father
works as a farm laborer but which would be quite differently placed if that
man's university degree and aspirations to be a poet were taken into
account. And there are increasing numbers of incomplete families whose
occupational/social-class patterns have been disrupted by the practical
and economic constraints of single parenthood. Nevertheless, whatever
the limitations of a social-class classification, the positive correlation between higher social class and more rapid linguistic development in children does hold *statistically*. Over large numbers, the relationship is strong
enough to show up despite individual discrepancies.

Neither the institution of this kind of research nor its findings reflect
the kind of value-judgment which has rightly brought discussion of social
class into disrepute. Nobody is saying: "Because you are working class,
your child will not talk as well as your boss's child talks." Rather they are
saying: "Certain modes of interaction with very young children have been
consistently found to be typical of working-class parents and not of middle-class parents. Children reared within that mode of interaction tend
to develop language more slowly and less richly than others." They are
statements of observed group likelihood not of individual prediction and
certainly not of indictment. What parents need to know, on an individual
level, is what are the modes of interaction which appear to limit or extend
a child's language acquisition or other cognitive skills.

Overall there seems to be a "verbal climate" which is beneficial to
early language development and more typical of middle-class than of
working-class families. Such a climate includes a great deal of spontaneous shared "talk," face-to-face with the infant, from the earliest months.
It includes an easy use of "motherese" such that the mother adapts her
own mode of speech to the infant's; together with a natural tendency to
expand on the infant's own communications rather than to withhold
response or to reply monosyllabically. It probably also includes a great
deal of mutual problem-solving—in play with gestures and words—and
a genuine pleasure in successful communication. In summary, one can
perhaps risk saying that the mother who enjoys words and communicat-

ing in words and who has a rich fund of language readily available within herself which she is accustomed to use, with or instead of action, in her relationships with other people, will easily be able to provide such an environment. Whether she will actually do so will then depend on whether the infant seems to her a suitable candidate for verbal kinds of communication. There are people (usually people with little experience of infants, but including some parents also) who find it unnatural to talk to babies, however voluble they may be with other people. Remarks like "She'll be company later on," or "I've nobody to talk to; you can't talk to a baby can you?" are commonplace. From observation it would seem that infants themselves often overcome such attitudes: their responses are so clearly sociable that parents find themselves "prattling away when we're on our own" although they sometimes add: "I'd feel an idiot if anybody else could hear me." But not every baby will manage to enrich his own environment in this way and not every small child will manage to override the kind of family communication system which is based on "shut up," on monologues or on inter-personal silence filled with half-heard noise from the media.

In Chapter Twenty-three we suggested that while much is known about the order and rate of language acquisition by children, very little is known about why and how language is acquired at all.

Two principal theories have been put forward. Language acquisition as a straightforward learning process has been described by B. F. Skinner [204]. He, and his many followers, believe that the child learns to *understand* language by a classical conditioning process, such that by endless repetition he comes to associate the sound of the word "dog" with the sight of a pictured or real dog, until eventually the word-sound comes to evoke the same behavior as the sight-impression. He believes that the child comes to *use* language by operant conditioning, his attempts at saying "dog" being reinforced by the mother or some other adult, and the strength of the reinforcement lending him the motivation to try.

Proponents of the other main theory, laid down by N. Chomsky [49, 50] and much elaborated by E. H. Lenneberg [140] and others, find the learning model naive and untenable. They argue for the existence of some kind of inherent "language-acquisition device." They do not claim that they have identified such a device, or that they can describe it, but that without it, language could not develop. Imitation and reinforcement could not, alone, account for the extraordinary rapidity with which a child learns his own language once he has begun. They could not alone account for his beginning to learn it—because you cannot reinforce behavior which has not begun to appear. Nor could they conceivably account for the child's learning not only of words but of grammar and syntax, which alone enable him both to understand and to speak sentences he has never heard before: to generate "new language" for himself.

Kagan is impatient of these classical theories yet propounds a theoretical formulation of his own which has some features of all of them. He believes that infants develop and learn, in all fields, by noticing "discrepancy" (that is, events which are unexpected or surprising, given the child's stage of memory-development and his previous experience). Discrepant events, once noticed, give rise to uncertainty in the child who will then strive, in whatever way is developmentally appropriate, to resolve the uncertainty and assimilate the discrepant event. Naming things is, he believes, a developmentally appropriate way for 1- to 2-year-olds to resolve particular uncertainties. He sees no reason to assume that language acquisition is a continuous process which has been going on within the child since birth. Rather he believes that the ability to name things can be seen as a new competence which the child now has available and will therefore use. He can use words and therefore he will do so when they are useful to him in assimilating events. The child notices the new shoes which his mother has put on his feet. The sight and feeling of those familiar feet, newly encased in leather, is certainly surprising ("discrepant" with his past knowledge and experience). He feels uncertain and the uncertainty stimulates in him a kind of excitement, a need to assimilate the experience. If he is ready to use words in this way he will announce "shoes!" and may be seen to relax, apparently satisfied.

But equally convincing interpretations of similar observed behaviors are made by other workers adopting quite different theoretical positions. Hazel Francis [85], for example, states:

> The foundation of language learning, the establishment of an agreed basis of verbal communication, . . . has its roots in the purposeful imitation of fragmentary speech patterns as the child learns to control his babbling and achieves not only the pay-off of communicative interaction but also of communicated meaning. . . . The second nine to twelve months of a child's life is a lengthy and fascinating period of beginning to be aware that vocalisations can achieve effects independently of other forms of bodily expression and of beginning to make sense of the sound patterning of speech.

For her, then, speech is a tool in the service of interpersonal communication rather than in individual mastery of the world's novelty.

It will be clear by now that the specialist literature in the development of language is complex and controversial. At the date of writing, the real answer to the question: "How and why is language acquired?" is "We do not know." From the practical point of view, language must, at least for the moment, remain a phenomenon which we can certainly describe and facilitate but for which we cannot, with any hope of consensus, account.

Children, at almost all ages, and especially in the second year, invariably understand more language than they can use. Infants may demonstrate that they understand a good deal that is said to them well before their first birthday. By the middle of the second year, the mother may report, "He understands everything you say to him," even though he may still only have a few words that he uses himself. But the actual degree of the child's *verbal,* as opposed to his general *social* understanding, is very difficult to assess. The infant may understand the *sense* of a given command, by combining verbal understanding with the context, the situation, and gestures so minute that the mother does not even realize she is making them. Perhaps the table is laid for lunch, and the mother has been cooking. She turns to the child (who can also smell food, and is probably hungry) and says, "Lunchtime now." The infant goes at once to the table, and holds up his arms to be lifted into his high chair. How much did he understand the words? I put this point to a mother, who scoffed. Experimentally, in exactly the situation I have described, she turned to the child and said, "Lunch not ready yet." The infant looked at her, looked at the table, looked back at her, and went on with his play. The mother was triumphant. But as she spoke to the child, she had shaken her head slightly; her whole demeanor had suggested a negative statement: she had not begun to move toward the child; she had not taken off her apron. All sorts of cues had been different. Interested, now, she came and played briefly with the child, and after a few minutes, being careful *not* to indicate the table, she said, "Now shall we have lunch?" The infant looked at her. He clearly knew she had asked him something; equally clearly he did not know what. He waited for her to cue him, and as she rose, holding out her hand to him and moving toward the table, he went, happily.

Of course at this level of understanding the mother is communicating with the infant, but she is doing it through a combination of his perceptions, not simply through his speech perception. A little later, he will understand one key word of her communication, but still need gestures to explain what has been said about it. If the mother says, "Give me the ball," the infant will pick up the ball, and he will wait. When she holds out her hand and says again, "Give me the ball," he will bring it to her. Clearly this level of communication between parent and child is extremely personal and subtle. It sheds some light on the language retardation which is so general among infants in inadequate institutional care, or those who are hospitalized or otherwise left among strangers. A stranger's cues are different from the mother's. Put those cues in a strange environment, and the world must suddenly appear utterly incomprehensible to a child who, in his own home, was just beginning to "understand." Often toddlers will not speak to strangers, and become extremely shy if the stranger tries to speak directly to them. This kind of perceptual difficulty may be a contributing factor. The stranger gets the context, the intonations, the facial expressions and the gestures "wrong." It is comic to hear the mother acting as interpreter for the stranger in such a situation. The visitor says, "What a pretty dress!" beaming down at the toddler. The toddler looks worriedly blank and puts a finger in her mouth. "She likes your pretty dress," says mother. Toddler beams, holds out her skirt, and smiles shyly.

Most infants begin to speak their first words at around a year—although, as we have seen, there is a very wide age range in language acquisition. These first words are almost invariably labels. They are the names for people, animals, or other highly significant objects in the child's immediate environment.

An unusual study [183], in which mothers with psychological training kept journals of their children's verbal development over several years, found that single words were produced in the following order of frequency: first, people's names, then animals' names, then names for food and drink. Once some of these names were in the children's repertoire, parts of the body, clothes, and everyday articles used in the home were named with equal frequency. The names for toys, furnishings and any objects outside the home appeared much less often, and later than any of these. No abstract nouns, those describing groups or concepts, such as size, weight or measure, appeared before 2 years in this sample. For all these children adjectives—whether as single words or as parts of two-word phrases—appeared after nouns, and the first adjectives were always those conveying a value judgment such as "nice," "naughty," or "pretty." The next category of adjectives to appear were those conveying sense impressions, such as "hot" or "cold."

The first words are sometimes standard ones, correct copies of the adult name. More often they are approximations of the adult word. Sometimes they are self-words—invented by the child. With such a variety of possible sounds, it is sometimes difficult to recognize a word for a word. It is probably safe to call a sound a word when the infant uses it consistently and exclusively, for a single object or class of objects. A "gaw" is a ball if it is always a ball, and never anything other than a ball.

Some authorities would say that "gaw" was a self-word for ball; others would say it was a word approximation, because it contains one sound in common with the standard word. H. Winitz and O. C. Irwin [224], using this last, generous, definition of word approximation, found the following shift between the three classes of utterance, between children who were studied at 13 months and again at 18 months.

First words, which are labels for things, are usually regarded, in a Skinnerian way, as nothing *more* than labels. The child is seen as simply learning that the name of this is "dog," the name of that is "John" and so forth. But observation of infants suggests that these first words have a more complex communicative purpose. The infant does not simply state, "Dog," as if to say, "That is a dog." Sometimes he states it in the way the linguists would call "declarative." But sometimes he uses the word as an emphatic. "Dog!" he says, expressing surprise, annoyance,

TABLE 16. SHIFT TOWARD STANDARD SPEECH FORMS EARLY IN THE SECOND YEAR

Speech classified as	13 months	18 months
Approximations	83%	56%
Standard	16%	38%
Self-language	1%	6%

delight at the dog's arrival. And he uses the word as a question too. "Dog?" he asks, perhaps looking at an animal, perhaps hearing a noise at the door.

Some people have denied that there is any communicative meaning to the varied intonations attached to early labeling words. They have maintained that the child learns the labels, but is also practicing the adult intonations and inflections of speech, just as he did when he jargoned at an earlier stage. The juxtaposition of intonation and label is, they argue, a chance one. P. Menyuk [157] believes, on the basis of her experiments, that the variation in intonation and inflection is both meaningful and deliberate on the infant's part. She makes the often neglected point that it is more effortful for the child to exclaim or to question than to declare. Why should he make the effort to say "Dog?" if he only wished to declare the presence and recognizability of "Dog"?

We all so readily accept that speech begins with single words that we seldom stop to ask ourselves why the infant should choose to begin in this way. Why does his speech not begin with phrases that he often hears repeated, such as "Night night darling" or "Upsadaisy baby"? If he is going to begin with single words, why does he choose the particular words he selects? We do not know. Menyuk speculates that the infant may only be able to store in his memory a single word, at this stage, not a word sequence. Certainly we know from experiments with the repetition of strings of numbers by older children that the capacity to store an increasing number in short-term memory increases with age. Certainly, too, the infant tends to select either a single-syllable word, or one syllable of a multi-syllable word, or a multi-syllable word that is repetitious (such as "dad-dad" or "ba-ba"). It may be that he also hears (or more correctly, auditorily perceives, which is to say *meaningfully* hears) only the isolated words, or the first or last or most stressed words of a sentence. These words may stand out for him from what is otherwise still a blur of talk.

Menyuk makes the point that the actual word the child selects is usually a "topic" word—the subject of conversation rather than what is said about that subject. He learns the word "dog" both because the dog is important to him, and because whatever we say about the dog, that word is the one consistent sound in a vast complexity of other sounds involved in: "I must put the dog out," "Where's the dog?," "Let's find the dog," and so on. In adult speech, we do not always stress, verbally, the topic word of a sentence. We may say: "Oh, for heaven's *sake* close that door." But when we speak to very young children most of us tend to stress the topic word without necessarily realizing we are doing it. We say: "Close the *door,* darling." And if we get no response we repeat: "The *door,* close the *door.*"

According to R. Griffiths's [99] norms for British babies, most infants will say three words by the end of the twelfth month—whether these are standard, approximations, or self-words. Four or five words will be clear by the fifteenth month and six or seven by the seventeenth month. In her sample progress was rather steady, giving nine words by the nineteenth month, twelve by the twentieth, and twenty by the end of the second year. While no doubt these were accurate norms for the words *observed* in her studies of infants, the actual number of words are very much lower than those suggested by others. Most agree that new words come very slowly at the beginning, so that the child may only acquire one new word a month between, say, 11 months and 15 months. But most also agree that there is a tremendous spurt in word acquisition around the middle of the year, so that the infant's spoken vocabulary may grow from say, twenty words at 18 months to more than 200 words at 21 months [141].

It is interesting to note, by comparing studies of the 1920s with those of the present day, that children of *all* ages appear to have larger vocabularies now than then. Perhaps this is a genuine gain from the advent of television; perhaps it is an artifact reflecting our greater interest in very young children, our greater readiness to listen to them with care. But between the difficulties of defining what we *mean* by a word, the difficulties of *evoking* those words in a test situation, the unreliability of mothers' reports of their children's words, and the enormous range of age at which language develops, the actual number of words spoken by a child in the second year is probably among the least valid and interesting measures of his language ability.

Somewhere around the middle of the second year, and almost invariably *after* he has learned at least a small number of single-word name-labels, the infant begins to put two words together: to speak in "phrases" rather than in single words. Just as we accept, without much thought, the fact that speech begins with single-word labels, so we accept this progression to two-word phrases. Yet they are not an obvious development. There is no *a priori* reason why these typical phrases *should* be the next stage in speech. Why not sentences?

The easy answer is that the infant begins to feel the need to communicate both more accurately and more economically. Certainly a two-word phrase allows him to do this. Suppose he has just finished a biscuit, and he wants another one, of a particular kind out of the variety in the box. In one-word communication he may have to say, as separate communication items: "bikkit!" "more?" "gimme!" He may be misunderstood at the first stage, his mother taking his first "bikkit" to be a comment on the one he has just consumed, rather than a demand for more. Clearly he is likely to get his biscuit more quickly and efficiently if he can start out by demanding "more bikkit."

But we have no reason to assume that the infant wants economy in communication. The desire to say things in the fewest and most telling number of words is a peculiarly adult one. The infant is in no hurry. Furthermore we have no reason to suppose that he feels the need for greater explicitness. Few of his early words are need-fulfilling ones, and he has managed to get what he wanted up to now with single words linked with gesture and context. Why should he suddenly find this combination unsatisfactory? Perhaps he does. Perhaps mothers who are consciously trying to make their infants speak become deliberately dense at this stage. Perhaps a greater contact with people from the outside world makes it incumbent on the infant to speak more explicitly. Certainly this sometimes happens. One small boy had reached the one-word stage when he had to be hospitalized with meningitis. His mother was with him all the time except during the most unpleasant procedure of a spinal tap. During the ten minutes of her exclusion from the room, the following development of communication took place, for the very first time:

"Mummy!"
"Want Mummy."
"Mummy *come.*"
"Want my mummy."
"Oh, Mummy come!"

There seemed little doubt, in this case, that the infant was experiencing, for the first important time, an apparent failure by the adult world to understand what he wanted. Under the extreme stress of a painful and frightening procedure, he produced more and more explicit speech. But most infant speech, as we have seen, is not need-fulfilling. Most two-word phrases are not produced under unpleasant stress, but in interest or excitement. The development from single words to two-word phrases must remain as mysterious as is the achievement of any words at all.

The lengthening of the child's utterances may occur as the result of the maturing of the vocal mechanisms, and the auditory memory span. The infant becomes able to notice and to retain not only the single "topic" words of sentences he often hears, but the words he hears used to describe them, or what they do.

The content of the two-word phrase is almost always of this kind. The child does not learn the word adjacent to the topic word in adult speech. He does not progress from "ball" to "*the* ball." He rather moves from "ball" to "nice ball" or "go ball" or "John ball." He puts together the nouns with which he started his naming, with main verbs and principal adjectives. He uses his new "second word" to amplify what he used to communicate via intonation and inflection only. Earlier he might watch the family dog depart rapidly through the park and say "Dog!" in tones of shocked or delighted surprise. Now he says, "Dog gone!"

The importance of this two-word stage is twofold. First it demonstrates the infant's ability, already stressed in Chapter Twenty-nine, to think about objects when they are not immediately present. A child who wanders around the room saying "Ted? Ted?" may be deduced to be thinking about finding his teddy bear; but no deduction is needed once he says "Ted gone?" or "Where ted?" His planning can be seen more clearly too. Seeing a forbidden ashtray on the table he proposes to climb on, he may at an earlier stage announce "Tray!" to which his mother is likely to reply, "Yes, ashtray, darling, don't touch." Now he can say "Tray up!'' making it quite clear that he wants his mother to pick the ashtray up out of harm's way. His beginning conceptualization becomes clearer too. Perhaps he is still at the stage where all animals are referred to as "pussy." But now he can make it clear that while he still does not have another *word* for non-cat animals, he sees, he perceives, that they are not all the same. *"Big* pussy!" he may announce when he meets a German shepherd in the park. His two-word phrases allow us to see something of his developing thinking. Probably they also help his thinking to develop. If he perceives the differences and similarities among things—which, as we have seen, is the basis of concept formation—those perceptions will be sharpened, and made more consistent, and easily remembered as he finds the words to label those differences and similarities.

The second vitally important thing about the two-word phrase stage is that it demonstrates the fact that the infant has already learned the basic rules of grammar and syntax in his language before he could do more than attach a few labels. He invariably gets the *sequence* of words right in the context of what he is trying to say. Talking directly to his brother, he says "naughty boy," not "boy naughty"; reporting that brother's wrong-doing to his mother, he says "boy naughty," not "naughty boy." Telling his mother that he has seen a truck through the window, he says "see truck." But trying to make her come and see it, he pulls her skirt saying, "truck, see!" His language is not a meaningless jumble but a tele-graphese, leaving out auxiliary verbs, articles, prepositions, and many word-endings. Only in certain consistent ways does he string words to-gether wrongly.

The grammatical mistakes that he does make are both logical (in the sense that they are wrong but logical deductions) and consistent from child to child. For example, the English-speaking infant tends to make all nouns plural by adding an S or Z sound to them, as in "shop/shops." He talks of "mans" and "childs" and "sheeps" and "shoeses." Similarly he puts all verbs into the past tense by adding a D sound, so that he says "goed" and "comed" as well as "jumped" and "laughed." Some word orders are consistently confused, too, usually where they involve insert-ing an extra word between two words which customarily come together. Most infants, for example, will request mother to "put on it" or to "pick up it." The passive of verbs is usually ignored. The "-ing" endings are simply left out, so that the child announces "I go," "I come," "Daddy run," and so on.

As we saw in Chapter Twenty-three, the role of the adult as a direct teacher of new words is extremely dubious. While there is no doubt that imitation plays a part in language as in other kinds of learning, it does not seem that direct imitation, at the time, plays a very large part.

This seems to hold true for more complex speech learning. The infant's two-word and later three-word telegraphese is singularly resist-ant both to the models offered by the ordinary adult speech he hears around him, and to direct attempts to teach him to expand it. S. M. Ervin-Tripp [76] set out to see whether, if they were given a model to copy, young children at this telegraphese stage of speech development would produce sentences that were more complex than their spontaneous speech. Had the infants been willing and able to repeat the more complex sentences offered to them, it would have demonstrated that imitation was at least one of the mechanisms by which new speech forms could be acquired. A few of the infants did imitate speech forms and structures which they only produced in their spontaneous speech some weeks or months later. But equally, some infants refused to imitate speech forms which they *were* already producing in their spontaneous speech. Most of the time the infants reproduced, out of the model given them, exactly that complexity of sentence structure which they were already using in spontaneous speech.

These results should not be surprising. The infant's telegraphese is his very own. His two-word and three-word phrases are not imitations of what he has heard adults say. What adult has said to a child, "See lots mans!" when watching a football game? The adult is likely to say, "See what a lot of men!" Compared in terms of sounds, the two sentences have very little in common.

It seems that the adults' role at this stage is not that of teacher or even model, but of provider of innumerable consistent examples of the rules of the grammar and syntax of the child's language. The child reproduces the sense of the sentence he hears, obeying the rules in so far as he has understood and generalized them, and reducing the complexity to the level he can manage to express. When mother wants to help father avoid yet another rough-and-tumble game, she says, "Daddy's having a little rest now." Hearing this, over and over again, enables the child to produce "Daddy have rest," rather than "have Daddy rest" or "rest have Daddy" or "Daddy rest have." But it does not enable him to reproduce the mother's sentence.

Mothers spend a good deal of time, at this stage of speech development, expanding their children's telegraphese into sentences. In one study [205] two mothers were observed with their infants, and it was found that they thus expanded no less than 30 percent of the utterances their children made. If, for example, the mother said something such as, "Now let's get your shoes on," the child would answer with part of her sentence, such as "shoes on," and the mother would expand the child's communication by repeating what she had said at the beginning. Or the infant would volunteer something like "out now" and the mother would reply, "You want to go out into the garden now."

In this experiment, the mother's expansions had little effect on the child's immediate responses. Only 1 percent of the time did the child answer with *any* elaboration of his original utterance, and even on those occasions it was usually only a different way of saying the same thing, still within the child's own telegraphese. For example he might say "gar-gar now" in response to the mother's expansion of his request to go into the garden.

But even while such expansions do not lead infants to copy more complex speech forms, they may still play a vital role in offering models for the child to add to his general linguistic thinking. Furthermore they often help the *mother* in her communication with the child. She expands or repeats what he has said in order to recode his telegraphese into her own language, and make sure she has understood him correctly. If she has not, he will correct her.

With somewhat older children, newly admitted to nursery groups at the age of 2 1/2–3, experiments have shown that deliberate expansions of everything the child says are less effective in increasing his verbal competence than a comparable period of talking and play with an adult. Once again such results tend to indicate that the adult's vital role in infant speech learning is not that of teacher but that of stimulus-provider. The more language the child hears, especially language which is directed at him, with appropriate facial and gesturing cues, the more language-models he has to use in his own language development. Seen from this point of view, the more direct attempts to teach him language, by correcting what he says, are, for him, boring. He has already grasped whatever he can say in telegraphese. He is not ready to say the same thing more correctly. He wants to say new things, different things. The expanded sentence and the corrected grammar will come, in their own good time, with his maturing.

In the meantime, those who need to understand the language of very young children can learn it just as they would learn a foreign tongue. Mothers pick it up by constantly interacting with the infant from the time he begins to babble to the time when he talks as she does, but many people whose professions bring them into close communication with infants have had no such experience. The dentist who must fill a milk tooth, the doctor who must give an injection, or find out what hurts, the nurse who must make sure the child knows mother will come soon, the stranger who finds a lost toddler and wants to know where he last saw his mother, all need to know how this early language works, and could all do their jobs more effectively if they could communicate with those who speak it. Parental interpreters are not always present when they are needed most.

31

FEARS AND PHOBIAS;

TEARS AND TANTRUMS

NOBODY CAN BE SURE that he understands what a toddler is thinking or feeling. It is difficult enough to know what a fully communicating adult thinks and feels, as opposed to what he wants us to believe he thinks or feels. Therefore when one writes about the emotions of toddlers, one lays oneself open to a charge of trying to get inside their skins, trying to pretend an insight which is really only guesswork.

The attempt is valid nevertheless, if it is based upon the *behavior* of infants. We cannot know exactly what they think, nor what they feel, but we can see how they behave. Where there is a high degree of consistency between one child and the next, it is reasonable to try and see what circumstances and what handling contribute to that behavior. This has been superbly done by J. Bowlby [35]. His trilogy *Attachment and Loss* [32, 33, 35] reviews comprehensively the research, from many disciplines, which contributes to this kind of understanding, as well as putting it into a psychoanalytic theoretical framework. In an ideal world, this great work would be read by everyone who dealt with infants and young children. Above all it should be read by anyone who cannot accept the idea that infants have, and suffer from, the kinds and degrees of emotion described in this brief chapter.

In the second year of life, as we hinted in Chapter Twenty-four, two related issues seem to dominate the toddler's relationship with his adult world. On the one hand he seeks ever-increasing personal independence and autonomy, resenting the power adults have over him, reacting negatively to coercion, wanting to go his own way, in his own time, for his own reasons. On the other hand he actively seeks more and more protection and support from his mother, fearing separation from her above all things, shying away from strangers, resenting any other people who take her time and attention from him. If he were capable of conceptualizing his relationship with his mother, an infant of this age would probably describe the ideal mother as one who had nothing to do all day but follow him around. She would never interfere with his activities but would do interesting things herself, in parallel with them, so that he could join in or pick up ideas when he wished. She would never coerce him into doing anything or even into giving her his attention, but she would always be there and ready to respond to his requests for attention and cooperation. Above all, she and all that she stood for in warmth, love, and security would always be on tap when the adventurer decided to take a short rest and be a baby again.

Life being what it is, both prongs of this situation get the toddler into emotional and practical trouble. The thwarting of his drive for independence, his developing ego, expose him to frustration, to anger, to hate. The thwarting of his desire for dependence, his need to cling to his mother, expose him to anxiety and fear. To complicate matters further, feeling angry makes him anxious and afraid, while feeling anxious and afraid makes him angry. His own emotions are his worst enemy. They are, as far as one can see, as strong at this age as they will ever be in his life. But he has not had the time to grow a protective skin over them. He has not enough experience to know how to deal with them; he cannot control himself.

Within this simplified framework one can see most of the fears and the furies of young children as revolving around twin poles: anxiety around separation, anger around the desire for autonomy. Too little care and protection and the infant's separation anxieties are touched off; too much and his desire for autonomy breaks out in anger. The exact balance which keeps him both unafraid and unfrustrated differs for every infant at every stage of his development. For many, it varies day by day and hour by hour. It is the sensing and acting out of this balance which describes sensitive mothering of a toddler. And it is the individuality of each infant's needs which makes continuous mothering so important. A child who is cared for by comparative strangers cannot be "understood" in this minute-by-minute way. A child whose care is shared with one or more mother-substitutes may benefit if one happens to be more sensitive to his needs than is the mother herself, but even he will have to change gear each time he changes caretaker. A child who actually loses a caretaker with whom he has been deeply involved, at this stage in his life, will probably mourn. In certain families in Britain, for example, "au pairs" come and go and are expected to do so. Nobody suffers deeply except, sometimes, the babies and toddlers whose relationships are rudely severed.

Every human being carries within himself a sort of reservoir of anxiety. Nobody is secure and happy, self-confident and self-approving, right through the layers of his personality. But as we grow up we learn all kinds of ways of dealing with our anxiety. We seek certain kinds of security, perhaps in relationships with other people, perhaps in our jobs, or our children. We learn to avoid situations which make us feel anxious, or to recognize specific anxieties so that they become known devils. We manipulate our environments and the people around us in all sorts of ways to keep ourselves comfortable. And when we fail, the drug industry provides the pills that tide millions of us over crises.

Toddlers are anxious however securely, lovingly, and sensitively they are reared. They have not developed many defenses against anxiety. The defenses which they do have are not in their own power; they are in the power of the adult world. As we have seen, many infants are anxious over separation from their mothers at night. By 1 year, most have developed specific defenses against that anxiety, such as sucking a pacifier, and cuddling a special piece of blanket. With those aids, the toddler's nighttime anxiety stays down at a tolerable level. But whether he gets those aids or not is in the hands of others. His mother may wash his blanket and not get it dry by bedtime. His father may decide he is too old for a pacifier and throw it away. The babysitter may not realize the importance of the precious objects; the jealous older child may hide them to make the baby cry.

The infant is vulnerable to anxiety when he is separated from his mothering-person in the daytime, too. His own defense against this is simple. He stays close to her. As we have seen, very few toddlers will voluntarily put themselves more than a certain distance away from the mother at any time, unless they are with another close person, who temporarily stands in for her. But once again this simple mechanism for staying anxiety-free is not in the toddler's own control. His mother goes out for the day leaving him with a neighbor, or she goes into the bathroom and locks the door between them. He can never be quite sure of being allowed to feel safe.

The infant begins to get anxious whenever his own emotions begin to get out of control. His mother can usually damp down his feelings before they reach the explosion point, but once again he cannot make her; he cannot usually even convey his need. All too often her response is the very opposite of what he needs. The more hysterical his laughter becomes, the more she tickles him. The angrier he gets, the crosser she becomes; the more demanding and clingy he gets, the more she pushes him away.

In some families, even the child's own anxious feelings are not allowed to be his own. Not only is he not able to arrange his own solutions to his anxieties, he is not even allowed to experience them. In one single hour spent in a children's public playground, I noted 38 instances of parents *telling* their toddlers what they did and did not feel, against all the evidence of the child's behavior and attempted words: "You don't mind him," "That's not too high for you," "You don't want to go home. . . ." Perhaps it was just a "manner of speaking." Perhaps the parents did not *mean* to imply that they knew better than the child what he felt. But how is the toddler supposed to know that? Is he supposed to be a mindreader? It must surely seem to him that his parents refuse outright to understand his feelings.

Some infants are clearly more anxious, overall, than others. They may function with anxiety always close beneath the surface, and many small fears always operative. Other children seem generally more phlegmatic. But all infants vary markedly in their anxiety levels from time to time. Anxiety tends to show itself in a general clinginess—apprehension about new things, new places, new people, a reluctance to explore and adventure—and in physiological tensions, with sleep difficulties, lack of appetite, and so forth. But it also manifests itself in actual specific fears.

Unfortunately where fears are concerned we tend to treat toddlers as if they were miniature versions of adults. When a child is afraid of something which many adults fear, he is usually sympathetically handled. Few parents will scoff at the toddler who wakes pale, trembling, and sweat-soaked from a nightmare. We all have nightmares. We know what they feel like. But when the toddler expresses a fear that seems to the adult to be simply silly, it is often treated with bossiness, irritation, or even shame. We forget that the toddler has an intrinsic fear of the strange; we forget that he does not have our experience or our knowledge to call on. Meeting his first tortoise, an 18-month boy reacted immediately with pure horror: "Way, way," he said, scarlet-faced. "It's a tortoise, darling," said his mother, picking it up and moving toward him. "Notty," wailed the toddler, exploding into tears and backing up against the wall. "Don't be silly, darling, it's a nice tortoise," said his mother, and she carried it right up to him, took his desperate flailing hand and forced him to touch it. "Ho'bble," screamed the child. The mother could not see that the child *could* be afraid of a tortoise. He had never met one before; had had no nasty experiences with tortoises; it made no noise. . . . Yet she herself disliked spiders. I wonder how many spiders had bitten or roared at her? And how she would have felt about somebody who forced one into her protesting hand to prove its harmlessness?

We are always out to *prove* something to our infants, when it comes to fear. Out to prove that fears are illogical (although we pander to our own, and accept politely those of other adults), out to prove that "you'll like it when you get used to it" as we plunge the screaming child into the swimming pool, or push him higher on the swing. Perhaps we need to rethink our attitudes to two separate issues: fearlessness and bravery. Fearlessness is simply not being afraid. It comes from not feeling fear. Logically, then, the less we frighten children, the more fearless they will be. Bravery is doing, or putting up with, what *does* frighten or hurt you. If that is what we are asking of our toddlers, then we should not pretend that we want them not to be afraid. Rather than "It's a nice tortoise, darling," we should be saying: "I know you think this tortoise is horrible and you would like it to go away, but I want you to touch it to show what a brave boy you are." Written out like that it looks silly. But logically it is the message that particular mother must have been conveying.

All toddlers have transient fears which arise unexpectedly, and may pass as quickly. But a great many acquire the focused fears which are usually called phobias. Sometimes the mother can date the beginning of a phobia, recounting the incident which touched it off. With hindsight, she says that the child must have been really terrified when that big dog knocked him down in the park, because he has been increasingly afraid of dogs ever since. But the degree of the child's disturbance may be quite out of proportion to that original incident. The child may have weathered far worse frights without any sequel. The phobia arises from his own inner state far more than from outward happenings. When his inner anxiety builds up a psychological pressure, it seeks an outlet; the child is vulnerable to fear. He will focus that fear on whatever frightening stimulus presents itself.

The frequency of actual phobias in the toddler population is difficult to assess because it is difficult to define. A child may be afraid of swinging on swings, without being made afraid by *seeing* swings. He may be afraid of dogs when they run or bark at him, without being afraid of dogs in the distance. Perhaps a phobia is most usefully discriminated from an ordinary fear if it is considered in terms of the effect which it has on the infant's ordinary life. An ordinary real fear will only affect his life when circumstances require him to meet the feared object. As long as he is not faced with the thing he fears, he does not think about it. As long as he can avoid or reject it, the rest of his life is unaffected. But a phobia works on the child through his new imagination. He is not only afraid when he meets a dog, he is afraid when he sees one, when he thinks about one, when he sees a picture of one. He not only avoids dogs when they are there, he constantly seeks to avoid going where they *may* be. In an extreme case, his whole life may be permeated with dogs, so that he must ride in his stroller in case there should be a dog in the street, cannot go in the park in case dogs should be there, cannot enjoy his picture book because there is a dog on the third page, cannot cuddle his toy monkey because it is suddenly a dog.

Among the 100 infants of 21 months studied by J. W. Macfarlane, L. Allen and M. P. Honzik [151], around 30 percent had acute specific fears. At 3 years old nearly 70 percent of the infants were affected. The most frequent fear was of dogs. After dogs came darkness and the bogies associated with it. Less frequent were snakes, and such specific alarming noises as fire-engine sirens or ambulance alarms. In C. M. Drillien's sample [66] of nearly 450 infants, the numbers experiencing acute specific fears for at least 6 months were assessed by social class and also by whether the care they were receiving was considered generally "good" or not. On that basis the range was enormous, with only 7 percent of children receiving good care in homes of social-class I or II being reported to have fears, while 53 percent of those receiving unsatisfactory care in social-class-IV homes were thus reported. Interestingly, Drillien's middle-class range—social-class III—reported acute fears in about 37 percent of infants irrespective of the judgment on standard of care; and that is close to Macfarlane's overall figure.

Kagan [120] and his colleagues studied both the observed and the reported fears of their sample of infants. Kagan believes that infants' fears —and the changes in their fears as they grow older—can be understood in terms of their natural tendency to be alarmed by objects or events which are unexpected, are impossible to relate to previous experience, and which cannot therefore be understood or coped with. When an 8-month baby is shown a jack-in-the-box he is likely to be afraid. Its "behavior" is totally unexpected; it is like nothing he has seen before and he cannot, so to speak, see what it is or how it works. But when a 2-year-old is shown the same toy he is likely to want to play with it. Whether or not he has ever seen anything similar he has had enough experience with toys to recognize this as part of that benign category; probably he can even see how it works and therefore how to tackle it himself. This theoretical explanation certainly fits much observable infant behavior. Most fears are focused on the strange, the unexpected, and the unmanageable. Few children, for example, are afraid of cars. They have been familiar to the child throughout his life and their behavior, today, is therefore predictable and orderly in terms of past experience. But many children are afraid of fire engines rushing through the streets, sounding alarms, and bringing the traffic to a standstill. Similarly I have never met a child who was afraid of bright lights being switched on but I have met many who were afraid of lightning.

Fears which arise because a child cannot understand or manage an object or event tend to die out naturally as his understanding grows. If he cannot actually comprehend lightning as a phenomenon, he will come to understand that it *is* a phenomenon and does not alarm others. Parents can therefore confidently expect their infants to "grow out of it" provided that "it" is a normal fear and not a phobia. The distinction is important. If the child is sufficiently mature, the departure of a fear can be hastened by rational explanations, demonstrations, and arranged experiences. But a phobia is, by definition, not realistic. To try to prove its irrationality to the young victim is often cruel and always useless.

Behavioral psychologists have developed methods of handling phobias in adults which are often highly effective. The adult, whose life is being ruined by a specific phobia, is very gradually "desensitized." First he is shown the feared object at a distance which allows him to stay calm and unafraid. Very gradually, day by day, the feared object is brought closer to him, always staying within his own limits of calm, never making him afraid, until eventually he can look at it and even touch it, without panic. Parents often try to do this kind of thing with their phobic toddlers. They argue that if they could just persuade the child to *touch* a nice warm cuddly dog, he would find out how silly it was to be afraid. Unfortunately such attempts are usually made from an adult's point of view rather than with a real understanding of the child's. An adult *knows* that fear of dogs is largely irrational. He knows that other people can live with dogs and that his own life would be much easier if he could stop being so afraid of them. A very young child knows none of these things. Such children can be desensitized, but the process needs to be far more gradual than most people realize. If he sees a dog in the distance today and does not panic, he has made a step forward. But this step will not make him able to pass within 6 feet of a dog tomorrow, and touch one next week. Attempts to force toddlers out of phobias or to force the pace when desensitizing them, invariably make matters worse. So if the problem is so acute that it is interfering with daily life, most parents would be well advised to ask for psychiatric help and advice in dealing with it. In less extreme cases most phobic toddlers will respond, slowly, to a general lessening of their overall level of anxiety, the level of anxiety which led to the phobia forming in the first place. Sometimes the infant is under a particular and identifiable stress. Perhaps a new babysitter has been introduced, or his mother has started to go out to work, or there is a new baby present or imminent, or a row going on about toilet training or giving up a bottle.

Often no obvious cause of this kind can be found. The infant has simply reached a stage where his development has got out of step with itself. He feels as we feel when we say: "I just don't seem to be able to cope at the moment." When we say that, we want somebody to take off us some of our responsibilities and problems, so that we can have the time and the energy to cope with the remaining ones and thus catch ourselves up. The same is true of the toddler. Perhaps he is trying to forge ahead on too many fronts at once. Perhaps he is at that stage of learning to walk where he falls down just *too* many times, has too many bumps and bruises. Perhaps he is fighting his mother for independence rather harder than his dependent-baby bit really likes—telling her to "let me!" when a bit of him would like her to do it for him. This kind of situation usually resolves if, for a while, the child is treated either as if he were a little younger than he is, or (which is really the same thing) as if he were slightly unwell. If the mother alters her handling in this direction, she need not know exactly what the trouble is. The infant has the opportunity to retrench on any one or on all fronts. And he will be quick to reassert himself when he has caught himself up again.

What will not help him become unafraid is fear. What will not reduce his anxiety level is making him anxious. The children whose lives are most beset and disordered by fears and phobias tend to be those whose parents decide that they are clingy because they are "spoiled" or that they are fearful because they are "sissy." Such a decision, followed by a toughening-up policy, can only leave the toddler more exposed to the anxiety he could not manage in the first place. The usual vicious circle is set up, with the child demanding more and more support, and the parents offering less and less, so that he demands even more and they offer even less. Things can reach such a pitch that the infant has hardly any time and energy left for exploring, for growing, for asserting himself. He cannot be the tough, adventurous child his parents want, because they keep him too busy filling his dependency needs.

With his anxiety running at a manageable level, and his fears tactfully handled, the toddler's other big problem area can come to the fore. Just as all toddlers, whatever their upbringing, must be at least a little anxious, so all must be at least a little frustrated. Just as the warmest parents cannot prevent their child feeling the anxious loneliness of independent life from time to time, so the most imaginative and permissive parents cannot prevent him feeling frustration. If they do not directly frustrate him, he will frustrate himself; objects will frustrate him; the world will frustrate him. Frustration is implicit in the very drives which ensure his development.

As we have seen, the infant has strong drives to practice each new ability as it comes within his developmental scope. When he can get on to his two legs, he must, however many times he falls down. When he can get the screw-top off the jar, he must, however much the process maddens him. The difficulties of what he must accomplish are so great that without a powerful self-perpetuating drive toward attainment he would give up. So when people stop him doing what he wants to do, he is frustrated; when he cannot manage what he sets himself to do he is frustrated; when objects will not behave as he intends them to, he is frustrated.

Just as individual children vary in their vulnerability to anxiety and to fears, so they vary in their vulnerability to frustration. Some infants seem always able to cope with it better than others. They vary, of course, from stage to stage and day to day, but they seem always basically philosophical, patient, ready to try again. Others seem to set themselves unattainable standards and to be thrown into despair by small setbacks.

The kind of frustration which causes most trouble between parents and child is the frustration of his basic autonomy as a person which is implicit in the socialization of his physiological functions during this year. The infant begins to feel himself to be a separate individual. He no longer accepts, unquestioningly, his mother's right of total control. He is liable to resent her insistence on his using a potty; on his eating certain foods, wearing certain clothes, going to bed at certain times; coming when he is called, going out when it suits her, coming home when she thinks it is time. Any situation involving control by an adult can become an autonomy issue at this stage in development. As soon as the infant feels himself harried, bullied, pressured, he reacts negatively. Yet as long as he feels that he is being allowed to control his own life, he will use that potty, eat the food, stay in bed, come, go, and love it [137]. Mothers need not only the usual virtues of tact and patience and humor, but also talent as actresses. The mother in a rush to get home must appear anything but hurried. Swoop the toddler into his stroller when he meant to walk and all hell will be let loose; but offer to be his horse and *pull* him home and he will probably ride with glee.

Frustrating objects are often educational. The child may get furious because he cannot fit a round peg into a square hole. Nevertheless it is a fact of solid geometry that such pegs will *not* fit square holes, and it is a fact which, if he is ready to fit any kind of peg into any kind of hole, the infant is ready to learn. But he need not be left to wrestle unaided. Just as the 6-year-old will fight her knitting until her temper is completely gone if mother does not tactfully lure her away into a romp in the garden, so the infant who is getting very frustrated with such a task needs help in concluding it, and then something easier to do for a while. Perhaps he even needs an easier version of the same toy, a big cardboard box with *big* holes for tennis balls and blocks, for example. There is frustration with objects which has a positive effect—spurring the child on to success and pleasure in his own achievement; and there is the negative kind which is self-defeating, making him angrier and angrier and less and less competent, until there is no hope of him succeeding and pleasing himself.

Often the behavior of objects is understood, but the child is frustrated by his own small size or unsteady gait. He may long to push the doll's carriage, but be unable to reach the handle; long to throw the football but be too unbalanced to manage its weight. There is little virtue and much grief in this kind of situation. As we have said before, children do not need, for their development or for their happiness, rooms full of expensive toys. But any equipment they are to have must fit them. To be shown a push-toy which is too high is as maddening for a child as a six-foot stove would be to his mother. To try and play ball with a real football is as sad as to try and play tennis with a baseball. If he cannot have a little carriage, or a baby-walker or small push-cart, and an inflatable beach ball or plastic football he is better off with none at all, until he is bigger.

Very few families manage to strike the balance between the amount of frustration which is reasonable and even developmentally useful, and the amount which is too much, all the time. The child is as liable to degrees of anger which are, to an adult, incomprehensible, as he is to puzzling degrees of fear. Even more infants have temper tantrums than have phobias. Hardly surprisingly, temper tantrums are most usual in active, energetic, determined children. Such children are very clear what they want to do, and they want to do a lot. They mind correspondingly much when they cannot, or are not allowed, to do it. In J. W. Macfarlane's sample [151] 60 percent of boys and 45 percent of girls had frequent tantrums at 21 months, while they were frequent in nearly 70 percent of the 3-year-olds. In C. M. Drillien's sample [66] a range over social class was reported similar to that for acute fears, with about 37 percent of the infants of the social-class-III families reporting frequent tantrums, while around 60 percent of the social-class-IV families experienced them. In the Newson survey [170] 14 percent of the study infants were already having very frequent tantrums at 1 year of age, while nearly half the sample were already having quite a few.

Temper tantrum is an unfortunate term. "Temper," in common parlance, is a derogatory word. We apologize for losing our tempers; speak scoffingly of people "getting in a real temper"; express our dislike of people by dismissing them as "thoroughly bad-tempered." Accordingly, an infant having a temper tantrum tends to be regarded as naughty, as giving way to something he should control. Yet in infants of this age group a temper tantrum is very close to an emotional blown fuse. It is what happens when the load of frustration within the child builds up to such a tension that only an explosive discharge can release it. A true tantrum is not within the toddler's control at all, and it is an event that is far more unpleasant for him than for his embarrassed or infuriated mother.

Tantrums take many forms. The most usual, the type with which most parents will have to cope at one time or another, is obvious, furious anger. It is this violent fury which tends to evoke answering anger in the adult and is therefore responsible for children having tantrums being classed as "naughty." The child combines screaming with violent physical activity. He may rush around, send things flying, bang into furniture and walls. He may throw himself down and roll and kick as if fighting unseen devils or, if he is confined in a high chair or car-seat, he may struggle frantically for release, totally careless of his own safety.

A very few parents will have to cope with what are commonly called "breathholding tantrums" [148]. These rare extremes have been well-described in a paper published in 1981 and entitled "Fits and Other Frightening or Funny Turns in Young Children" [27]. While this paper is primarily designed to help doctors to distinguish between medically unimportant "fits" and those, such as various forms of epilepsy, which require treatment, it is nevertheless salutary reading for anyone dealing with tantrums. It makes it clear that whether a tantrum ends in a furious parent smacking a child, or in a terrified parent thinking the child is dead, is a matter of physiological chance. A few infants react to "a hurt to . . . body or . . . ego" by holding their breaths until they turn bluish-gray and may become unconscious or even have a "fit." A few react to "a sudden frightening event which is often, but not always, painful" by becoming pale, limp, and unconscious. Such children naturally elicit the very greatest concern from adults yet the emotions which cause such dramas are no more painful for the child than the emotions which evoke "ordinary" tantrums in the majority of toddlers. *Any* infant who is having a tantrum is, for the moment, lost to the world. He is not open to exhortation, to scolding, to shouts, to smacks. He is overwhelmed by his own internal anger. Probably he is also terrified by it. He seems to feel that he would like to kill everyone and destroy everything. Can he know that he cannot? Over the years he has to learn that it is safe to be angry, that feelings and words cannot physically injure people or things. But at this stage he cannot know these things. His anger must feel hideously all-powerful.

The mother's job is to prevent him hurting himself or anybody or anything else. The child must not, at all costs, recover himself to discover proof that he is dangerous. A smashed vase, a lump on his head, a scratch down his mother's face are all likely to be seen as proof of his horrible power, and evidence that even his mother cannot control him. So it may be best for his mother to hold him, on the floor, secure in her arms. As he calms down, he finds himself close to her. He finds, often with touching amazement, that everything is quite unchanged by the storm. Slowly he relaxes; the screams subside into sobs; the furious monster reverts to a pathetic baby who has frightened himself silly.

Unfortunately toddlers often do not find the world unchanged by the storm. Anger tends to provoke anger, and many mothers lose their tempers to match the child, giving shout for shout. Fifty percent of the mothers in the Newson survey got angry and punished their year-old babies for having tantrums. While the storm is on, punishment and anger are totally ineffective. When it is over, they will only increase the child's feeling that the world is an aggressive and dangerous place, with himself one of its angriest and most dangerous occupants.

Many mothers find tantrums both alarming and socially embarrassing. I have known mothers reach a point where they would not take their child into a store in case he threw a tantrum for sweets; I have known others treat their child with saccharine sweetness whenever there were visitors present, hoping to avert trouble.

Such attitudes are disastrous. A child who finds that the horrific experience of a genuine, uncontrollable tantrum actually serves as a way of controlling his mother, and getting what he wants, would not be human if he did not move toward the semi-voluntary tantrums typical of mishandled 4-year-olds. Such a child "works himself up" on purpose, to a point where he genuinely loses control.

The child must see, from the very first outburst, that tantrums are horrible for him, and have absolutely nothing to do with getting what he wants. He needs comfort and love afterward, but he should never get sweets or anything else he might see as a reward. His behavior must have changed nothing, either in his favor, or against him.

Along with making sure that the child achieves nothing by his outburst, the mother needs also to be very sure that he had to be driven into such a fury of frustration in the first place. Handling toddlers takes infinite patience and tact. Mothers cannot be patient and tactful all of the time, but the frequency of tantrums will at this stage very directly reflect how much of the time they do manage it. Very few issues are worth a direct clash. Safety, cruelty, and reasonable peace for everybody are obvious issues, but even these can usually be dealt with by diversion and friendly talk. The child need seldom be backed into a corner from which he can only explode in rage. The mother needs to ask herself, "Why can't he? Do I really mind if he does?" The mother's mouth may be open to say "No" when, just in time, she realizes that the issue does not really matter.

Yesterday I watched an 18-month boy ask his mother to open his sandbox. She said, "No; nearly bathtime." The child tried to pull the cover off himself. She removed him. He fought away, tried again, could not manage, and exploded. When he would accept comfort again, the mother said to me, "I didn't realize he wanted to *that* much," and opened the sandbox. If she was going to give in, eventually, she would have done much better to have accepted the child's first request.

Tantrums teach a child nothing good or useful. They are essentially unconstructive, as well as unpleasant for all concerned. Yet just as some parents feel that frightened children must be "toughened up" (thus making them more liable to fear), so some parents feel that angry children must be "shown they can't have it all their own way" (thus making them more liable to frustration). The child's own increasing competence deals with both his dependence and anxiety and his independence and frustration, in time. When he is big enough, and brave enough, and can manage his own body and emotions and everyday objects easily enough, he will not need so much reassurance, and he will not meet such continual frustration. When he can talk freely, about what he is thinking and imagining as well as what is there in front of him, he will be able to accept reassuring *words* in lieu of some of his mother's continual physical closeness, and remonstrating words instead of physical restrictions. Once he can understand a little more about how the world works, distinguish a little more clearly between fantasy and reality, he will be able to see the illogic of his fears, the logic of the restrictions imposed upon him.

The calmer, the smoother, the happier he is kept, while he does this vital growing up, the more inclined he will be, at 3 or 4, to use his new abilities in what we regard as a socialized manner. He has already come an extraordinarily long way since we first opened the parcel 2 years ago.

BIBLIOGRAPHY
INDEX

BIBLIOGRAPHY

1. Ainsworth, M. D. S. "The Development of Infant-Mother Attachment," in *Review of Child Development Research*, vol. III, ed. B. M. Caldwell and H. N. Ricciuti. Russell Sage Foundation, 1967.
2. ———. *Infancy in Uganda. Infant Care and the Growth of Attachment*. Baltimore: Johns Hopkins University Press, 1967.
3. Ainsworth, M. D. S.; Bell, S. M.; and Stayton, D. J. "Infant-Mother Attachment and Social Development," in *The Integration of a Child into a Social World*, ed. M. P. Richards. New York: Cambridge University Press, 1974.
4. Ainsworth, M. D. S.; Blehar, M. C.; Waters, E.; and Wall, S. *Patterns of Attachment in the Strange Situation and at Home*. Hillsdale, NJ: Lawrence Erlbaum, 1978.
5. Ainsworth, M. D. S., and Salter, "Social Development in the First Year of Life: Maternal Influences on Infant-Mother Attachment," Geoffrey Vickers Lecture, London, 1975.
6. Ainsworth, M. D. S. and Wittig, B. A. "Attachment and Exploratory Behaviour of One Year Olds in a Strange Situation," in *Determinants of Infant Behaviour*, vol. IV, ed. B. Foss. New York: Barnes & Noble, 1969.
7. Ames, L. B.; Gillespie, C.; Haines, J.; and Ilg, F. *The Child from One to Six*. London: Hamish Hamilton, 1980.
8. Anderson, J. W. "Attachment Behaviour Out of Doors," in *Ethological Studies of Child Behaviour*, ed. N. Burton Jones. New York: Cambridge University Press, 1972.
9. Atherton, D. J.; Sewell, M.; Soothill, J. F.; Wells, R. F.; and Chilvers, C. *Lancet*, vol. I, 1978.
10. Atkinson, J. "New Tool Pin-Points Focusing Faults in Babies," *New Scientist*, April 24, 1980.
11. ———; Braddick, O.; and Howland, H. *Vision Research*, 19, 1980.
12. Azrin, N., and Fox, R. *Toilet Training in Less Than a Day*. New York: Simon & Schuster, 1974.
13. Bahna, S. L., and Heiner, D. C. *Allergies to Milk*. New York: Grune & Stratton, 1980.
14. Barltrop, D. "Artificial Milks in Neonatal Nutrition," *The Practitioner*, 212, no. 1270, 1974.
15. Basedon. *American Journal of Public Health*, 64, no. 8, 1974.
16. Bassler, L. S. "Hemiplegia of Early Onset and the Faculty of Speech, with Special Reference to the Effects of Hemispherectomy," *Brain*, 85, 1962.
17. Bax, M. "Sleep Disturbance in the Young Child," *British Medical Journal*, May 10, 1980.
18. Bayley, N. "Mental Development Index," in *Carmichael's Manual of Child Psychology*, ed. P. H. Mussen. New York: John Wiley, 1970.
19. ———. "Mental Growth During the First Three Years. A Developmental Study of Sixty-One Children by Repeated Tests," *Genetic Psychology Monograph*, 14, 1933.

20. Bell, R. Q. "Detection of Cross-Stage Relations Between Transition Periods in Which the Form of Behaviour Differs Markedly: A Longitudinal Study of the Newborn and Preschool Periods," *Monograph of the Society for Research in Child Development*, 36, 1971.

21. Bernstein, B. "A Public Language: Some Sociological Implications of a Linguistic Form," *British Journal of Sociology*, 10, 1959.

22. Blatz, W. E. *Human Security. Some Reflections.* Toronto: University of Toronto Press, 1966.

23. Boersma, E. R. "Changes in Fatty-Acid Composition of Body Fat Before and After Birth in Tanzania: An International Comparative Study," *British Medical Journal*, March 31, 1979.

24. Bolland, J., and Miller, H. E. *Personality and Psychotherapy*, 1966.

25. Boniface, D., and Graham, P. "The Three Year Old and His Attachment to a Special Soft Object," *Journal of Child Psychology and Psychiatry*, 20, no. 3, 1979.

26. Bourne, G. H. *Progress in Ape Research.* New York: Academic Press, 1977.

27. Bower, B. "Fits and Other Frightening or Funny Turns in Young Children," *The Practitioner*, 225, March 1981.

28. Bower, T. "Competent Newborns," in *Child Alive*, ed. R. Lewin. London: Maurice Temple, Ltd., 1975.

29. ———. *Development in Infancy.* San Francisco: W. H. Freeman, 1974.

30. ———. "Object Perception in Infants," *Perception*, 1, 1972.

31. ———. "The Object in the World of the Infant," *Scientific American*, October 1971.

32. Bowlby, J. *Attachment.* London: Penguin Books, 1971.

33. ———. *Loss: Sadness and Depression.* New York: Basic Books, 1980.

34. ———. *Maternal Care and Mental Health.* World Health Organization, 1951. Available as *Child Care and the Growth of Love.* Baltimore: Penguin Books, 1965.

35. ———. *Separation: Anxiety and Anger.* New York: Basic Books, 1973.

36. Bradley, Hoskisson J. *What Is This Thing Called Sleep?* London: Davis Poynter, 1976.

37. Brazelton, T. B. "A Child-Oriented Approach to Toilet-Training," *Pediatrics*, 29, 1962.

38. Brooke, O. G. "Infant Feeding, the Perennial Problem," *The Practitioner*, 221, 1978.

39. ———., et. al. "Vitamin D Supplements in Pregnant Asian Women: Effects on Calcium Status and Fetal Growth," *British Medical Journal*, March 15, 1980.

40. Bruner, J. S. "Early Social Interactions and Language Acquisition," in *Studies in Mother-Infant Interaction*, ed. H. R. Schaffer. New York: Academic Press, 1977.

41. ———, and Koslowski, B. "Visually Adapted Constituents of Manipulatory Action," *Perception*, 1, 1972.

42. Bullowa, M.; Jones, L. G.; and Duckert, A. "The Acquisition of a Word," *Language and Speech*, 7, 1964.

43. Burt, C.; Miller, E.; and Moodie, W. *How the Mind Works.* New York: Appleton-Century-Crofts, 1934.

44. Burton, L.; White, B.; and Held, R. "Plasticity of Sensorimotor Development in the Human Infant," in *The Causes of Behaviour: Readings in Child Development and Educational Psychology*, ed. J. R. Rosenblith and W. Allinsmith. Boston: Allyn & Bacon, 1966.

45. Caffey, J. "On the Theory and Practice of Shaking Infants: Its Potential Residual Effects of Permanent Brain Damage and Mental Retardation," *American Journal of Diseases of Children*, 124, August 1972.

46. Carr, J. *Helping Your Handicapped Child.* London: Penguin Books, 1980.

47. Caudill, W., and Weinstein, H. "Childcare and Infant Behaviour in Japanese and American Urban Middle Class Families," in *Yearbook of the International Sociological Association*, ed. R. Konig and R. Hill, 1966.

48. Chess, T. A.; Birch, H. G.; and Hertzig, M. E. *Behavioral Individuality in Early Childhood.* New York: New York University Press, 1964.

49. Chomsky, N. *Aspects of the Theory of Syntax.* Cambridge, MA: MIT Press, 1969.

50. ———. *Syntactic Structures.* Atlantic Highlands, NJ: Humanities Press, 1957.
51. Cobb, J. *Babyshock.* London: Hutchinson & Co., Ltd., 1980.
52. Committee on Medical Aspects of Food Policy. "Artificial Foods for the Young Infant: Report of the Working Party on the Composition of Foods for Infants and Young Children," H.M.S.O., 1980.
53. ———. "Recommended Daily Amounts of Food Energy and Nutrients for Groups of People in the United Kingdom," H.M.S.O., 1979.
54. David, M., and Appell, G. "Mother-Child Relations," in *Modern Perspectives in International Child Psychiatry,* ed. J. G. Howells. New York: Brunner/Mazel, 1971.
55. Davie, R.; Butler, N.; and Goldstein, H. *From Birth to Seven.* London: Longman, 1972.
56. Decarie, T. G. *The Infant's Reaction to Strangers.* New York: International Universities Press, 1974.
57. Department of Health and Social Security. "Present-Day Practice in Infant Feeding," H.M.S.O., 1974.
58. ———. *Recommended Daily Amounts of Food Energy and Nutrients for Groups of People in the United Kingdom.* H.M.S.O., 1979.
59. ———. "Rickets and Osteomalacia," H.M.S.O., 1980.
60. Desmond, A. *The Ape's Reflection.* New York: Dial Press, 1979.
61. Dickerson, J. W. T., and Fehily, A. M. "Bizarre and Unusual Diets," *The Practitioner,* 222, May 1979.
62. Dimson, S. B. "Toilet Training and Enuresis," *British Medical Journal,* 2, 1959.
63. Dodwell, P. C.; Muir, D.; and DiFranco, D. "Responses of Infants to Visually Presented Objects," *Science,* 194, October 8, 1976.
64. Dollard, J., and Miller, N. E. *Personality and Psychotherapy.* New York: McGraw-Hill, 1950.
65. Doman, G. *Teach Your Baby to Read.* New York: Doubleday, 1975.
66. Drillien, C. M. *The Growth and Development of the Prematurely Born Infant.* Baltimore: Williams & Wilkins, 1964.
67. Dunn, J., and Richards, M. "Observations in the Neonatal Period," in *Studies in Mother-Infant Interaction,* ed. H. R. Schaffer. New York: Academic Press, 1977.
68. ———. "Patterns of Early Interaction," in *Studies in Mother-Infant Interaction,* ed. H. R. Schaffer. New York: Academic Press, 1977.
69. Eid, E. E. "Follow Up Study of the Physical Growth of Children Who Had Excessive Weight Gain in the First Six Months," *British Medical Journal,* 2, 1970.
70. Eimas, P. *Perception and Psychophysics,* 18, 1976.
71. Eisenberg, R. B. "Auditory Behaviour in the Human Neonate: A Preliminary Report," *Journal of Speech and Hearing Research,* 7, 1964.
72. ———. "Auditory Behaviour in the Human Neonate: Methodological Problems and the Logical Design of Research Procedures," *Journal of Auditory Research,* 5, 1965.
73. ———. "Habituation to an Acoustic Pattern as an Index of Differences Among Human Neonates," *Journal of Auditory Research,* 6, 1966.
74. ———. "Stimulus Significance as a Determinant of Newborn Responses to Sound," *Paper to the Society for Research in Child Development,* New York, 1967.
75. Erikson, E. *Childhood and Society.* New York: W. W. Norton, 1950.
76. Ervin-Tripp, S. M. "Imitations and Structural Changes in Children's Language," in *New Directions in the Study of Language,* ed. E. Lenneberg. Cambridge, MA: MIT Press, 1964.
77. Escalona, S. K. *The Roots of Individuality.* Chicago: Aldine, 1968.
78. ———, and Corman, H. "The Evaluation of Piaget's Hypothesis Concerning the Development of Sensori-Motor Intelligence: Methodological Issues," *Paper to the Society for Research in Child Development,* New York, 1967.
79. Fagen, J. W.; Rovee, C. K; and Kaplan, M. G. "Psychophysical Scaling of Stimulus Similarity in Three Month Infants," *Journal of Experimental Child Psychology,* 22, 1976.

80. Fallot, Mary B.; Boyd, John L., III; and Oski, Frank A. "Breast-Feeding Reduces the Incidence of Hospital Admissions for Infants," *Pediatrics*, 65, 1980.
81. Fantz, R. L. "Pattern Discrimination and Selective Attention as Determinants of Perceptual Development from Birth," in *Perceptual Development in Children*, ed. A. H. Kidd and J. L. Rivoire. New York: International Universities Press, 1966.
82. Flavell, J. H. *The Developmental Psychology of Jean Piaget.* New York: Van Nostrand Reinhold, 1963.
83. Formby, D. "Maternal Recognition of the Infant's Cry," *Developmental Medicine and Child Neurology*, 9, 1967.
84. Fox, *et al. Science*, 207, 1980.
85. Francis, H. *Language in Childhood.* New York: St. Martin's Press, 1975.
86. Frank, L. K. *On the Importance of Infancy.* New York: Random House, 1966.
87. Gairdner, D. "The Fate of the Foreskin," *British Medical Journal*, 1, 1949.
88. Galaburda, A. M.; LeMay, M.; Kemper, T. L.; and Geschwind, N. "Right-Left Asymmetries in the Brain," *Science*, 199, 1978.
89. Gardner, R. A., and Gardner, B. C. "Teaching Sign Language to a Chimpanzee," *Science*, 165, 1969.
90. Geber, M., and Dean, R. F. A. "Gesell Tests in African Children," *Pediatrics*, 20, 1957.
91. Gerrard, J. W., ed. *Food Allergy.* Springfield, IL: Charles C. Thomas Publishing, 1980.
92. Geschwind, N., and Levitsky, W. "Human Brain: Left-Right Asymmetries in the Temporal Speech Region," *Science*, 161, 1968.
93. Gesell, A. *The First Five Years of Life.* New York: Harper & Row, 1940.
94. ———. *Infancy and Human Growth.* New York: Macmillan, 1928.
95. ———. "The Ontogenesis of Infant Behaviour," in *Manual of Child Psychology*, ed. L. Carmichael. New York: John Wiley, 1946.
96. ———, and Amatruda, C. S. *Developmental Diagnosis.* Scranton, PA: Hoeber, 1947.
97. Gewirtz, H. B., and Gewirtz, J. L. "Visiting and Caretaking Patterns for Kibbutz Infants: Age and Sex Trends," *American Journal of Orthopsychiatry*, 39, 1968.
98. Gewirtz, J. L. "Mechanisms of Social Learning: Some Roles of Stimulation and Behaviour in Early Development," in *Handbook of Socialisation Theory and Research*, ed. D. A. Goslin. Skokie, IL: Rand McNally, 1968.
99. Griffiths, R. *The Abilities of Babies.* Mystic, CT: Verry Lawrence, 1954.
100. Guthrie, L. "Teething," *British Medical Journal*, 2, 1908.
101. Halverson, H. M. "An Experimental Study of Prehension in Infants by Means of Systematic Cinema Records," *Genetic Psychology Monograph*, 10, 1932.
102. Harlow, H. F. "The Nature of Love," *American Psychologist*, 13, no. 673, 1958.
103. Haynes, H.; White, B. L.; and Held, R. "Visual Accommodation in Human Infants," *Science*, 148, 1965.
104. Heinstein, M. *Child Rearing in California.* Bureau of Maternal and Child Health, State of California Department of Public Health, 1966.
105. Helfer, R. E., and Kempe, H. C. *The Battered Child.* Chicago: University of Chicago Press, 1968.
106. Herbst, J. "Gastro-Intestinal Reflux," *Journal of Pediatrics*, 98, no. 6, 1981.
107. Howard, A. N., and McLean Baird, I., eds. *Nutritional Deficiencies in Modern Society.* (Based on a symposium held by the Food Education Society in 1972.) Newman Books, 1973.
108. Huenemann, R. "Environmental Factors Associated with Pre-School Obesity," *Journal of the American Dietary Association*, 64, 1974.
109. Illingworth, R. S. *The Development of the Infant and Young Child.* Baltimore: Williams & Wilkins, 1970.
110. ———. "Evening Colic in Infants: A Double Blind Trial of Dicyclomine Hydrochloride," *Lancet*, 2, 1959.
111. ———. *The Normal Child: Some Problems of the Early Years and Their Treatment*, 7th edition. Edinburgh: Churchill, Livingston, 1979.

112. ———. "Three-Months Colic," *Archives of Diseases in Childhood,* 29, 1954.

113. Irwin, O. C. "Language and Communication," in *Handbook of Research Methods in Child Development,* ed. P. H. Mussen. New York: John Wiley, 1960.

114. Jelliffe, E. B., and Jelliffe, E. F. P. "Human Milk," *New England Journal of Medicine,* 297, 1977.

115. Joint Committee of the Royal College of Obstetricians and Gynaecologists and the Population Investigation Committee. *Maternity in Great Britain.* Oxford: Oxford University Press, 1948.

116. Jorup, S. "Colonic Hyperperistalsis in Neurolabile Infants," *Acta paediatrica* (Uppsala) 41, supp. 85, 1952.

117. Kaffman, N., and Elizur, E. "Infants Who Became Enuretics: A Longitudinal Study of 161 Kibbutz Children," *Monograph of Social Research in Child Development,* 42, no. 2, 1971.

118. Kagan, J. "Do Infants Think?," *Scientific American,* March 1972.

119. ———. "On the Need for Relativism," *American Psychologist,* 22, 1967.

120. ———, Kearsley, R., and Zelazo, P. *Infancy: Its Place in Human Development.* Cambridge, MA: Harvard University Press, 1978.

121. Kagan, J.; Klein, R. E.; Finley, G. E.; Rogoff, B.; and Nolan, E. *A Cross-Cultural Study of Cognitive Development.* Unpublished ms. Harvard University, 1977.

122. Kagan, J., and Lewis, M. "Studies of Attention," *Merrill-Palmer Quarterly,* 2, 1965.

123. Kagan, J., *et al. Change and Continuity in Infancy.* New York: John Wiley, 1971.

124. Kessen, W.; Williams, E. J.; and Williams J. P. "Selection and Test-Response Measures in the Study of the Human Newborn," *Child Development,* 32, 1961.

125. Kimura, D. "Functional Asymmetry of the Brain in Dichotic Listening," *Cortex,* 3, 1967.

126. Kinney, D., and Kagan, J. "Infant Attention to Auditory Discrepancy," *Child Development,* 47, 1976.

127. Klaus, M. H., and Kennel, J. H. *Maternal-Infant Bonding.* St. Louis: C. V. Moshu, 1976.

128. Klein, R. E.; Irwin, M. H.; Engle, P. L.; and Yarborough, C. "Malnutrition and Mental Development in Rural Guatemala," in *Advances in Cross-Cultural Psychology,* ed. N. Warren. New York: Academic Press, 1977.

129. Kleitman, N., and Engelmann, T. G. "Sleep Characteristics of Infants," *Journal of Applied Physiology,* 6, 1953.

130. Knobloch, H. "Precocity of African Children," *Pediatrics,* 22, 1958.

131. Knox, C. "Cerebral Processing of Nonverbal Sounds in Boys and Girls," *Neuropsychologia,* 8, 1970.

132. Kopelman, P. G.; Pilkington, T. R. E.; White, N.; and Jeffcoate, S. L. "Evidence for the Existence of Two Types of Massive Obesity," *British Medical Journal,* January 12, 1980.

133. Kotelchuk, M.; Zelazo, P.; Kagan, J.; and Spelke, E. "Infant Reactions to Parental Separations When Left with Familiar and Unfamiliar Adults," *Journal of Genetic Psychology,* 126, 1972.

134. Lakdawala, Dr., and Widdowson, E. M. *Lancet,* I, no. 167, 1977.

135. Lakin, M. "Personality Factors in Mothers of Excessively Crying (Colicky) Babies," *Monograph of the Society for Research in Child Development,* 22, 1957.

136. La Leche League International. "The Womanly Art of Breastfeeding," 1981.

137. Leach, P. J. "A Critical Study of Literature Concerning Rigidity," in *Thought and Personality,* ed. P. B. Warr. Baltimore: Penguin, 1971.

138. ———. *Your Baby and Child.* New York: Alfred A. Knopf, 1978.

139. ———. *Who Cares? A New Deal for Mothers and Their Small Children.* London: Penguin, 1979.

140. Lenneberg, E. H. *Biological Foundations of Language.* New York: John Wiley, 1967.

141. ———. "The Natural History of Language," in *Genesis of Language,* ed. F. Smith and G. A. Miller. Cambridge, MA: MIT Press, 1966.

142. ———. "Speech as a Motor Skill with Special Reference to Non-Aphasic Disorders," in *The Acquisition of Language*, ed. U. Bellugi and R. W. Brown, *Monograph of the Society for Research in Child Development*, 29, 1964.

143. Lewis, C. *Growing Up with Good Food*. London: George Allen & Unwin, 1981.

144. Lewis, M., and McGurk, H. "Evaluation of Infant Intelligence Scales," *Science*, 178, 1972.

145. Liberman, A. *Perception and Psychophysics*, 18, 1976.

146. Liddiard, M. *The Mothercraft Manual: An Outline of the Work of Sir Truby King*. Edinburgh: Churchill, 1928.

147. Lipsitt, L. P. "The Development of Human Behaviour: Theoretical Considerations for Future Research," in *The Biopsychology of Development*, ed. E. Tobach, L. Aronson, and E. Shaw. New York: Academic Press, 1971.

148. Livingston, S. "Breath-Holding Spells in Children," *Journal of the American Medical Association*, 212, 1970.

149. MacAdam, D. W., and Whitaker, H. A. "Language Production: Electroencephalographic Localization in the Normal Human Brain," *Science*, 172, 1971.

150. Macfarlane, J. W. "Olfaction in the Development of Social Preferences in the Human Neonate," in *Parent-Infant Interaction*. CIBA Foundation Symposium, 33, Amsterdam, 1975.

151. ———; Allen, L.; and Honzik, M. P. *Behaviour Problems of Normal Children*. Berkeley: University of California Press, 1954.

152. Main, M. B. "Analysis of a Peculiar Form of Reunion Behaviour in Some Day-Care Children: Its History and Sequelae in Children Who are Home-Reared," in *Social Development in Childhood: Day-Care Programs and Research*. Baltimore: Johns Hopkins University Press, 1977.

153. Martin, J. "Infant Feeding 1975: Attitudes and Practise in England and Wales." Office of Population Censuses and Surveys, Social Survey Division, H.M.S.O., 1978.

154. McCarthy, D. "Affective Aspects of Language Learning," in *Perceptual Development in Children*, ed. A. H. Kidd and J. L. Rivoire. New York: International Universities Press, 1966.

155. McCarthy, D.; Douglas, J.; and Mogford, C. "Circumcision in a National Sample of Four-Year-Old Children," *British Medical Journal*, 2, 1952.

156. McGurk, H. "Visual Perception in Young Infants," in *New Perspectives in Child Development*, ed. B. Foss. London: Penguin Books, 1974.

157. Menyuk, P. *The Acquisition and Development of Language*. Englewood Cliffs, NJ: Prentice-Hall, 1971.

158. Ministry of Agriculture, Fisheries and Food. *Manual of Nutrition*. London: H.M.S.O., 1970.

159. Moore T., and Ucko, L. E. "Nightwalking in Early Infancy," *Archives of Diseases in Childhood*, 32, 1957.

160. Morgan, G. A.; and Ricciuti, H. N. "Infants' Response to Strangers During the First Year of Life," in *Determinants of Infant Behaviour*, vol. IV, ed. B. Foss. New York: Barnes & Noble, 1969.

161. Moss, H. A. "Sex, Age and State as Determinants of Mother-Infant Interaction," *Merrill-Palmer Quarterly*, 13, 1967.

162. ———, and Robson, K. S. "Maternal Influence on Social/Visual Behaviour," *Child Development*, 39, 1968.

163. ———, "The Relation Between the Amount of Time Infants Spend in Various States and the Development of Visual Behaviour," *Child Development*, 41, 1970.

164. ———, and Pedersen, F. "Determinants of Maternal Stimulation of Infants and Consequences of Treatment for Later Reactions to Strangers," *Developmental Psychology*, 1, 1969.

165. Mowrer, O. H. "Hearing and Speaking: An Analysis of Language Learning," *Journal of Speech and Hearing Disorders*, 23, 1960.

166. Muellner, S. R. "Obstacles to the Treatment of Primary Enuresis," *Journal of the American Medical Association*, 178, 1961.

167. Mura Jun Ichi. "The Sounds of Infants," *Studia Phonologica*, 3, 1963–64.

168. Nakazima, S. "A Comparative Study of the Speech Developments of Japanese and American English in Childhood," *Studia Phonologica*, 2, 1962.

169. Newson, J., and Newson, E. *Four Years Old in an Urban Community*. Chicago: Aldine, 1968.

170. ———. *Infant Care in an Urban Community*. Chicago: Aldine, 1963.

171. O'Connor, N., and Hermelin, B. "Cognitive Deficits in Children," *British Medical Bulletin*, 27, no. 3, 1971.

172. Osofsky, J. D., and Danzger, B. "Relationships Between Neonatal Characteristics and Mother-Infant Interaction," *Developmental Psychology*, 10, 1974.

173. Papousek, H., and Papousek, M. "Mothering and the Cognitive Head Start," in *Structures in Mother-Infant Interaction*, ed. H. R. Schaffer. New York: Academic Press, 1977.

174. Paradise, J. L. "Maternal and Other Factors in the Etiology of Infantile Colic," *Journal of the American Medical Association*, 197, 1966.

175. Pavenstedt, E. *The Drifters: Children of Disorganized Lower Class Families*. Boston: Little, Brown, 1967.

176. Petre-Quadens, O., and Schlag, J. B., eds. *Basic Sleep Mechanisms*. London: Academic Press, 1974.

177. Piaget, J. *The Construction of Reality in the Child*. New York: Basic Books, 1954.

178. ———. *The Origins of Intelligence in the Child*. New York: International Universities Press, 1966.

179. Poskitt. "Nutrition in Childhood," in *Topics in Pediatrics*, ed. B. Wharton. Pitman Medical, 1980.

180. Prechtl, H. F. R. "Problems of Behavioural Studies in the Newborn Infant," in *Advances in the Study of Behaviour*, vol. I, ed. D. S. Lehrman and R. A. Hinde. New York: Academic Press, 1965.

181. ———, and Stemmer, C. J. "The Choreiform Syndrome in Children," *Developmental Medicine and Child Neurology*, 4, 1962.

182. Premack, A., and Premack, D. "Teaching Language to an Ape," *Scientific American*, October 1972.

183. Przetacznikowa, M. "Study in the Use of the Longitudinal Method for Investigating the Verbal Behaviour of Children of Pre-School Age," in *Determinants of Behavioural Development*, ed. F. J. Moenks, *et al.* New York: Academic Press, 1972.

184. Rheingold, H. L. "The Development of Social Behaviour in the Human Infant," *Monograph of the Society for Research in Child Development*, 31, 1966.

185. Robertson, J., and Robertson, J. *A Series of Films, and Written Guides, on the Response of Young Children of Previous Good Experience to Separation from the Mother, When the Substitute Care Meets, or Fails to Meet, Their Emotional Needs*. Tavistock Institute of Human Relations, London; New York University Film Library, 1967, 1968, 1969.

186. Rosenzweig, M. "Effects of Environment on the Development of Brain and Behaviour," in *The Biopsychology of Development*, ed. E. Tobach, L. Aronson, and E. Shaw. New York: Academic Press, 1971.

187. ———; Bennett, E.; and Diamond, M. "Brain Changes in Response to Experience," *Scientific American*, February 1972.

188. Ross, G.; Kagan, J.; Zelazo, P.; and Kotelchuk, M. "Separation Protest in Infants in Home and Laboratory," *Developmental Psychology*, 11, 1975.

189. Ross, H. S., and Goldman, B. D. "Infants' Sociability Towards Strangers," *Child Development*, 48, 1977.

190. Sander, L. W.; Stechler, G.; Julia, M.; and Burns, P. "Early Mother-Infant Interaction and Twenty-Four-Hour Patterns of Activity and Sleep," *Journal of the American Academy of Child Psychiatry*, 9, 1970.

191. Scaife, M., and Bruner, J. S. "The Capacity for Joint Visual Attention in the Infant," *Nature*, 253, 1975.
192. Schaefer, E. S., and Bayley, N. "Maternal Behaviour, Child Behaviour and Their Intercorrelations from Infancy Through Adolescence," *Monograph of the Society for Research in Child Development*, 28, 1963.
193. Schaffer, H. R. "Activity Level as a Constitutional Determinant of Infantile Reaction to Deprivation," *Child Development*, 37, 1966.
194. ———. *Mothering*. London: Open Books, 1977.
195. ———, ed. *Studies in Mother-Infant Interaction*. New York: Academic Press, 1977.
196. Schaffer, H. R., and Emerson, P. E. "The Development of Social Attachments in Infancy," *Monograph of the Society for Research in Child Development*, 29, 1964.
197. ———. "Patterns of Response to Physical Contact in Early Human Development," *Journal of Child Psychology and Psychiatry*, 5, 1964.
198. Scopes, J. W. "Metabolic Rate and Temperature Control in the Newborn Baby," *British Medical Bulletin*, January 22, 1966.
199. Scott, J. P. "Critical Periods in Behavioural Development," *Science*, 138, 1962.
200. Seglow, J.; Kellmer; Pringle, M.; and Wedge, P. *Growing Up Adopted*. National Foundation for Educational Research, 1972.
201. Shukla, A.; Forsyth, H. A.; Anderson, C.; and Marway, S. M. "Some Aspects of Infant Nutrition in the First Year of Life: A Field Study in Dudley, Worcs, England," *British Medical Journal*, 4, 1972.
202. Sime, M. *Read Your Child's Thoughts: Pre-School Learning Piaget's Way*. London: Thames & Hudson, 1980.
203. Simner, M. "Response of the Newborn Infant to the Cry of Another Infant," *Paper to the Society for Research in Child Development*, New York, 1969.
204. Skinner, B. F. *Verbal Behavior*. New York: Appleton-Century-Crofts, 1957.
205. Slobin, D. I. "Some Thoughts on the Relation of Comprehension to Speech," *Paper to American Speech and Hearing Association*, San Francisco, 1964.
206. Smith, A. *The Body*. New York: Walker & Co., 1968.
207. Spitz, R., and Cobliner, W. G. *The First Year of Life*. New York: International Universities Press, 1966.
208. Spock, B. *Baby and Child Care*. New York: Dutton, 1976.
209. ———. *Dr. Spock Talks with Mothers*. Boston: Houghton Mifflin, 1961.
210. Stevenson, O. "The First Treasured Possession," *Psychoanalytic Study of the Child*, 9, 1954.
211. Stott, L. S., and Ball, R. S. "Infant and Pre-School Mental Tests: Review and Evaluation," *Monograph of the Society for Research in Child Development*, 30, 1965.
212. Taitz, L. S. "Infantile Overnutrition Among Artificially Fed Infants in the Sheffield Region," *British Medical Journal*, 1, 1972.
213. Tanner, J. M.; Whitehorse, R. H.; and Takaishi, H. "Standards from Birth to Maturity for Height, Weight, Height Velocity and Weight Velocity: British Children," *Archives of Diseases in Childhood*, 41, no. 613, 1966.
214. Thomas, A., and Chess, S. *Temperament and Development*. New York: Brunner/Mazel, 1977.
215. Trevarthen, C. "Basic Patterns of Psychogenic Change in Infancy," Proceedings of OECD Conference, "Dips in Learning," March 1975.
216. ———. "Descriptive Analyses of Infant Communicative Behaviour," in *Studies in Mother-Infant Interaction*, ed. H. R. Schaffer. New York: Academic Press, 1977.
217. Tripp, J. H.; Francis, D. E. M.; Knight, J. A.; and Harries, J. T. "Infant Feeding Practises: A Cause for Concern," *British Medical Journal*, September 22, 1979.
218. Valman, H. B. "The First Year of Life: Weaning," *British Medical Journal*, March 29, 1980.
219. Von Békésy, G., and Rosenblith, W. "The Mechanical Properties of the Ear," in *Handbook of Experimental Psychology*, ed. S. S. Stevens. New York: John Wiley, 1951.

220. Watson, J. B. *Psychological Care of Infant and Child.* New York: W. W. Norton, 1928.
221. Weisberg, P. "Social and Nonsocial Conditioning of Infant Vocalisations," *Child Development,* 34, 1963.
222. White, B. L. *The First Three Years of Life.* New York: Avon, 1978.
223. White B.; Castle, P.; and Held, R. "Observations on the Development of Visually Directed Reaching," *Child Development,* 35, 1964.
224. Winitz, H., and Irwin, O. C. "Syllabic and Phonetic Structures of Infants' Early Words," *Journal of Speech and Hearing Research,* 1, 1958.
225. Wolff, P. H. "The Natural History of Crying and Other Vocalisations in Early Infancy," in *Determinants of Infant Behaviour,* vol. IV, ed. B. Foss. New York: Barnes & Noble, 1969.
226. ———. "Observations on the Early Development of Smiling," in *Determinants of Infant Behaviour,* vol. II, ed. B. Foss. New York: Barnes & Noble, 1963.
227. Yarrow, L. J. "The Development of Focused Relationships During Infancy," in *Exceptional Infant,* vol. I, ed. J. Hellmuth. New York: Brunner/Mazel, 1969.
228. ———. "Separation from Parents During Early Childhood," in *Review of Child Development Research,* vol. I, ed. M. L. Hoffman and L. W. Hoffman. Russell Sage Foundation, 1964.
229. Zelazo, N.; Zelazo, P.; and Kolb, S. " 'Walking' in the Newborn," *Science,* 176, April 1972.

INDEX

A NOTE ABOUT THE AUTHOR

Penelope Leach was educated at Cambridge University and the London School of Economics, where she received her Ph.D. in social psychology for a study of the effects of different kinds of upbringing and discipline on personality development. She has lectured at the London School of Economics on psychology and child development, and for four years ran a study, under the auspices of Britain's Medical Research Council, of the effects of babies on their parents. She is vice president of the Pre-School Playgroups Association and the Health Visitors' Association, has served on the committee of the Developmental Section of the British Psychological Society, and is the author of *Your Baby and Child, Your Growing Child,* and *The First Six Months.* She is married to an energy specialist, and they have two children.

A NOTE ON THE TYPE

This book was set, via computer-driven cathode ray tube, in a type face called Baskerville. The face is a reproduction of types cast from molds made for John Baskerville (1706–75) from his designs. John Baskerville's original face was one of the forerunners of the type style known as "modern face" to printers—a "modern" of the period A.D. 1800.

This book was composed, printed, and bound by Haddon Craftsmen, Inc., Scranton, Pennsylvania.

Typography and binding based on a design by Christine Aulicino.